BLACKPOO

For Refere

Vol. 2

INTERNATIONAL

COLLATION

OF

TRADITIONAL

AND

FOLK MEDICINE

NORTHEAST
ASIA

Part II

International Collation of Folk and Traditional Medicine

Managing Board:
(Chairman)   **Byung Hoon Han**, *Natural Products Research Institute, Seoul National University, Korea*

Norio Aimi, *Faculty of Pharmaceutical Sciences, Chiba University, Japan*

Kin Fai Cheng, *Department of Chemistry, The University of Hong Kong, Hong Kong*

Guo-Wei Qin, *Shanghai Institute of Materia Medica, Chinese Academy of Sciences, China*

Fumin Zhang, *UNESCO Office, Jakarta, Indonesia*

Vol. 1:   Northeast Asia Part I
eds. Takeatsu Kimura (Editor-in-Chief), Paul P. H. But, Ji-Xian Guo, Chung Ki Sung

Vol. 2:   Northeast Asia Part II
eds. Paul B. H. But (Editor-in-Chief), Takeatsu Kimura, Ji-Xian Guo, Chung Ki Sung

Vol. 3:   Northeast Asia Part III
eds. Chung Ki Sung (Editor-in-Chief), Takeatsu Kimura, Paul P. H. But, Ji-Xian Guo

Vol. 4:   Northeast Asia Part IV
eds. Ji-Xian Guo (Editor-in-Chief), Takeatsu Kimura, Paul P. H. But, Ji-Xian Guo, Chung Ki Sung

INTERNATIONAL

COLLATION

OF

TRADITIONAL

AND

FOLK MEDICINE

Editor-in-Chief

Paul P. H. But
The Chinese University of Hong Kong

Editors

Takeatsu Kimura
Daiichi College of Pharmaceutical Sciences

Ji-Xian Guo
Shanghai Medical University

Chung Ki Sung
Chonnam National University

NORTHEAST ASIA

Part II

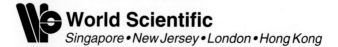
World Scientific
Singapore • New Jersey • London • Hong Kong

Published by

World Scientific Publishing Co. Pte. Ltd.
P O Box 128, Farrer Road, Singapore 912805
USA office: Suite 1B, 1060 Main Street, River Edge, NJ 07661
UK office: 57 Shelton Street, Covent Garden, London WC2H 9HE

Library of Congress Cataloging-in-Publication Data
Northeast Asia / editor-in-chief, Paul P. H. But; editors, Takeatsu Kimura, Ji-Xian Guo, Chung Ki Sung.
    p.   cm. -- (International collation of traditional and folk medicine ; vol. 2)
    "A project of UNESCO."
    Includes bibliographical references and index.
    ISBN 981023130X
    1. Materia medica, Vegetable -- East Asia.   2. Medicinal plants -- East Asia.
  3. Traditional medicine -- East Asia.   I. Kimura, Takeatsu.   II. UNESCO.
  III. Series.
    [DNLM: 1. Medicine, Herbal.   2. Plants, Medicinal -- chemistry.
  3. Plant Extracts -- therapeutic use.   4. Drug Design.
  5. International Cooperation.   WB 925 N874 1996]
  RS180.E18N67   1997
  615'.321'095--dc20
  DNLM/DLC   96-4659
  for Library of Congress   CIP

British Library Cataloguing-in-Publication Data
A catalogue record for this book is available from the British Library.

Printed in Singapore by Uto-Print

FOREWORD

The plant floras in China, Hong Kong, Japan, and Korea - located nearly in the same temperature zone - share much similarity with the result that traditional folk medical experiences in this region are comparable in nature. Nonetheless, since folk medical experience in different countries have been developed rather independently each with a long history, both similarities and differences coexist in traditional folk medical knowledge from different countries.

Folk medical knowledge may be regarded as clinical experience obtained naturally. However, part of the experience might be mythical reflecting regional differences in culture. The task of separating fact from myth and isolating placebo-effects from objective bioactivity in folk and traditional medicines is a difficult one. We believe that when folk medical experiences derived from the same plant are collated comparatively the real medical effects associated with plant bioactivity will emerge. From this perspective, an international collation of folk medical knowledge should help in establishing objective and reliable medical experience.

The search for bioactive components from plants as a source of lead compounds in drug development, is a major endeavor in phytochemical research. This book is aimed at assisting phytochemists to identify the plant species which most likely contain bioactive components of interest and which may warrant further investigation.

The folk medical knowledge of each entry in the book includes the botanical and local names of the drug, special processing involved, method used for administration, apparent folk medical efficacy in each country, contra-indications and side effects. Also included is the information concerning modern scientific data relating to the associated chemistry and pharmacology as well as references to the available literature.

This second volume continues to cover the outcome generated by the "international collaborating project" propelled by the Regional Network for the Chemistry of Natural Products in Southeast Asia, operated by the United Nations Educational, Scientific and Cultural Organization (UNESCO). The Ministry of Education, Republic of Korea has kindly provided financial support for this ongoing project. On behalf of the Managing Board, I am most grateful to Professor Paul But, the *Editor-in-Chief* of volume II, and other members of the editorial board who undertook the painstaking job of making a literature survey, as well as writing and editing this volume. My sincere gratitude is also extended to the UNESCO Office, Jakarta (ROSTSEA) and the Korea National Commission for UNESCO for their valuable help in the planning and organizing this project.

Byung Hoon Han, Prof., PhD.
Chairman, Managing Board

CONTENTS

EXPLANATIONS AND ABBREVIATIONS

Plant Name
Two hundred important medicinal plants are presented in this volume. The sequence of the plant families follows the classification and arrangement of plant families of Engler's system[1] and the sequence of the individual species in a family follows the alphabetical order of their scientific names. Synonyms are shown as (=). Each representative vernacular name is shown in Roman script followed by an abbreviation of a country/region name. [2]Chinese characters of the herb and plant names are shown in the "Chinese Character Index." Related plants are shown in similar manner.

Part
Pharmacopoeias which adopt a particular herb are shown in abbreviations. [3]Local drug names are the standard or representative vernacular names for that particular herb.

Processing
Procedures for processing the crude drug.

Method of Administration
Routes of administration and preparation methods.

Folk Medicinal Use
Names of diseases or symptoms treated with the herb, followed by an abbreviation of the country which uses the herb for that purpose.

Contra-indications and Side Effects
Warnings for conditions to be avoided in the application of a particular herb and adverse reactions that may be induced by the herb.

Scientific Research
Chemical components and pharmacology reported before 1993 are summarized.

Literature
Format of the literature citation is as follows: First author, *journal title or book title* (in italics), **year** (boldface), volume, and first page.

201. *Gelidium amansii* **Lamouroux** (Gelidiaceae)

Shi-hua-cai (C), Makusa (J), U-mu-ga-sa-ri (K)

Herb
Local Drug Name: Shi-hua-cai (C), Ten-gusa (J), Cheon-cho (K).
Processing: Dry under the sun (C, K).
Method of Administration: Oral (decoction: C, K, agar: J).
Folk Medicinal Uses:

          1) Chronic constipation (C, J).
          2) Ascariasis (C).
          3) Psoriasis (K).
          4) Carbuncle (K).
          5) Suppurative otitis (K).
          6) Diarrhea (K).
          7) Dysentery (K).
          8) Measles (K).
          9) Jaundice (K).

Scientific Research:
Chemistry
    1) Polysaccharides: agarose, agaropectin [1–3, 5, 9–13].
    2) Aminosulfonic acids: taurine, N,N-dimethyltaurine [4].
    3) Inorganics: gallium [7], Ca, K, Na, Mg, Fe, Cu, Zn, S [8].
    4) Enzymes: fructose diphosphate aldolase [6].
    5) Polyamines: putrescine, spermidine, 1,3-diaminopropane, norspermidine, norspermine
       [12].
Pharmacology
    1) Tropic effects of kidneys and tibia [8].

Literature:
[1] Araki, C.: *Proc. Int. Seaweed Symp., 5th, Halifax, N. S.* **1965**, 3.
[2] Fuse, T.: *Nippon Nogei Kagaku Kaishi* **1969**, 43, 292.
[3] Fuse, T. *et al.*: *Nippon Nogei Kagaku Kaishi* **1969**, 43, 621.
[4] Miyazawa, K. *et al.*: *Nippon Suisan Gakkaishi* **1969**, 35, 1215.
[5] Akahane, T. *et al.*: *Nippon Nogei Kagaku Kaishi* **1968**, 42, 740.
[6] Ikawa, T. *et al.*: *Proc. Int. Seaweed Symp., 7th* **1971**, 526.
[7] Yamamoto, T. *et al.*: *Nippon Kaiyo Gakkai-Shi* **1976**, 32, 182.
[8] Kisu, Y. *et al.*: *Seikatsu Kagaku Kenkyusho Kenkyu Hokoku,* **1980**, 13, 9.
[9] Nakamura, T. *et al.*: *Kyushu Joshi Daigaku Kiyo* **1977**, 13, 23.
[10] Yoon, H. S. *et al.*: *Han'guk Susan Hakhoechi* **1985**, 18, 37.
[11] Yoon, H. S. *et al.*: *Pusan Susan Taehak Yongu Pogo, Chayon Kwahak,* **1984**, 24, 27.
[12] Hamana, K. *et al.*: *J. Biochem.(Tokyo)* **1982**, 91, 1321.
[13] Whyte, J. N. C. *et al.*: *Carbohydr. Res.* **1985**, 140, 336.

                     [C.K. Sung]

202. *Cordyceps sinensis* (Berk.) Sacc. (Hypocreaceae)

Dong-chong-xia-cao (C), Dung-chung-har-cho (H), To-chu-ka-so-kin (J),
Dong-chung-ha-cho (K)

Fruiting body with moth larva body (CP)
Local Drug Name: Dong-chong-xia-cao (C), Dung-chung-har-cho (H), To-chu-ka-so (J),
Dong-chung-ha-cho (K).
Processing: Collect in early summer while the fruiting body just emerges above the ground
and before the spores are released, dry partially in the sun, remove the
attached fibrous matter and other impurities, and dry in the sun or at a low
temperature (C, K).
Method of Administration: Oral (decoction: C, H, J, K).
Folk Medicinal Uses:
1) Chronic cough and asthma (C, H, K).
2) Hemoptysis in phthisis (C).
3) Impotence and seminal emissions with aching of loins and knees (C, H, J, K).
4) Weakness (H, K).

Scientific Research:
Chemistry
1) Nucleosides: uracil, uridine, adenine, adenosine, thymine, thymidine, rigosylhypoxanthine, hypoxanthine [1–4].
2) Amino acids: glutamic acid, phenylalanine, proline, histidine, alanine, etc. [5–6].
3) Steroids: ergosterol, $5\alpha,8\alpha$-epidioxy-5α-ergosta-6,22-dien-3β-ol, cholesterol palmitate [7].
4) Phospholipids: phosphatidylcholine, phosphatidylinositol, phosphatidylserine, phosphatidic acid, phosphatidylethanolamine, etc. [8].
5) Polyamines: 1,3-diaminopropane, putrescine, cadaverine, homospermidine, spermine [9].
6) Sugars: mannitol (cordycepic acid), mycose [1], galactomannan [10].
7) Organic acids: stearic acid [1], palmitic acid [7], oleic acid, linoleic acid.
8) Trace elements: Mg, Fe, Ca, P, etc. [11–12].
9) Others: fluoride [13].
Pharmacology
1) Bronchiectasic effect [14–15].
2) Calmative effect [15].
3) Androgen-like effect [15].
4) Effect on cardiovascular system [14–16].
5) Anticancer effect [17].
6) Psyctic effect [18].
7) Effect on glycometabolism and lipometabolism [18–19].
8) Antiinflammatory effect [19].
9) Intensive effect on adrenocortial funtion [19–20].
10) Radiation protective effect [20].
11) Expectorant effect and asthma preventing effect [16].
12) Antihypertensive effect [22].
13) Immunoenhancing effect [20, 23–24].
14) Cholesterol-lowering effect [25].

15) Analgesic effect [26].
16) Antiherpes effect [27].
17) Antidiabetic effect [28].
18) Inhibitory effect on ileum [29].
19) Inhibitory effect on womb.
20) Antibacterial effect.
21) Protective effect against nephrotoxicity [30–32].

Literature:
[1] Lu, R. J. *et al.*: *Yaoxue Tongbao* **1981**, 16, 567.
[2] Xu, W. H. *et al.*: *Zhongyao Tongbao* **1983**, 13(4), 34.
[3] Jiang, P.: *Xibei Yaoxue Zazhi* **1987**, (12), 43.
[4] Xu, W. H. *et al.*: *Zhongyao Tongbao* **1988**, 13, 226.
[5] Huang, R. Y. *et al.*: *Zhongcaoyao* **1980**, 11, 135.
[6] Huang, Y. M. *et al.*: *Zhongchenyao Yanjiu* **1983**, (5), 25.
[7] Xiao, Y. Q. *et al.*: *Zhongyao Tongbao* **1983**, 8(2), 32.
[8] Xu, Y. M. *et al.*: *Tianran Chanwu Yanjiu Yu Kaifa* **1992**, 4(2), 29.
[9] Zhu, C. L. *et al.*: *Zhongcaoyao* **1993**, 24(2), 71.
[10] Miyazaki, T. *et al.*: *Chem. Pharm. Bull.* **1977**, 25, 3324.
[11] Gui, X. G. *et al.*: *Fujian Zhongyiyao* **1982**, 2(2), 32.
[12] Xia, Y. C. *et al.*: *Zhongchenyao Yanjiu* **1985**, (10), 29.
[13] Sakai, T. *et al.*: *Shoyakugaku Zasshi* **1985**, 39, 165.
[14] Zhang, S. S. *et al.*: *Yaoxue Xuebao* **1958**, 6(3), 142.
[15] Zhang, S. S. *et al.*: *Yaoxue Tongbao* **1981**, 16, 139.
[16] Zhao, Y. *et al.*: *Guangxi Zhongyiyao* **1984**, 7(1), 48.
[17] Jiang, P. *et al.*: *Qinghai Yiyao* **1982**, (3), 23.
[18] Bao, T. T. *et al.*: *Zhongcaoyao* **1983**, 14, 224.
[19] Tang, R. J. *et al.*: *Zhongcaoyao* **1985**, 16, 489.
[20] Zang, Q. Z. *et al.*: *Zhongcaoyao* **1985**, 16, 306.
[21] Lou, Y. Q. *et al.*: *Zhongcaoyao* **1986**, 17, 209.
[23] Chen, D. M. *et al.*: *Zhongxiyi Jiehe Zazhi* **1985**, 5, 45.
[24] Du, D. J. *et al.*: *Zhongyao Tongbao* **1986**, 11(7), 51.
[25] Soma, G. *et al.*: *Eur. Pat. Appl.* EP 462,021 (cl. A61 K 37/20) 18 Dec **1991**, JP. Appl.
    90/155, 425, 15 Jun **1990**; 36pp.
[26] Soma, G. *et al.*: *Eur. Pat. Appl.* EP 472,467 (cl. A61 K 37/20) 26 Feb **1992**, JP. Appl.
    90/218, 599, 20 Aug **1990**; 48pp.
[27] Soma, G. *et al.*: *Eur. Pat. Appl.* EP 462,020 (cl. A61 K 37/20) 18 Dec **1991**, JP. Appl.
    90/155, 426, 15 Jun **1990**; 36pp.
[28] Soma, G. *et al.*: *Eur. Pat. Appl.* EP 462,022 (cl. A61 K 37/20) 18 Dec **1991**, JP. Appl.
    90/155, 428, 15 Jun **1990**; 34pp.
[29] Ikumoto, T. *et al.*: *Yakugaku Zasshi* **1991**, 111, 504.
[30] Tian, J. *et al.*: *Zhonghua Shenzangbing Zazhi* **1991**, 7, 142.
[31] Tian, J. *et al.*: *Zhongxiyi Jiehe Zazhi* **1991**, 11, 547.
[32] Zhen, F. *et al.*: *Zhongxiyi Jiehe Zazhi* **1992**, 12, 288.
[30] Zhuang, Y.Z.. *et al.*: *Zhonghua Shenzangbing Zazhi* **1996**, 12, 300.

[J.X. Guo]

203.   *Lentinus edodes* **(Berk.) Sing.** (Polyporaceae)
[*=Cortinellus edodes* Ito et Imai]

Xiang-gu (C), Dung-gwoo (H), Shiitake (J), Pyo-go-beo-seot (K)

Fruiting body
Local Drug Name: Xiang-gu (C), Dung-gwoo (H), Ko-jin (J), Pyo-go-beo-seot (K).
Processing: Dry under the sun (C, H, K).
Method of Administration: Oral (decoction or as food: C, H, J, K).
Folk Medicinal Uses:
          1) Hypertension (C, H, J).
          2) Hyperlipemia (H, J).
          3) Weakness after child birth (K).

Scientific Research:
  Chemistry
    1) Polysaccharides: lentinan [1, 4, 21].
    2) Cyclic methylene polysulfides: lenthionine [3, 5, 8, 14, 30].
    3) Lentysine [6–7].
    4) Vitamins: vitamin D [9], thiamine [16].
    5) Purine derivatives: deoxyeritadenine [15], 4-(6-amino-9H-purin-9-yl)-3-hydroxy-
        butyric acid [17], eritadenine [17–19, 22],.
    6) Amino acids [20]: glutamic acid [23].
    7) Flavor compounds: 1-octen-3-ol [23], octanol, *cis*-2-octen-1-ol, furfuryl alcohol,
        1,2,4-trithiolane, dimethylsulfide, 1-methylthiodimethyldisulfide [28].
    8) Nucleosides: 5'-GMP [23].
    9) Alkanes: C_{18} - C_{28} [28].
    10) Nucleic acid: DNA [29].
    11) Sterols: ergosterol [30].
  Pharmacology
    1) Antitumor effect (polysaccharides) [1, 10, 12–13, 21].
    2) Plasma cholesterol lowering effect (eritadenin) [2, 18–19, 22, 24–27], (lentysine) [7],
        (lentinacin) [11].
    3) Hypolipidemic effect (lentysine) [6].

Literature:
[1] Chihara, G. *et al.*: *Cancer Res.* **1970**, 30, 2776.
[2] Kaneda, T. *et al.*: *J. Nutr.* **1966**, 90, 371.
[3] Wada, S. *et al.*: *Eiyo To Shokuryo* **1968**, 20, 355.
[4] Yoshida, T. *et al.*: *Hakko Kogaku Zasshi* **1968**, 46, 125.
[5] Morita, K. et al: *Japan.* 67 20,319, 11 Oct. **1967**, Appl. 15 Oct. **1965**; 3 pp.
[6] Rokujo, T. *et al.*: *Life Sci.* **1970**, 9, 379.
[7] Michi, K. *et al.*: *Eiyo To Shokuryo* **1970**, 23, 218.
[8] Morita, K. *et al.*: *Japan.* 70 18,459, 24 Jun. **1970**, Appl. 28 Jul. **1966**; 2 pp.
[9] Fujita, A. *et al.*: *Vitamin* 1969, 40, 129.
[10] Chihara, G. *et al.*: *Nature* **1969**, 222, 687.
[11] Chibata, I. *et al.*: *Experientia* **1969**, 25, 1237.
[12] Komatsu, N. *et al.*: *Ger. Offen.* 1,915,687, 16 Oct. **1969**, Japan Appl. 28 Mar. 1968-14
    Oct. **1968**; 15 pp.

[13] Fukuoka, F.: *Fr. Demande* 2,020,160, 10 Jul. **1970**, Japan Appl. 08 Oct. 1968-15 Mar. **1969**; 13 pp.

[14] Morita, K. *et al.*: *Chem. Pharm. Bull.* **1967**, 15, 988.

[15] Saito, Y. *et al.*: *Tetrahedron Lett.* **1970**, (56), 4863.

[16] Kikuchi, M. *et al.*: *Shokubutsugaku Zasshi* **1968**, 81, 328.

[17] Itoh, H. *et al.*: *Experientia* **1973**, 29, 271.

[18] Kamiya, T. *et al.*: *Tetrahedron* **1972**, 28, 899.

[19] Kamiya, T. *et al.*: *J. Heterocycl.* **1972**, 9, 359.

[20] Pyo, M. Y. *et al.*: *Hanguk Yongyang Hakhoe Chi* **1975**, 8, 47.

[21] Chihara, G. *et al.*: *Japan.* 72 37,002, 18 Sep. **1972**, Appl. 69 26,023, 04 Apr. **1969**; 5 pp.

[22] Tokita, F. *et al.*: *Mushroom Sci.* **1972**, 8, 783.

[23] Dijkstra, F. Y.: *Z. Lebensm.-Unters. Forsch.* **1976**, 160, 401.

[24] Amano, M. *et al.*: *Eiyo To Shokuryo* **1971**, 24, 428.

[25] Tokuda, S. *et al.*: *Eiyo To Shokuryo* **1972**, 25, 608.

[26] Tokuda, S. *et al.*: *Eiyo To Shokuryo* **1971**, 24, 477.

[27] Tokuda, S. *et al.*: *Eiyo To Shokuryo* **1973**, 26, 113.

[28] Kameoka, H. *et al.*: *Nippon Nogei Kagaku Kaishi* **1976**, 50, 185.

[29] Kuo, M. *et al.*: *Mushroom Sci.* **1972**, 8, 441.

[30] Ono, T. *et al.*: *Eiyo To Shokuryo* **1973**, 26, 547.

[C.K. Sung]

204. *Calvatia gigantea* (Batsch ex Pers.) Lloyd (Lycoperdaceae)

Da-ma-bo (C), Mar-boot (H)

Related plants: *C. lilacina* (Mont.et Berk.) Lloyd: Zi-se-ma-bo (C); *Lasiosphaera fenzlii* Reich.: Tuo-pi-ma-bo (C); *L. nipponica* (Kawam.) Kobayashi: Oni-fusube (J).

Sporophore (CP)
Local Drug Name: Ma-bo (C), Mar-boot (H), Ba-botsu (J).
Processing: Eliminate foreign matter, and break to pieces (C).
Method of Administration: Oral (decoction: C, H, J); Topical (decoction: C).
Folk Medicinal Uses:
        1) Sore throat, cough and hoarseness of voice caused by wind-heat in the lung (C, H).
        2) Epistaxis and traumatic bleeding by external use (C, H).

Scientific Researches:
Chemistry
  1) Lipoid compound [1].
  2) Enzyme [2–4].
  3) Amino acid [5].
  4) Phosphate.
  5) Nitrogen compound: urea [6].
  6) Others: calvatic acid [7].

Pharmacology
  1) Antibacterial effect [8].
  2) Styptic effect [9].
  3) Anticancer effect [10].

Literatures:
[1] Ronald, B. *et al.*: *Comp. Biochem. Physiol.* **1964**, 11, 263.
[2] Mel'nichuk, G. G. *et al.*: *Ukr. Bot. Zh.* **1979**, 36, 243.
[3] Galiotou-Panayotou, M. *et al.*: *Appl. Microbiol. Biotechnol.* **1988**, 28, 543.
[4] Komninos, T.: *Biotechnol. Bioeng.* **1988**, 32, 939.
[5] Wang, L. *et al.*: *Shipin Kexue (Beijing)* **1985**, 61, 10.
[6] Stijve, T. *et al.*: *Dtsch. Lebensm-Rundsch* **1988**, 8, 248.
[7] Umezawa, H. *et al.*: *J. Antibiot.* **1975**, 28, 87.
[8] Cao, R. L. *et al.*: *Zhonghua Pifuke Zazhi* **1957**, 5, 286.
[9] Dept. of Stomatology, Shanghai Second Medical College: *Zhonghua Kouqiangke Zazhi* **1960**, 8(3), 143.
[10] "*Zhongyao Zhi*" **1994**, 5, 771.

[J.X. Guo]

205.   *Usnea diffracta* **Vain.**   (Usneaceae)

Jie-song-luo (C), Yokowa-saruogase (J), Song-ra (K)

Herb
Local Drug Name: Song-luo (C), Sho-ra (J), Song-ra (K).
Processing: Dry under the sun (C, J, K).
Method of Administration: Oral (decoction: C, J, K); Topical (powder or decoction: C).
Folk Medicinal Uses:
              1) Scrofula (J, K).
              2) Swelling (J, K).
              3) Pulmonary tuberculosis (C).
              4) Chronic bronchitis (C).
              5) Infectious wound (C: topical).
              6) Melena (J).
              7) Epistaxis (J).
              8) Scalds (J).
              9) Menostasis (K).
              10) Cardiac disease (K).

Scientific Research:
Chemistry
  1) Acids: *d*-usnic acid, diffractaic acid [1].
  2) Fatty acids: linoleic acid, oleic acid, arachidonic acid [2–3].
  3) Sterols: $\Delta^{5,7}$-sterol, ergosterol [3].
Pharmacology
  1) Antiinflammatory effect (*d*-usnic acid) [1].

2) Analgesic effect [4].
3) Antipyretic effect [4].

Literature:
[1] Otsuka, H. *et al.*: *Takeda Kenkyusho Ho* **1972**, 31, 247.
[2] Yamamoto, Y. *et al.*: *J. Gen. Appl. Microbiol.* **1974**, 20, 83.
[3] Mitsuhashi, T. *et al.*: *Tokyo Gakugei Daigaku Kiyo, Dai-4-Bu* **1974**, 26, 110.
[4] Okuyama, E. *et al.*: *Planta Med.* **1995**, 61, 113.

[C.K. Sung]

206.   *Selaginella tamariscina* **Spring**   (Selaginellaceae)

Juan-bai (C), Guan-park (H), Iwahiba (J), Bu-cheo-son (K)

Herb (CP)
Local Drug Name: Juan-bai (C), Guan-park (H), Kan-paku (J), Gwon-baek (K).
Processing: Dry under the sun (C, J, K), stir-fry until charred black (C).
Method of Administration: Oral (decoction: C, H, J, K).
Folk Medicinal Uses:
    1) Amenorrhea (C, H, K).
    2) Uterine bleeding and atony (C, H).
    3) Melena (H, K).
    4) Menoxenia (J, K).
    5) Dysmenorrhea (C).
    6) Mass formation in the abdomen (C).
    7) Spitting of blood (C, H: carbonized drug).
    8) Hemorrhoids (H).
    9) Hemostyptic (K).
    10) Itching (K).
    11) Traumatic injury (K).
    12) Acute gastritis (K).
    13) Abdominal pain (K).
    14) Prolapse of rectum (C, H).
    15) Hematochezia (C, H).
Contraindications: Pregnancy.

Scientific Research:
Chemistry
    1) Flavonoids: lutein, hinokiflavone [1], amentoflavone [2–3], cryptomerin B,
        isocryptomerin [3].
    2) Steroids: 3β-cholesterol [1].
Pharmacology
    1) Cytotoxic effect [2].

Literature:
[1] Shin, D. I. *et al.*: *Yakhak Hoechi*, **1994**, 38, 683.

[2] Lee, I. R. *et al.*: *Saengyak Hakhoechi* **1992**, 23, 132.
[3] Shin, D. I. *et al.*: *Saengyak Hakhoechi* **1991**, 22, 207.

[C.K. Sung]

207.   *Equisetum hiemale* **L.**   (Equisetaceae)

Mu-zei (C), Muk-chark (H), Tokusa (J), Sok-sae (K)

Herb (CP)
Local Drug Name: Mu-zei (C), Muk-chark (H), Moku-zoku (J), Mok-jeok (K).
Processing: Remove withered stems and remaining roots, cut into sections, and dry (C, K).
Method of Administration: Oral (decoction: C, H, J, K).
Folk Medicinal Uses:
    1) Conjunctival congestion caused by wind-heat (C, H).
    2) Lacrimation induced by irritation of the wind (C).
    3) Nebula (C, H).
    4) Intestinal hemorrhage (J, K).
    5) Hemorrhoidal bleeding (J).
    6) Menorrhagia (J).
    7) Large intestinal catarrh (K).
    8) Ophthalmia (K).
    9) Prolapse of anus (K).

Scientific Research:
Chemistry
    1) Flavonoids: herbacetin-3-β-D-(2-*O*-β-D-glucopyranosido-glucopyranoside)-8-β-D-
        glucopyranoside, gossypetin-3-β-D-(2-*O*-β-D-glucopyranosido-glucopyranoside)-
        8-β-D-glucopyranoside [1], kaempferol-3,7-diglucoside, kaempferol-3-digluco-
        side-7-glucoside, kaempferol-3-glucoside-7- diglucoside [2].
    2) Alkaloids: palustrine [3], nicotine [4].
    3) Organic acids: caffeic acid, ferrulic acid [4].
    4) Sugars: glucose, fructuse [5].
    5) Silicon compounds [6].
    6) Trace elements: K, Ca, Mn, N, S, P [7].
Pharmacology
    1) Antihypertensive effect [3].
    2) Toxic reaction [8].
    3) Weak inhibitory effect on aldose reductase [9].

Literature:
[1] Geiger, H. *et al.*: *Z. Naturforsch. B: Anorg. Chem., Org. Chem.* **1982**, 37B, 504.
[2] Saleh, N. A. M. *et al.*: *Phytochemistry* **1972**, 11, 1095.
[3] Phillipson, J. D.: *J. Pharm. Pharmacol.* **1960**, 12, 506.
[4] Heynauer, R.: *Chemotaxonomie der Pflanzen* **1962**, 1, 251.
[5] Kientzler, L. *et al.*: *Bull. Soc. Lorraine Sci.* **1962**, 2, 34.
[6] Hartley, R. D. *et al.*: *J. Exp. Bot.* **1972**, 23, 637.

[7] Saint-Paul, A.: *Plant. Med. Phytothec.* **1980**, 14(2), 73.
[8] Kingsbury: *Plants of the U.S. & Canada* **1964**, 116.
[9] Matsuda, H. *et al.*: *Biol. Pharm. Bull.* **1995**, 18, 463.

[J.X. Guo]

208.   *Lygodium japonicum* **Swartz**   (Schizaeaceae)

Hai-jin-sha (C), Hoi-gum-sar (H), Kanikusa (J), Sil-go-sa-ri (K)

Spore (CP)
  Local Drug Name: Hai-jin-sha (C), Hoi-gum-sar (H), Kai-kin-sha (J), Hae-geum-sa (K).
  Processing: Dry under the sun (C, K).
  Method of Administration: Oral (decoction: C, H, J, K).
  Folk Medicinal Uses:
                1) Acute urinary tract infection (C, H, J).
                2) Urolithiasis (C, J).
                3) Gonorrhoea (J, K).
                4) Hematuria (C).
                5) Chyluria (C).
                6) Urethral pain with difficult urination (C).
                7) Leukorrhea (H).
                8) Edema (H).
                9) Enteritis (H).
               10) Eczema (H).

Herb
  Local Drug Name: Hoi-gum-sar-teng (H).
  Processing: Dry under the sun (H).
  Method of Administration: Oral (decoction: H).
  Folk Medicinal Uses:
                1) Urinary tract infection and stones (H).
                2) Nephritis edema (H).
                3) Common cold (H).
                4) Fever (H).
                5) Epidemic encephalitis (H).
                6) Hepatitis (H).
                7) Enteritis (H).
                8) Dysentery (H).
                9) Parotitis (H).
               10) Mastitis (H).
               11) Bronchitis (H).

Scientific Research:
  Chemistry
    1) Flavonoids: low-polymeric flavonols, kaempferol [1].
    2) Phenolic acids: chlorogenic acid, neochlorogenic acid, caffeic acid [1].

9

3) Tannins [1].
4) Fatty acids: palmitic, stearic, oleic, linoleic acid, (+)-8-hydroxyhexadecanoic acid [2].
5) Plant hormones: (+)-*cis,trans*-abscisic acid [2].
Pharmacology
1) Antimicrobial effect.

Literature:
[1] Vaudois, B. *et al.*: *Bull. Soc. Bot. Fr.* **1976**, 123, 219.
[2] Yamane, H. *et al.*: *Agric. Biol. Chem.* **1980**, 44, 1697.

[C.K. Sung]

209.   *Cibotium barometz* **(L.) J.Sm.**   (Dicksoniaceae)

Jing-mao-gou-ji (C), Gum-moe-gau-jak (H), Taka-warabi (J), Gu-cheok (K)

Rhizome (CP)
Local Drug Name: Gou-ji (C), Gau-jak (H), Ku-seki (J), Gu-cheok (K).
Processing: 1) Eliminate foreign matter, wash clean, soften thoroughly, cut into thick slices, and dry (C, K).
            2) Scald the slices with sand until inflated, and after cooling remove all hair (C).
Method of Administration: Oral (decoction: C, H, J, K).
Folk Medicinal Uses:
            1) Weakness and aching of the back and loins (C, H, J, K).
            2) Limpness of the legs (C, J).
            3) Rheumatic arthralgia (C, H, J, K).
            4) Hemiplegia (H).
            5) Enuresis (H).
            6) Polyuria (H).
            7) Nocturnal emission (H).
            8) Leukorrhea (H).
            9) External bleeding (using hair as topical treatment: H).

Scientific Research:
Chemistry
1) Phenol: aspidinol [1].
2) Pterosin derivatives: pterosin Y, isohistopterosin A, etc. [2].
3) Tannins [3].
4) Phytochromes [3].
5) Trace elements [4].
Pharmacology
1) Styptic effect [5].

Literature:
[1] *"Quanguo Zhongcaoyao Huibian"* **1975**, Vol. 1, 530.
[2] Murakami, *et al.*: *Phytochemistry* **1980**, 19, 1743.
[3] Hoppe, H. A.: *Drogenkunde* **1958**, 219.

[4] Xi, Y. Y. *et al.*: *Shanxi Daxue Xuebao, Ziran Kexueban* **1990**, 13, 334.

[5] Dept. of Surgery, Second Hospital of the Second Military Medical University: *Zhonghua Waike Zazhi* **1962**, 10, 507.

[J.X. Guo]

210. *Pteridium aquilinum* (L.) Kuhn. var. *latiusculum* Underw.
(Pteridaceae)

Jue (C), Warabi (J), Go-sa-ri (K)

Herb
Local Drug Name: Jue (C), Ketsu-sai (J), Gweol (K).
Processing: Dry under the sun (C, J, K), or use in fresh (C).
Method of Administration: Oral (decoction: C, J, K).
Folk Medicinal Uses:

            1) Dysentery (C, K).

            2) Beri-beri (J, K).

            3) Acute gastritis (K).

            4) Dermatopathy (J, K).

            5) Fever (C).

            6) Jaundice due to damp-heat pathogen (C).

            7) Hypertension (C).

            8) Anasarca (J).

            9) Tuberculosis (K).

          10) Malaria (K).

Side Effects: Mutagenicity.

Scientific Research:
Chemistry

    1) Norsesquiterpene glucoside: ptaquiloside [1, 3, 5, 7, 9].

    2) *p*-Hyroxystyrene glycosides: ptelatoside A, B [4, 6].

    3) Phenylpropanoids: 5-*O*-caffeoylshikimic acid [10].

    4) 1-Indanone derivatives: pterosins [11, 13, 16–17, 19–21, 23–27].

    5) Steroids: ponasteroside A [28].

    6) Organic acids: shikimic acid, quinic acid [15].

    7) Polysaccharides [2].

    8) Amino acids: glutamic acid, phenylalanine, glutamine [18].

    9) Free sugars: glucose, fructose [22].

Pharmacology

    1) Carcinogenic effect [8, 12, 14].

    2) Antithiamine effect [10].

Literature:
[1] Kigoshi, H. *et al.*: *Tennen Yuki Kagobutsu Toronkai Koen Yoshishu* **1992**, 34, 376.

[2] Watson, M. B. *et al.*: *Phytochemistry* **1990**, 29, 3815.

[3] Ojika, M. *et al.*: *Tetrahedron* **1987**, 43, 5261.

[4] Ojika, M. *et al.*: *Tetrahedron* **1987**, 43, 5275.

[5] Ojika, M. *et al.*: *J. Nat. Prod.* **1985**, 48, 634.

[6] Ojika, M. *et al.*: *Chem. Lett.* **1984**, (3), 397.

[7] Niwa, H. *et al.*: *Tetrahedron Lett.* **1983**, 24, 5371.

[8] Hirono, I. *et al.*: *Tennen Yuki Kagobutsu Toronkai Koen Yoshishu*, **1983**, 26, 9.

[9] Niwa, I. *et al.*: *Tetrahedron Lett.* **1983**, 24, 4117.

[10] Fukuoka, M.: *Chem. Pharm. Bull.* **1982**, 30, 3219.

[11] Kuroyanagi, M.: *Chem. Pharm. Bull.* **1979**, 27, 731.

[12] Fukuoka, M. *et al.*: *J. Pharmacobio-Dyn.* **1978**, 1, 324.

[14] Yoshihara, K. et al: *Chem. Pharm. Bull.* **1978**, 26, 2346.

[15] Nakamura, H. *et al.*: *Nippon Nogei Kagaku Kaisi* **1975**, 49, 665

[16] Kuroyanagi, M. *et al.*: *Chem. Pharm. Bull.* **1979**, 27, 592.

[17] Hikino, H. *et al.*: *Phytochemistry* **1976**, 15, 121.

[18] Nakamura, H. *et al.*: *Nippon Nogei Kagaku Kaishi* **1974**, 48, 573.

[19] Kuroyanagi, M. *et al.*: *Chem. Pharm. Bull.* **1974**, 22, 2762.

[20] Kuroyanagi, M. *et al.*: *Chem. Pharm. Bull,* **1974**, 22, 723.

[21] Fukuoka, M. *et al.*: *Chem. Pharm. Bull.* **1972**, 20, 2282.

[22] Nakamura, H. *et al.*: *Nippon Kagaku Kaishi* **1972**, 46, 313.

[23] Yoshihara, K. *et al.*: *Chem. Pharm. Bull.* **1972**, 20, 426.

[24] Hikino, H. *et al.*: *Chem. Pharm. Bull.* **1972**, 20, 210.

[25] Hikino, H. *et al.*: *Chem. Pharm. Bull.* **1971**, 19, 2424.

[26] Yoshihira, K. *et al.*: *Chem. Pharm. Bull.* **1971**, 19, 1491.

[27] Hikino, H.. *et al.*: *Chem. Pharm. Bull.* **1970**, 18, 1488.

[28] Hikino, H. *et al.*: *Tetrahedron* **1969**, 25, 3909.

[C.K. Sung]

211.   *Dryopteris crassirhizoma* **Nakai**   (Aspidiaceae)

Chu-jin-lin-mao-jue (C), Oshida (J), Gwan-jung (K)

Rhizome
Local Drug Name: Guan-zhong (C), Men-ma (J), Gwan-jung (K).
Processing: Dry under the sun (C, J, K).
Method of Administration: Oral (decoction: C); Ether extract (J, K).
Folk Medicinal Uses:
        1) Taeniasis (J, K).
        2) Hookworm (C, J, K).
        3) Prevention of measles and epidemic encephalitis B (C).
        4) Influenza (C).
        5) Dysentery (C).
        6) Endometrorrhagia (C).
        7) Ascariasis (C).
        8) Oxyuriasis (C).
Contraindication: Use with caution in pregnancy (C).

Scientific research:
Chemistry
    1) Phloroglucin derivatives: filicin, flavaspidic acid, filmarone, aspidin, albaspidin, aspidinol, filixinic acid, desaspidin [1-2].

2) Triterpenoids: fern-7-ene, neohop-12-ene, fern-9(11)-ene, hop-22(29)-ene, neohop-13(18)-ene, dryocrassyl acetate, fern-9(11)-en-12-one, isoadiantone, 17αH-trisnorhopanone, hydroxyhopane, dryocrassol, hopene, diplopterol, diploptene, adiantone, hopanol-29, neriifoliol, filicene, trisnorhopane [3].

3) Phenolic compounds: catechol tannin, leucocyanidin, caffeic acid, four chlorogenic acids, coumarylquinic acid and rutin [4], lignins [5], benzoic acid [6].

Literature:

[1] Hisada, S. *et al.*: *Yakugaku Zasshi* **1961**, 81, 301; 1207.

[2] Penttila, A. *et al.*: *J. Pharm. Pharmacol.* **1961**, 13, 531.

[3] Shiojima, K. *et al.*: *Phytochemistry* **1990**; 29, 1079; *Chem. Pharm. Bull.* **1994**, 42, 377.

[4] Laurent, S.: *Compt. Rend.* **1961**, 253, 703.

[5] Sogo, M. *et al.*: *Mokuzaishi.* **1962**, 8, 112; **1966**, 12, 96.

[6] Yasunaga, K. *et al.*: *Nogeishi.* **1962**, 36, 802.

[T. Kimura]

212.   *Cycas revoluta* **Thunb.**   (Cycadaceae)

Su-tie (C), Soe-tid (H), Sotetsu (J), So-cheol(K)

Seed

Local Drug Name: Su-tie (C), Soe-tid (H), Cheol-su-gwa (K).

Processing: Dry under the sun (C, K).

Method of Administration: Oral (decoction: C, H, J, K); Topical (J).

Folk Medicinal Uses:

> 1) Hemostatic (J, K).
> 2) Pleurisy (J, K).
> 3) Hypertension (C, H).
> 4) Menstrual disorder (J).
> 5) Traumatic injury (J).

Side Effects: Toxic.

Leaf

Local Drug Name: Su-tie-ye (C), Tid-shue-yip (H).

Processing: Dry under the sun (C, H).

Method of Administration: Oral (decoction: C, H).

Folk Medicinal Uses:

> 1) Hemorrhagic (C, H).
> 2) Gastritis (C, H).
> 3) Peptic ulcer (C, H).
> 4) Hypertension (C, H).
> 5) Neuralgia (C, H).
> 6) Amenorrhea (C, H).
> 7) Cancer (C, H).

Side effect: Toxic.

Scientific Research:
Chemistry
  1) Glycoside: cycasin [1, 7–8], neocycasins [6].
  2) Polyamines: putrescine [2].
  3) Fatty acids: 5,9,12,15-18:4, 5,11-20:2, 5,11,14-20:3 [3].
  4) Vitamins: vitamin C [4].
  5) β-D-glucosidase [5].
Pharmacology
  1) Carcinogenic effect [9].
  2) Anticancer effect [10].

Literature:
  [1] Kobayashi, A. *et al.*: *Kagoshima Daigaku Nogakubu Gakujutsu Hokoku* **1971**, 21, 129.
  [2] Matsumoto, T. *et al.*: *Nippon Nogei Kagaku Kaishi* **1982**, 56, 209.
  [3] Takagi, T. *et al.*: *Lipids* **1982**, 17, 716.
  [4] Ying, W. *et al.*: *Linchan Huaxue Yu Gongye* **1982**, 2, 42.
  [5] Yagi, F. *et al.*: *J. Biochem.(Tokyo)* **1985**, 97, 119.
  [6] Yagi, F. *et al.*: *Agric. Biol. Chem.* **1985**, 49, 1531.
  [7] Tadera, K. *et al.*: *Agric. Biol. Chem.* **1985**, 49, 2827.
  [8] Nishida, K. *et al.*: *Bull. Agric. Chem. Soc. Japan* **1956**, 20, 74.
  [9] Gusek, W. *et al.*: *Beitr. Pathol. Anat. Allg. Pathol.* **1969**, 139, 199.
  [10] Arikawa, T.: *Igaku Kenkyu* **1961**, 31, 833.

[C.K. Sung]

213.   *Abies holophylla* **Max.**   (Pinaceae)

Shan-song (C), Jeon-na-mu (K)

Leaf
  Local Drug Name: Shan-song (C), Jeon-na-mu-ip (K).
  Processing: Dry under the sun (K).
  Method of Administration: Oral (decoction, K).
  Folk Medicinal Uses:
                1) Leukorrhea (K).
                2) Contusion (K).
                3) Hemiplegia (K).
                4) Rheumatism (C).

Scientific Research:
Chemistry
  1) Essential oils (fir oil) [1]: α-pinene, camphene, bornyl acetate, santene, tricyclene, β-pinene, myrcene, Δ^3-carene, limonene, perillene, linalool, camphor, borneol, *p*-cymen-α-ol, verbenone, *trans*-carveol, 2-isopropyl-5-methyl-anisole, *d*-carvone, bornyl acetate, terpinyl acetate, geranyl acetate, fenchyl acetate, γ-muurolene, α-muurolene, β-bisabolene, α-terpinene, α-terpineol, [1–3].
  2) Nucleic acids (pollen): RNA, DNA, lipid, P, N [4].

14

Literature:

[1] Kolenikova, R. D. *et al.*: *Dev. Food Sci.* **1988**, 18, 601.
[2] Yan, Z.: *Zhongcaoyao* **1988**, 19, 53.
[3] Li, S.: *Linchan Huaxue Yu Gongye* **1982**, 2(4), 36.
[4] Lee, K. Y. *et al.*: *Korean J. Biochem.* **1976**, 8, 13.

[C.K. Sung]

214.   *Pinus densiflora* Sieb. et Zucc.   (Pinaceae)

Chi-song (C), Akamatsu (J) So-na-mu (K)

Related plants: *Pinus thunbergii* Parl.; Kuromatsu (J) and other species of *Pinus* (C).

Balsam
Local Drug Name: Song-xiang (C), Sei-sh -shi (J), Saeng-song-ji (K).
Processing: Dry under the sun.
Method of Administration: Topical (paint, plaster: C, J, K).
Folk Medicinal Uses:
        1) Rheumatism (J, K).
        2) Neuralgia (J, K).
        3) Eczema (C).
        4) Carbuncle (C).
        5) Traumatic bleeding (C).
        6) Burns (C).

Essential oil (CP, JP)
Local Drug Name: Song-jie-you (C), Terebin-yu (J), Te-re-bin-yu (K).
Processing: Steam distillation of the balsam (C, J, K).
Method of Administration: Topical (paint: C, J, K).
Folk Medicinal Uses:
        1) Rheumatism (C, J, K).
        2) Neuralgia (J, K).
        3) Myalgia (C).

Leaf
Local Drug Name: Song-zhen (C), Song-yeop (K).
Processing: Raw or dry (K).
Method of Administration: Oral (decoction: C, K); Topical (decoction: C; fresh juice: K).
Folk Medicinal Uses:
        1) Toothache (K).
        2) Cough (K).
        3) Gonorrhoea (K).
        4) Apoplexy (K).
        5) Gingivitis (K).
        6) Influenza (C).
        7) Rheumatism (C).

8) Swelling (C).
9) Hypertension (C).
10) Neurasthenia (C).
11) Frost bite (C).
12) Nyctalopia (C).

Scientific research:
 Chemistry
   1) Monoterpenes: l-α-pinene, l-β-pinene, dipentene, limonene, terpinene[1].
   2) Diterpenes: abietic acid [6].
   3) Polysaccharides: glucomannan [7–9].
 Pharmacology
   1) Inhibition of cough reflex (essential oil) [2].
   2) Secretion of respiratory tract (essential oil) [3].
   3) Antibacterial effect (essential oil) [4-5].

Literature:
[1] Nagasawa, T. *et al.*: *Koryo* **1961**, 62, 53.
[2] Misawa, M. et al: *Oyo Yakuri* **1990**, 39, 81.
[3] Boyd, E. M. *et al.*: *Am. J. Med. Sci.* **1946**, 211, 602.
[4] Okazaki, K. *et al.*: *Yakugaku Zasshi* **1952**, 72, 1131.
[5] Chalchat, J. C. *et al.*: *Planta Med.* **1985**, 285.
[6] Okada, K. *et al.*: *Bull. Chem. Soc.* **1994**, 67, 807.
[7] Koshojima, T. *et al.*: *Bull. Agr. Chem. Japan* **1960**, 24, 687.
[8] Koshojima, T. *et al.*: *Bull. Agr. Chem. Japan* **1961**, 25, 706
[9] Koshojima, T. *et al.*: *Mokuzai Kenkyu* **1960**, 14.

[T. Kimura]

215.   *Juniperus chinensis* **L.**   (Cupressaceae)
         [=*Sabina chinensis* (L.) Antoine]

Yuan-bai (C), Ibuki (J), Hyang-na-mu (K)

Leaf
 Local Drug Name: Yuan-bai (C), Hoe-yeop (K).
 Processing: Dry under the sun (C, K), or use in fresh (C).
 Method of Administration: Oral (decoction: K); Topical (decoction: C).
 Folk Medicinal Uses:
           1) Common cold caused by wind and cold (C).
           2) Pulmonary tuberculosis (C).
           3) Urinary infection (C).
           4) Urticaria (C).
           5) Dysentery (K).
           6) Hemorrhage (K).
           7) Leukorrhea (K).
           8) Rheumatic arthritis (C).

Scientific Research:

Chemistry

    1) Sterols: sitosterol, campesterol [1].

    2) Lignins [2].

    3) Polyprenols: betulaprenol [3].

    4) Hydrocarbons [4].

    5) Polyphenols: [4].

    6) Essential oils: sabinyl acetate, bornyl acetate [5–6].

    7) Monoterpenes [7].

    8) Fatty acids [1].

Literature:

[1] Endo, S. *et al.*: *Tokyo Gakugei Daigaku Kiyo, Dai-4-bumon* **1984**, 36, 49.

[2] Kutsuki, H. *et al.*: *Phytochemisty* **1982**, 21, 267.

[3] Ibata, K. *et al.*: *Phytochemistry* **1984**, 23, 2517.

[4] Carr, M. E. *et al.*: *JAOCS, J. Am. Oil Chem. Soc.* **1986**, 63, 1460.

[5] Fournier, G. *et al.*: *J. Pharm. Belg.* **1990**, 45, 293.

[6] Fournier, G. *et al.*: *Plant. Med. Phytother.* **1990**, 24, 158.

[7] Van den Dries, J. M. A. *et al.*: *Flavour Fragrance J.* **1989**, 4, 59.

[C.K. Sung]

216.   *Juniperus rigida* **Sieb. Zucc.**   (Cupressaceae)

Du-song (C), Nezu (J), No-gan-ju-na-mu (K)

Seed

Local Drug Name: Du-song (C), To-sho-jitsu (J), Du-song-sil (K).

Processing: Dry under the sun (C, K).

Method of Administration: Oral (decoction: C, K).

Folk Medicinal Uses:

          1) Rheumatic arthralgia (C).

          2) Cystitis (J).

          3) Nephropathy (J).

          4) Edema (J).

          5) Gout (J).

          6) Colic (J).

          7) Toothache (K).

Scientific Research:

Chemistry

    1) Sesquiterpenes: allo-cedrol [1].

    2) Diterpenes: 3β-hydroxysandaracopimaric acid [2].

Literature:

[1] Tomita, B. *et al.*: *Phytochemistry* **1973**, 12, 1409.

[2] Doi, K. *et al.*: *Phytochemistry* **1972**, 11, 841.

[C.K. Sung]

217.   *Taxus cuspidata* Sieb. et Zucc.   (Taxaceae)

Dong-bei-hong-dou-shan (C), Ichi-i (J), Ju-mok (K)

Bark
  Local Drug Name: Ja-sam-pi (K).
  Processing: Dry under the sun (K).
  Method of Administration: Oral (decoction: K).
  Folk Medicinal Uses:
             1) Menostasis (K).
             2) Swelling (K).
             3) Nephritis (K).
             4) Cancer (K).

Leaf
  Local Drug Name: Dong-bei-hong-dou-shan (C), Ichi-i-yo (J), Il-wi-yeop (K).
  Processing: Dry under the sun (J, K).
  Method of Administration: Oral (decoction: J, K).
  Folk Medicinal Uses:
             1) Menstrual disorder (C, J).
             2) Diabetes (C, J).
             3) Swelling (C).

Scientific Research:
  Chemistry
       1) Cyanogenic glucosides: dhurrin, taxiphyllin [1].
       2) Proanthocyanidins [2]: monomeric 3-flavanols [5].
       3) Ecdysteroids: makisterone A [3], taxisterone [10].
       4) Acyclic polyols [4].
       5) Tannins [2].
       6) Phenolic β-glucosides: syringin, coniferin [6].
       7) Lignans: isotaxiresinol, isolariciresinol [7].
       8) Polyprenols: betulaprenol [8], dolichol [9].

Literature:
  [1] Rosen, M. A. *et al.*: *J. Biol. Chem.* **1975**, 250, 8302.
  [2] Samejima, M. *et al.*: *Tennen Yuki Kagobutsu Toronkai Koen Yoshishu, 22nd*, **1979**, 331.
  [3] Burns, B. G. *et al.*: *Can. J. Chem.* **1977**, 55, 1129.
  [4] Wallaart, R. A. M.: *Proc. K. Ned. Akad. Wet., Ser. C* **1981**, 84, 465.
  [5] Samejima, M. *et al.*: *Mokuzai Gakkaishi* **1982**, 28, 67.
  [6] Terazawa, M. *et al.*: *Mokuzai Gakkaishi* **1984**, 30, 322.
  [7] Zhou, Y. *et al.*: *Zhongcaoyao* **1982**, 13, 1.
  [8] Ibata, K. *et al.*: *Phytochemistry* **1984**, 23, 2517.
  [9] Ibata, K. *et al.*: *Eur. Pat. Appl. EP* 95,133, 30 Nov. 1983, Appl. 82/87,049, 21 May 1982;
        52 pp.
  [10] Nakano, K. *et al.*: *Phytochemistry* **1982**, 21, 2749.

[C.K. Sung]

218. *Juglans mandshurica* **Maxim. var.** *sieboldiana* **Makino**
(Juglandaceae)

He-tao-qiu (C), Oni-gurumi (J), Wang-ga-rae-na-mu (K)

Related plant: *Juglans mandshurica* Maxim. He-tao-qiu (C)

Seed
Local Drug Name: He-tao-qiu (C), Ko-to-nin (J), Haek-do-chu-rwa (K).
Processing: Air dry (C, J, K).
Method of Administration: Oral (decoction: C, J, K).
Folk Medicinal Uses:
       1) Constipation (C, J, K).
       2) Cough (C, J, K).
       3) Weakness (C).
       4) Lumbago (C).
       5) Emission (C).
       6) Impotence (C).
       7) Lithangiuria (C).
       8) Hypogalactia (C).
       9) Allergy (K).
       10) Ancylostomiasis (K).
       11) Acute gastritis (K).

Scientific research:
Chemistry
  1) Steroid: sitosterol [1].
  2) Acids: gallic acid, ellagic acid [1].

Literature:
[1] Kondo, T. *et al.*: *Mokuzaishi* **1956**, 2, 221.

[T. Kimura]

219. *Juglans sinensis* **Dode** (Juglandaceae)

Ho-du-na-mu (K)

Related Plant: *Juglans mandshurica* Marium. var. *sieboldiana* Makino: Oni gurumi (J)

Seed
Local Drug Name: Ko-to-nin (J), Ho-do-in (K).
Processing: Dry under the sun (K).
Method of Administration: Oral (decoction: J, K).
Folk Medicinal Uses:
       1) Cough (J, K).
       2) Whooping cough (J, K).
       3) Arteriosclerosis (J).

4) Ancylostomiasis (K).
5) Syphilis (K).
6) Tympanitis (K).
7) Prolapsus ani (K).
8) Scrofula (K).
9) Pile (K).
10) Tooth caries (K).
Contraindications: Watery stool.

Scientific Research:
Chemistry
1) Gangliosides [1].

Literature:
[1] Kim, H. S. *et al.*: *Han'guk Saenghwa Hakhoechi* **1992**, 25, 429.

[C.K. Sung]

220.   *Betula platyphylla* **Suk.**   (Betulaceae)
         B. platyphylla **Suk. var.** *japonica* **Hara**

Bai-hua (C), Shira-kaba (J), Ja-jak-na-mu (K)

Bark
Local Drug Name: Hua-mu-pi (C), Hwa-pi (K).
Processing: Dry under the sun (K).
Method of Administration: Oral (decoction, K).
Folk Medicinal Uses:
1) Internal disease (K).
2) Weakness (K).
3) Febrile disease (C).
4) Expectoration (C).
5) Cough (C).

Scientific Research:
Chemistry
1) Triterpenes: $3\alpha,12\beta,20(S),24$-tetrahydroxydammar-25-ene, betulin, lupeol, oleanolic acid, $3\alpha,12\beta,20(S),25$-tetrahydroxy-dammar-23-ene, oleanolic acid acetate, betulin 3-caffeate, betulinic acid β-caffeate [1, 7].
2) Diarylheptanoids: platyphyllin, platyphyllonol [2].
3) Phenols: betuloside, platyphylloside [5-6] betuligenol [2], paeonol, antiarolaldehyde, vanillin, syringaldehyde, 2-hydroxy-5-(3-hydroxybutyl) benzaldehyde [4].
4) Polysaccharides: birch xylan [3].
5) Sterols: β-sitosterol [7].
6) Hydrocarbons: hexadecane, octadecane, eicosane, dodecane, tetracosane [7].
Pharmacology
1) Antifungal effect [4].

Literature:

[1] Ohta, A. *et al.*: *Phytochemistry* **1972**, 11, 3037.
[2] Terazawa, M. *et al.*: *Mokuzai Gakkaishi* **1973**, 19, 47.
[3] Shimizu, K. *et al.*: *Mokuzai Gakkaishi* **1976**, 22, 51.
[4] Yokota, M. *et al.*: *Yakugaku Zasshi* **1978**, 98, 1607.
[5] Miyake, M.: *Mokuzai Gakkaishi* **1984**, 30, 329.
[6] Ohta, S. *et al.*: *Bull. Chem. Soc. Jpn.* **1985**, 58, 2423.
[7] Ohara, S. *et al.*: *Mokuzai Gakkaishi* **1986**, 32, 266.

[C.K. Sung]

221.　　　　　*Quercus acutissima* **Carruth**　　(Fagaceae)

Ma-li (C), Kunugi (J), Sang-su-ri-na-mu (K)

Fruit
Local Drug Name: Ma-li (C), Sang-sil (K).
Processing: Dry under the sun (C, K).
Method of Administration: Oral (decoction: C, K).
Folk Medicinal Uses:
　　　　　　1) Mastitis (C, K).
　　　　　　2) Diarrhea (K).
　　　　　　3) True psoriasis (K).
　　　　　　4) Dysentery (K).
　　　　　　5) Panaritium (K).
　　　　　　6) Gonorrhoea (K).
　　　　　　7) Gastropathy (K).
　　　　　　8) Cathartic (K).
　　　　　　9) Ascariasis (K).

Bark
Local Drug Name: Ma-li (C), Boku-so (J), Sang-mok-pi (K).
Processing: Dry under the sun (J, K).
Method of Administration: Oral (decoction: C, K).
Folk Medicinal Uses:
　　　　　　1) Diarrhea (C, J).
　　　　　　2) Hemorrhoids (J).
　　　　　　3) Gonorrhoea (K).
　　　　　　4) Mastitis (K).
　　　　　　5) Panaritium (K).
　　　　　　6) Arthritis (K).

Scientific Research:
Chemistry
　　1) Tannins [1]: ellagic acid.
　　2) Proteins [2].
　　3) Amino acids [2].
　　4) Mineral and trace elements [2].

21

Pharmacology
1) Antioxidative effect (ellagic acid) [3].

Literature:

[1] Ishimaru, K. *et al.*: *Phytochemistry* **1987**, 26, 1147.
[2] Liu, P.: *Beijing Linxueyuan Xuebao* **1984**, (4), 36.
[3] Hosono, A. *et al.*: *Agric. Biol. Chem.* **1991**, 44, 1397.

[C.K. Sung]

222.   *Quercus myrsinaefolia* **Bl.**   (Fagaceae)
[=*Cyclobalanopsis myrsinaefolia* (Bl.) Oerst.]

Xiao-ye-qing-gang (C), Shirakashi (J), Ga-si-na-mu (K)

Fruit
Local Drug Name: Zhu-zi (C), Sho-shi (J), Myeon-sil (K).
Processing: Dry under the sun (J, K).
Method of Administration: Oral (decoction: J, K).
Folk Medicinal Uses:
1) Gallstone (J, K).
2) Urinary calculus (J).
3) Galactagogue (K).
4) Weakness (C, K).
5) Diarrhea (C).

Scientific Research:
Chemistry
1) Terpenoids [1].
2) Steroids [1].

Literature:

[1] Hui, W.-H. *et al.*: *J. Chem. Soc., Perkin Trans.* I **1977**, (8), 897.

[C.K. Sung]

223.   *Celtis sinensis* **Pers.**   (Ulmaceae)

Po-shu (C), Paeng-na-mu (K)

Related plant: *Celtis sinensis* Pers. var. *japonica* (Planch.) Nakai: Enoki (J).
Bark
Local Drug Name: Po-shu-pi (C), Boku-ju-hi (J), Bak-su-pi (K).
Processing: Dry under the sun (K), use in fresh (C).

Method of Administration: Oral (decoction, C, J, K).
Folk Medicinal Uses:
>1) Lumbago (C, J).
>2) Irregular menstruation (J, K).
>3) Gastric disease (J, K).
>4) Abdominal pain (K).

Leaf
Local Drug Name: Po-shu-ye (C), Bak-su-yeop (K).
Processing: Dry under the sun (C, K).
Method of Administration: Oral (decoction: K); Topical (paste: C).
Folk Medicinal Uses:
>1) Lacquer sore (C).
>2) Urticaria (J).
>3) Eczema (K).

Scientific Research:
Chemistry
>1) Cellulose [2].

Pharmacology
>1) Antifeedant effect [1].

Literature:
[1] Numata, A. *et al.*: *Chem. Pharm. Bull.* **1984**, 32, 325.
[2] Chao, S. C. *et al.*: *Tai-Wan Sheng Lin Yeh Shih Yen So Lin Wu Chu Ho Tso Shih Yen Pao Kao* **1971**, No. 14, 26 pp.

[C.K. Sung]

224. *Ulmus davidiana* Planch. var. *japonica* (Rehder) Nakai (Ulmaceae)

Haru-nire (J), Neu-reup-na-mu (K)

Bark
Local Drug Name: Yu-hi (J), Nang-yu-pi (K).
Processing: Dry under the sun (J, K).
Method of Administration: Oral (decoction: J, K).
Folk Medicinal Uses:
>1) Ringworm (J).
>2) Tinea (J).
>3) Edema (J).
>4) Furuncle (K).
>5) Inflammation (K).
>6) Boil (K).
>7) Bruise (K).
>8) Constipation (K).
>9) Granulating (K).

10) Eruption (K).
11) Hemorrhoid (K).
12) Mastitis (K).

Scientific Research:
Chemistry
   1) Triterpenes: friedelin, epifriedelanol, taraxerol [1].
   2) Catechin and catechin glycosides: uldavioside [2].
   3) Minerals: Ca, Mg, K [3–4].

Literature:
[1] Hong, N. D. *et al.*: *Saengyak Hakhoechi* **1990**, 21, 201.
[2] Son, B. H. *et al.*: *Arch. Pharmacal Res.* **1989**, 12, 219.
[3] Tomioka, E.: *Hokkaido Nogyo Shikenjo Kenkyu Hokoku*, **1978**, 123, 89.
[4] Tomioka, E. *et al.*: *Hokkaido Nogyo Shikenjo Kenkyu Hokoku* **1978**, 123, 79.

[C.K. Sung]

225. *Eucommia ulmoides* Oliv.   (Eucommiaceae)

Du-zhong (C), Doe-chung (H), To-chu (J), Du-chung (K)

Bark (CP)
Local Drug Name: Du-zhong (C), Doe-chung (H), To-chu (J), Du-chung (K).
Processing: 1) Scrap off the remains of the coarse outer layer, wash clean, cut into pieces or slivers, and dry (C, K).
             2) Stir-fry slices with salt-water until charred and the rubber threads shredded (C).
Method of Administration: Oral (decoction: C, H, J, K).
Folk Medicinal Uses:
             1) Dificiency condition of 'kidney' with lumbago and lack of strength (C, H, J, K).
             2) Threatened abortion (C, H, J, K).
             3) Hypertension (C, H, J, K).
             4) Impotence (J, K).

Leaf
Local Drug Name: To-chu-yo (J).
Processing: Drug under the sun (J).
Method of Administration: Oral (Tea: J).
Folk Medicinal Uses:
             1) General weakness (J).
             2) Lumbago (J).
             3) Hypertension (J).

Scientific Research:
Chemistry
   1) Liganans: pinoresinol-di-β-D-glucoside [1, 27], *d*-medioresinol di-*O*-β-D-glucopy-ranoside, *d*-pinoresinol-*O*-β-D-glucopyranoside, liriodendrin [2], *l*-olivil 4',4"-di-

O-β-D-glucopyranoside, *d*-medioresinol 4'-*O*-β-D-glucopyranoside (eucommin A), *d*-1-hydroxypinoresinol 4',4"-di-*O*-β-D-glucopyranoside, *d*-syringaresinol *O*-β-D-glucopyranoside [3], *d*-1-hydroxypinoresinol 4"-*O*-β-D-glucopyranoside, *d*-1-hydroxypinoresinol 4'-*O*-β-D-glucopyranoside, *dl*-erythro-guaiacylglycerol, *dl*-threo-guaiacylglycerol, *d*-cycloolivil, *l*-olivil [4], *l*-olivil 4"-*O*-β-D-glucopyranoside, hedyotol C 4",4"'-di-*O*-β-D-glucopyranoside (guaiacylglycerol-β-medioresinol ether 4",4"'-di-O-β-D-glucopyranoside), *l*-olivil 4'-*O*-β-D-glucopyranoside [5], erythro-dihydroxydehydrodiconiferyl alcohol and its thero-isomer [6], syringylglycerol-β-syringaresinol ether 4",4"'-di-*O*-β-D-glucopyranoside, citrusin B, dehydrodiconiferyl alcohol, 4,γ'-di-*O*-β-D-glucopyranoside [7], *d*-epipino-resinol [8].

2) Iridoids: eucommiol, eucommioside I, genipaside, aucubin, geniposidic acid [5], ulmoside (aucubigenin-1β-isomaltoside) [9].

3) Polysaccharides: eucomman A [10], eucomman B [11].

4) Phospholipid composition: phosphatidylcholine, lysophosphatidylcholine [12].

5) Organic acids: chlorogenic acid [13], vanillic acid [14].

6) Triterpenes: betulin, betulic acid, ursolic acid [14].

7) Steroids: β-sitosterol [14], daucosterol [15].

8) Aliphatic compounds: nonacosane, *n*-triacontanol [14], ulmoprenol [16].

9) Votatile components: 4 acids, 11 alcohols, 9 aldehydes, 4 esters, 3 ketones, 16 hydrocarbons, lactone [17].

10) Rubber: gutta-percha [18].

11) Trace elements: Zn, Mn, Cu, Fe, Ca, P, Pb [19].

12) Terpene: loliolide [26].

Pharmacology

1) Antihypertensive effect [13, 20] (pinoresinol-di-β-D-glucoside, aucubin, chlorogenic acid).

2) Antiinflammatory effect [21].

3) Sedative effect [22].

4) Analgesic effect [22].

5) Immunoregulatory effect [23–24, 26].

6) Inhibitory effect on heart cAMP phosphodiesterase (*d*-syringaresinol dipyranoside, *d*-pinoresinol di-*O*-β-D-glucopyranoside, *d*-1-hydroxypinoresinol 4',4"-di-*O*-β-D-glucopyranoside) [25].

7) Anticomplementary effect (*d*-syringaresinol monoglucoside, *d*-medioresinol monoglucoside, *d*-epipinoresinol, genipin) [8].

8) Reticuloendothelial system potentiating effect (eucomman A, eucomman B).

Literature:
[1] Charles, J. S. *et al.*: *J. Amer. Chem. Soc.* **1976**, 5412.
[2] Deyama, T. *et al.*: *Chem. Pharm. Bull.* **1983**, 31, 2993.
[3] Deyama, T. *et al.*: *Chem. Pharm. Bull.* **1985**, 33, 3651.
[4] Deyama, T. *et al.*: *Chem. Pharm. Bull.* **1986**, 34, 523.
[5] Deyama, T. *et al.*: *Chem. Pharm. Bull.* **1986**, 34, 4933.
[6] Deyama, T. *et al.*: *Chem. Pharm. Bull.* **1987**, 35, 1785.
[7] Deyama, T. *et al.*: *Chem. Pharm. Bull.* **1987**, 35, 1803.
[8] Oshima, Y. *et al.*: *J. Ethnopharmacol.* **1988**, 23, 159.
[9] Biamo, A. *et al.*: *Gazz. Chim. Ital.* **1978**, 108, (1–2), 17; *Tetrahedron* **1974**, 30, 4117.
[10] Gonda, R. M. *et al.*: *Chem. Pharm. Bull.* **1990**, 38, 1966.
[11] Tomoda, M. *et al.*: *Phytochemistry* **1990**, 29, 3091.
[12] Xu, Y. M. *et al.*: *Tianran Chanwu Yanjiu Yu Kaifa* **1992**, 4(2), 29.

[13] Li, J. S. *et al.*: *Zhongyao Tongbao* **1986**, 11, 489.

[14] Li, D. *et al.*: *Zhiwu Xuebao* **1986**, 28, 528.

[15] Xu, J. W. *et al.*: *Zhiwu Xuebao* **1989**, 31, 132.

[16] Horii, Z. *et al.*: *Tetrahedron Lett.* **1978**, (50), 5015.

[17] Jang, H. J. *et al.*: *Han'guk Nonghwa Hakhoechi* **1990**, 33, 116.

[18] Liu, S. T. *et al.*: *Zhongguo Zhongyao Zazhi* **1989**, 14, 596.

[19] Wang, Z, X.: *Kexue Tongbao* **1951**, 2, 468.

[20] Fan, W. H. *et al.*: *Yaoxue Tongbao* **1979**, (9), 404.

[21] Xu, S. L. *et al.*: *Zhongcaoyao* **1982**, 13, 264.

[22] Chen, J. M. *et al.*: *Zhongcaoyao* **1986**, 17(3), 30.

[23] Xu, S. L. *et al.*: *Zhongcaoyao* **1983**, 14(8), 27.

[24] Xu, S. L. *et al.*: *Zhongcaoyao* **1985**, 16(9), 15.

[25] Deyama, T. *et al.*: *Chem. Pharm. Bull.* **1988**, 36, 435.

[26] Okada, N. *et al.*: *Phytochemistry* **1994**, **37**, 281.

[27] Sha, Z.F. *et al.*: *Yaoxue Xuebao* **1986**, 21, 708.

[J.X. Guo & T. Kimura]

226.   *Broussonetia kazinoki* Sieb. et Zucc.   (Moraceae)

Xiao-gou-shu (C), Kouzo (J), Dak-na-mu (K)

Root bark

Local Drug Name: Gu-pi-shu (C), Gu-pi-ma (K).

Processing: Dry under the sun (C, K).

Method of Administration: Oral (decoction: C, J, K).

Folk Medicinal Uses:

         1) Edema (J, K).

         2) Abdominal pain (J, K).

         3) Wart (K).

         4) Leukorrhea (K).

         5) Boil (K).

         6) Traumatic injury (C).

         7) Lumbago (C).

Scientific Research:

  Chemistry

    1) Isoprenyl flavans: kazinol E, H [1].

    2) Isoprenyl 1,3-diphenylpropanes: kazinol C, D, F, G, H [1], J, L, M, N [3].

    3) Isoprenyl spiro compounds: kazinol P [2].

    4) Fibers [4].

  Pharmacology

    1) Antimicrobial effect [5].

Literature:

[1] Ikuta, J. *et al.*: *Chem. Pharm. Bull.* **1986**, 34, 1968.

[2] Kato, S. *et al.*: *Heterocycles* **1986**, 24, 2141.

[3] Kato, S. *et al.*: *Chem. Pharm. Bull.* **1986**, 34, 2448.

[4] Saito, Y. *et al.*: *Nenpo - Fukui-ken Kogyo Shikenjo* **1979**, 53, 179.
[5] Shirata, A. *et al.*: *Sanshi Shikenjo Hokoku* **1982**, 28, 707.

[C.K. Sung]

227.   *Cannabis sativa* **L.**   (Moraceae)

Da-ma (C), Die-mar (H), Asa (J), Sam (K)

Fruit (CP)
Local Drug Name: Huo-ma-ren (C), For-mar-yun (H), Ma-shi-nin (J), Ma-ja-in (K).
Processing: 1) Eliminate foreign matter (C, K).
              2) Stir-fry until yellowish and scented (C).
Method of Administration: Oral (decoction: C, H, J, K).
Folk Medicinal Uses:
            1) Constipation due to deficiency of blood and intestinal fluid (C, H, J, K).
            2) Acute gastritis (K).
            3) Leukorrhea (K).

Leaf
Local Drug Name: Ma-yeop (K).
Processing: Eliminate foreign matter, dry (K).
Method of Administration: Oral (decoction: K).
Folk Medicinal Uses:
            1) Pleurisy (K).
            2) Eczema (K).
            3) Tinea (K).
            4) Dysentery (K).

Scientific Research:
Chemistry
    1) Fatty acids: saturated fatty acids, oleic acid, linoleic acid, linolenic acid [1].
    2) Alkaloids: trigonelline, L-*d*-isoleucin betaine, muscarine [2].
    3) Amides: cannabisin A, grossamide, *N-trans*-caffeoyltyramine, *N-trans*-feruloyltyra-
        mine, *N-p*-coumaroyltyramine [3], cannabisin B, cannabisin C, cannabisin D [4].
    4) Phenols: cannabinol, cannabidiol [5].
    5) Vitumine: vitamin B1 [6].
    6) Proteins and Enzymes [7].
Pharmacology
    1) Effect of causing hypothermia and motor incoordination (feruloyltyramine, *p*-
        couma-royltyramine) [8].
    2) Cataleptogenic effect (*p*-coumaroyltyramine) [8].

Literature:
[1] *Dictionary of Applied Chemistry* (Thorep) 4Ed., 6, 203.
[2] Bercht, C. A. L. *et al.*: *Phytochemistry* **1973**, 12, 2457.
[3] Sakakibara, I. *et al.*: *Phytochemistry* **1991**, 30, 3013.

[4] Sakakibara, I. *et al.*: *Phytochemistry* **1992**, 31, 3219.
[5] Li, F. C. *et al.*: *Shanxi Yiyao Zazhi* **1978**, (6), 33.
[6] Yang, E. F. *et al.*: *Chin. J. Physiol.* **1940**, 15(1), 9.
[7] Berger, C. L. *et al.*: *C. R. Seances, Acad. Sci. Ser. III, Sci Vie* **1982**, 295, 397.
[8] Yamamoto, L. *et al.*: *Pharmcol. Biochem. Behav.* **1991**, 40, 465.

[J.X. Guo]

228. *Ficus carica* **L.** (Moraceae)

Wu-hua-guo (C), Moe-far-gwor (H), Ichijiku (J), Mu-hwa-gwa (K)

Fruit
Local Drug Name: Wu-hua-guo (C), Moe-far-gwor (H), Mu-ka-ka (J), Mu-hwa-gwa (K).
Processing: Dry under the sun (C, K), or use in fresh (C).
Method of Administration: Oral (decoction: C, J, K).
Folk Medicinal Uses:
       1) Cough and wheezing (C, K).
       2) Swelling and pain in throat (C, J).
       3) Constipation (C, H, J).
       4) Hemorrhoid (C, H, K).
       5) Pharyngitis (H).
       6) Asthma (H).
       7) Ring-worm (K).
       8) Neuralgia (K).
       9) Anemia (K).
      10) Incontinentia alvi (K).

Leaf
Local Drug Name: Wu-hua-guo-ye (C); Moe-far-gwor-yip (H), Ichijiku-yo (J).
Processing: Dry under the sun (C, J) or collect fresh latex (J).
Method of Administration: Oral (decoction: C, H), bathing (decoction: J); Topical (fresh
            latex: J).
Folk Medicinal Uses:
       1) Hemorrhoidal diseases (H, J).
       2) Tuberculous cervical lymphadenopathy (H).
       3) Women's diseases (J, bathing).
       4) Neuralgia (J, bathing).
       5) Wart (J, topical).
       6) Diarrhea (C).
       7) Carbuncle (C).

Root
Local Drug Name: Wu-hua-guo-gen (C), Moe-far-gwor-gun (H).
Processing: Dry under the sun (C, H).
Method of Administration: Oral (decoction: C, H).
Folk Medicinal Uses:
       1) Tuberculous cervical lymphadenopathy (H).

2) Hemorrhoid (H).
3) Diarrhea (C).
4) Carbuncle (C).

Scientific Research:
Chemistry
1) Triterpenes: calotropenyl acetate, lupeol acetate, oleanolic acid [1].
2) Anthocyanins: cyanidin 3-rhamnoglucoside, cyanidin 3,5-diglucoside, cyanidin 3-monoglucoside, pelargonidin 3-rhamnoglucoside [2, 36].
3) Coumarins: psoralen, bergapten [4–7, 10–13, 16], psoberan [15], schaftoside, isoschaftoside [18], umbelliferone, scopoletin [28–29], xanthotoxin, xanthotoxol, marmesin [26].
4) Flavonoids: epirutin, quercetin, isoquercitrin [28].
5) Volatiles: germacrene D, (Z)-3-hexenol, (Z)-3-hexenyl acetate, methyl salicylate [17, 37].
6) Polysaccharides [19].
7) Amines: serotonin [25].
8) Pigments: carotenoids, β-carotene, lutein [39].
9) Lipids [41–42].
10) Oligopeptides [44].
11) Enzymes: proteinases (ficins A, B, C, D. S) [3, 8–9, 14, 43], esterase, acid phosphatase [22–23], endo-β-N-acetylglucosaminidase [32–34].
12) Miscellaneous: benzaldehyde [24], sorbic acid [30].
Pharmacology
1) Antithrombogenicity (tree sap) [21].
2) Carcinostatic effect (benzaldehyde) [24].
3) Corrosion inhibition (water extract) [27].
4) Elastolytic effect (ficin) [31].
5) Antiinflammatory effect (ethanol extract of leaf) [35].
6) Angiotensin I-converting enzyme inhibition (oligopeptides) [38].
7) Antihypertensive effect (oligopeptides) [44].
8) Toxicities against larvae (methanol extract) [20].

Literature:
[1] Ahmed, W. *et al.*: *Fitoterapia* **1990**, 61, 373.
[2] Puech, A. A. *et al.*: *J. Food Sci.* **1975**, 40, 775.
[3] Sugiura, M. *et al.*: *Chem. Pharm. Bull.* **1975**, 23, 1969.
[4] Damjanic, A. *et al.*: *Planta Med.* **1974**, 26, 119.
[5] Akacic, B.*et al.*: *Acta Pharm, Jugoslav.* **1972**, 22(2), 55.
[6] Eidler, Ya. I. *et al.*: *Khim. Prir. Soedin.* **1975**, 11, 349.
[7] Vigorov, L. I. *et al.*: *Dokl. Akad. Nauk SSSR* **1973**, 208, 1484.
[8] Sugiura, M. *et al.*: *Nippon Yakurigaku Zasshi* **1973**, 69 409.
[9] Sugiura, M. *et al.*: *Biochim. Biophys. Acta* **1974**, 350 38.
[10] Yarosh, E.A. *et al.*: *Khim. Prir. Soedin.* **1971**, 7, 521.
[11] Marciani, S. *et al.*: *Atti 1st. Veneto Sci., Lett. Arti, Cl. Sci. Mat. Nat.* **1974**, 132, 275.
[12] Caporale, G. *et al.*: *Atti 1st. Veneto Sci., Lett. Arti, Cl. Sci. Mat. Nat.* **1974**, 132, 457.
[13] Fedorin, G. F. *et al.*: *Rastit. Resur.* **1975**, 11, 372.
[14] Sugiura, M. *et al.*: *Yakugaku Zasshi* **1973**, 93, 63.
[15] Kadyrova, F. R. *et al.*: *Khim. Prir. Soedin.* **1975**, 11, 91.
[16] Innocenti, G. *et al.*: *Farmaco, Ed. Sci.* **1982**, 37, 475.

[17] Buttery, R. G. *et al.*: *J. Agric. Food Chem.* **1986**, 34, 820.

[18] Siewek, F. *et al.*: *Z. Naturforsch., C: Biosci.* **1985**, 40C, 8.

[19] Arifkhodzhaev, Kh. A. *et al.*: *Khim. Prir. Soedin.* **1983**, (2), 229-30

[20] Mori. M.: *Nippon Sanchigaku Zasshi* **1981**, 50, 320.

[21] Sharma, C. *et al.*: *Bull. Mater. Sci.* **1985**, **7**, 75.

[22] Valizadeh, M.: *Biochem. Genet.* **1977**, 15, 1037.

[23] Valizadeh, M. *et al.*: *C. R. Hebd. Seances Acad. Sci., Ser. D* **1978**, 286, 1881.

[24] Takeuchi, S. *et al.*: *Agric. Biol. Chem.* **1978**, 41, 1449.

[25] Stachelberger, H. *et al.*: *Qual. Plant. -Plant Foods Hum. Nutr.* **1977**, 27, 287.

[26] El-Khrisy, E. A. M. *et al.*: *Fitoterapia* **1980**, 51, 269.

[27] Ibrahim, M. E. *et al.*: *Metalloberflaeche* **1981**, 35, 134.

[28] Karryev, M. O. *et al.*: *Akad. Nauk Turkm. SSR, Ser. Biol.Nauk* **1981**, (1), 65.

[29] Ashy, M. A. *et al.*: *Pharmazie* **1981**, 36, 297.

[30] Iwaida, M. *et al.*: *Eisei Shikensho Hokoku* **1976**, 94, 62.

[31] Gonashvili, M. Sh.: *Sb. Tr. Gruz. Zootekh.-Vet. Uchebno-Issled. Inst.* **1975**, 39, 162.

[32] Li, Su-Chen *et al.*: *Biochim. Biophys. Acta* **1981**, 660, 278.

[33] Ogata-Arakawa, M. *et al.*: *J. Biochem. (Tokyo)* **1977**, 82, 611.

[34] Chien, Su-Fang *et al.*: *Biochem. Biophys. Res. Commun.* **1977**, 76, 317.

[35] Shibata, M. *et al.*: *Shoyakugaku Zasshi* **1976**, 30, 62.

[36] Duro, F. *et al.*: *Quad. Merceol.* **1977**, 16, 37.

[37] Jennings, W. G.: *Food Chem.* **1977**, 2, 185.

[38] Maruyama, S. *et al.*: *Agric. Biol. Chem.* **1989**, 53, 2763.

[39] Kakhniashvili, T. A. *et al.*: *Khim. Prir. Soedin.* **1986**, (4), 508-9

[40] Kim, J. P. *et al.*: *Han'guk Sikp'um Kwahakhoechi* **1986**, 187, 270.

[41] Kolesnik, A. A. *et al.*: *Subtrop. Kul't* **1988**, (3), 117-20

[42] Kolesnik, A. A. *et al.*: *Khim. Prir. Soedin.* **1986**, (4), 423-7

[43] Cormier, F. *et al.*: *Biotechnol. Lett.* **1989**, 11, 797.

[44] Maruyama, S. *et al.*: *Jpn. Kokai Tokkyo Koho* JP **02,282,394** [90,282,394].

[C.K. Sung]

229.   *Humulus japonicus* **Sieb. et Zucc.**   (Moraceae)
[=*H. scandens* (Lour.) Merr.]

Lu-cao (C), Luet-cho (H), Kanamugura (J), Hwan-sam-deong-gul (K)

Herb
Local Drug Name: Lu-cao (C), Luet-cho (H), Ritsu-so (J), Yul-cho (K).
Processing: Dry under the sun (C, H, J, K).
Method of Administration: Oral (decoction: C, H, J, K); Topical (paste: C).
Folk Medicinal Uses:
        1) Dysuria (C, H, K).
        2) Edema (J).
        3) Tuberculosis (C, H).
        4) Hemorrhoids (H).
        5) Scrofula (H).
        6) Stomachache (K).

7) Gonorrhea (K).
8) Bone-fracture (K).
9) Gastroenteritis (C).
10) Dysentery (C).
11) Fever caused by common cold (C).
12) Nephritis (C).
13) Cystitis (C).
14) Urinary tract calculus (C).
15) Eczema (C).
16) Carbuncle (C).
17) Snakebite (C).

Fruit
Local Drug Name: Kanamugura (J).
Processing: Dry under the sun (J).
Method of Administration: Oral (decoction: J); Topical (paste with vinegar: J).
Folk Medicinal Uses:
1) Dyspepsia (J).
2) Abcess (J) .

Scientific Research:
Chemistry
1) Essential oils: β-humulene, caryophyllene, α-copaene, α-selinene, β-selinenes, γ-cadinene, caryophyllene oxide, humulene epoxide, benzyl alcohol, phenethyl alcohol [1].
2) Fatty acids: linoleic acid, linolenic acid [2].
Pharmacology
1) Antibacterial effect [3]
Literature
[1] Naya, Y. *et al.*: *Bull. Chem. Soc. Jap.* **1970**, 43, 3594.
[2] Koyama, Y. *et al.*: *Yukagaku* **1970**, 19, 251.
[3] *Quanguo Zhongcaoyao Huibian* **1975**, 1, 834.

[C.K. Sung]

230.   *Santalum album* **L.**   (Santalaceae)

Tan-xiang (C), Tarn-heung (H), Byakudan (J), Dan-hyang-na-mu (K)

Heartwood (CP)
Local Drug Name: Tan-xiang (C), Tarn-heung (H), Byaku-dan (J), Dan-hyang (K).
Processing: Dry under the sun, eliminate foreign matter, cut into slices or saw into small sections, and then split to small pieces (C, J, K).
Method of Administration: Oral (decoction: C, H, J, K).
Folk Medicinal Uses:
1) Abdominal pain (C, H, J, K).
2) Epigastric pain with anorexia (C).

31

3) Angina pectoris in coronary heart disease (C).
4) Vomiting (H).

Scientific Research:
Chemistry
1) Triterpenes: urs-12-en-3β-yl palmitate [1–3].
2) Sesquiterpenes [4]: santalol [5–6].
3) Steroids: β-sitosterol [2].
4) Fatty acids [2].
5) Tannins [2].
6) Substituted cyclohexanes [7].
7) Proteins: hydroxy proline-containing protein [8].
8) Amino compounds [9–10]: γ-L-glutamyl-S-(*trans*-1-propenyl)-L-cysteine sulfoxide [11].
9) π-Tricyclene derivatives [12].
Pharmacology
1) Analgesic effect (alcohol extract) [13].
2) Antiinflammatory effect (alcohol extract) [13].
3) Antifungal effect (oils) [14].
4) Insect growth inhibitory effect (urs-12-en-3β-yl palmitate) [1, 3].
5) Bacteriostatic effect [15].

Literature:
[1] Shankaranarayana, K. H. *et al.*: *Phytochemistry* **1980**, 19, 1239.
[2] Narayana, K. H. *et al.*: *Curr. Sci.* **1980**, 49, 198.
[3] Shankaranarayana, K. H. *et al.*: *J. Entomol. Res.* **1979**, 3, 116.
[4] Adams, D. R. *et al.*: *Phytochemistry* **1975**, 14, 1459.
[5] Brunke, E. J. *et al.*: *Tetrahedron Lett.* **1980**, 21, 2405.
[6] Brunke, E. J. *et al.*: *Liebigs Ann. Chem.* **1982**, (6), 1105.
[7] Shaffer, G. W. *et al.*: *Ger. Offen.* 2,804,075, 03 Aug. **1978**, US Appl. 764,668, 01 Feb. **1977**; 28 pp.
[8] Mani, U. V. *et al.*: *Biochem. J.* **1974**, 141, 147.
[9] Radhakrishnan, A. N.: *J. Sci. Ind. Res.* **1974**, 33, 461.
[10] Radhakrishnan, A. N.: *Biochem. Rev.* **1973**, 44, 1.
[11] Kuttan, R. *et al.*: *Biochemistry* **1974**, 13, 4394.
[12] Mookherjee, B. D. *et al.*: U.S. 3,944,621, 16 Mar. **1976**, Appl. 556,862, 10 Mar. **1975**; 32 pp.
[13] Melin, G.: Fr. Demande, FR 2,474,866, 07 Aug. **1981**, Appl. 80/2,102, 31 Jan. **1980**; 4 pp.
[14] Dikshit, A. *et al.*: *Fitoterapia* **1984**, 55, 171.
[15] Beylier, M. F.: *Perfum. Flavor.* **1979**, 4, 23.

[C.K. Sung]

231.   *Bistorta manshuriens* **Komarov** (Polygonaceae)
[=*Polygonum manshuriens* V. Peter]

Beom-ggo-ri (K)

Rhizome
Local Drug Name: Ken-jin (J), Gweon-sam (K).
Processing: Dry under the sun (K).
Method of Administration: Oral (decoction: J, K).
Folk Medicinal Uses:
        1) Swelling (J).
        2) Diarrhea (K).

Scientific Research:
Chemistry
   1) Amino acids [1].

Literature:
[1] Sugahara, T. *et al.*: *Joshi Eiyo Daigaku Kiyo* **1989**, 20, 77.

                                    [C.K. Sung]

232.   *Polygonum cuspidatum* **Sieb. et Zucc.** (Polygonaceae)
         [=*Reynoutria elliptica* M., *R. japonica* Houtt.]

Hu-zhang (C), Foo-cheung (H), Itadori (J), Ho-jang-geun (K)

Root and Rhizome (CP)
Local Drug Name: Hu-zhang (C), Foo-cheung (H), Ho-jang-geun (K).
Processing: Eliminate foreign metter, wash clean, soften thoroughly, cut into slides, and dry
        (C,K).
Method of Administration: Oral (decoction: C, H, J, K); Topical (decoction or ointment: C).
Folk Medicinal Uses:
        1) Constipation (H, J, K).
        2) Burns (H, K).
        3) Menostasis, menoxenia (J, K).
        4) Cough (J, K).
        5) Urethritis (H, K).
        6) Arthralgia (C).
        7) Jaundice caused by damp-heat (C).
        8) Amenorrhea (C, H).
        9) Mass formation in the abdomen (C).
       10) Carbuncles and sores (C).
       11) Hepatitis (H).
       12) Enteritis, dysentery (H).
       13) Tonsillitis, pharyngitis (H).
       14) Bronchitis (H).
       15) Nephritis (H).
       16) Vaginitis (H).
       17) Snake bites (H).
       18) Scalds (H).
       19) Traumatic injury (H, K).

20) Rheumatism (K).
21) Icterus (K).
22) Ulcer (K).
23) Gonorrhoea (K).
24) Pleurisy (K).
25) Leukorrhea (K).
Contraindications: Pregnancy (C).

Scientific Research:
Chemistry
1) Anthraquinones: physcion, chrysophanol [1], emodin [1, 10], fallacinol, citreorosein, questin, questinol [2], emodin 8-*O*-β-D-glucopyranoside, physcion 8-*O*-β-D-glucopyranoside [3].
2) Stilbens: resveratrol, piceid [4], 3,4',5-trihydroxystilbene, 3,4',5-trihydroxystilbene 3-*O*-β-D-glucoside [8], bisade, 2,3,4',5'-tetrahydroxystilbene [9].
3) Naphthoquinones: 2-methoxy-6-acetyl-7-methyljuglone [2].
4) Coumarins: 7-hydroxy-4-methoxy-5-methylcoumarin [2].
5) Chromones: 2,5-dimethyl-7-hydroxy-chromone [2].
6) Tannins: catechin [3].
7) Phenolic acids: protocatechuic acid [2].
8) Steroids: β-sitosterol glucoside [8].
9) Organic acids: oxalic acid [7].
Pharmacology
1) Inhibition of deposition of triglyceride and cholesterol (resveratrol, piceid) [5].
2) Inhibition of lipid peroxidation induced by ADP (resveratrol, piceid) [6].
3) Anti-leukemic effect [10].

Literature:
[1] Tsukida, K. *et al.*: *J. Pharm. Soc. Jpn.* **1954**, 74, 379.
[2] Kumura, Y. *et al.*: *Planta Med.* **1983**, 48, 164.
[3] Murakami, T. *et al.*: *Chem. Pharm. Bull.* **1968**, 16, 2299.
[4] Nonomura, S. *et al.*: *Yakugaku Zasshi* **1963**, 83, 899.
[5] Arichi, H. *et al.*: *Chem. Pharm. Bull.* **1982**, 30, 1766.
[6] Kimura, Y. *et al.*: *Planta Med.* **1983**, 49, 51.
[7] Kojima, K. *et al.*: *Shoyakugaku Zasshi* **1984**, 38, 138.
[8] Chi, H. J. *et al.*: *Saengyak Hakhoechi* **1986**, 17, 73.
[9] Osaka Yakuhin Kenkyusho K. K.: *Jpn. Kokai Tokkyo Koho* JP **60 09,455**, 18 Jan. **1985**, Appl. 83/116,639, 27 Jan. **1983**; 3 pp.
[10] Yeh, S. F. *et al.*: *Planta Med.* **1988**, 54, 413.

[C.K. Sung]

233.   *Portulaca oleracea* L.   (Portulacaceae)

Ma-chi-xian (C), Mar-chee-yin (H), Suberi-hiyu (J), Soe-bi-reum (K)

Herb (CP)
Local Drug Name: Ma-chi-xian (C), Mar-chee-yin (H), Ba-shi-ken (J), Ma-chi-hyeon (K).

Processing: Eliminate foreign matter, wash clean, soften briefly, cut into sections, and dry
under the sun (C), dry under the sun (K).
Method of Administration: Oral (decoction: C, H, J, K); Topical (paste of fresh herb: C).
Folk Medicinal Uses:
1) Dysentery (C, H: use fresh, J, K).
2) Insect-bite (C, J, K).
3) Gonorrhoea (J, K).
4) Appendicitis (H, K).
5) Boil (C, K).
6) Eczema (C, H: topical).
7) Erysipelas (C).
8) Hematochezia (C).
9) Abnormal uterine bleeding (C).
10) Snake-bite (C).
11) Mastitis (H).
12) Hemorrhoid (C, H, J).
13) Furunculosis (H: topical).
14) Melena (J).
15) Gingivitis (J).
16) Urticaria (K).
17) Tineapedis (K).
18) Swelling (K).
19) Psoriasis (K).
20) Neuralgia (K).
21) Foot-spasm (K).
Contraindications: Pregnancy.

Scientific Research:
Chemistry
1) Acylated betacyanins: oleracin I, II [1].
2) Protein [2–3].
3) Amino acids: phenylalanine, valine, alanine, tyrosine, aspartate, glutamate, aspartate
[3].
4) Vitamins: nicotinic acid, tocopherol [2], ascorbic acid [4].
Pharmacology
1) Antibiotic effect.
2) Stimulation of the uterus (water and alcohol extract).

Literature:
[1] Imperato, F.: *Phytochemistry* **1975**, 14, 2091.
[2] Tashbekov, I.: *Rastit. Resur.* **1977**, 13, 361.
[3] Mirajkar, P. B. *et al.*: *Curr. Trends Life Sci.* **1984**, 11, 95.
[4] Bruno, S. *et al.*: *Boll.-Soc. Ital. Biol. Sper.* **1980**, 56, 2067.

[C.K. Sung]

234.   *Gypsophila oldhamiana* **Miquel**   (Caryophyllaceae)

Xia-cao (C), Dae-na-mul (K)

Root
 Local Drug Name: Shan-yin-chai-hu (C), Gin-sai-ko (J), Eun-si-ho (K).
 Processing: Dry under the sun (C, K).
 Method of Administration: oral (decoction: C, J, K).
 Folk Medicinal Uses:
>   1) Hectic fever due to yin deficiency (C).
>   2) Long-standing malaria (C).
>   3) Infantile malnutrition with fever (C).
>   4) General weakness (J).
>   5) Sputum (K).

Scientific Research:
 Chemistry
   1) Saponin [1].
 Pharmacology
   1) Decrease the volume and fragility of red blood cell [1].

Literature:
 [1] Lee, S. W. *et al.*: *Yakhak Hoechi* **1989**, 33, 15.

[C.K. Sung]

235.   *Melandrium firmum* **Rohrbach**   (Caryophyllaceae)

Jian-ying-nu-lou-cai (C), Fushiguro (J), Jang-gu-chae (K)

Seed
 Local Drug Name: Ying-ye-nu-lou-cai (C), Wang-bul-ryu-haeng (K).
 Processing: Dry under the sun (C, K).
 Method of Administration: Oral (decoction: C, K).
 Folk Medicinal Uses:
>   1) Gonorrhea (K).
>   2) Galactagogue (C, K).
>   3) Cuts (K).
>   4) Boils (K).
>   5) Scabies (K).
>   6) Pharyngitis (C).
>   7) Otitis media (C).

Scientific Research:
 Chemistry
   1) Flavonoids: linarin, schaftoside [1].
   2) Sapogenins [2].

Literature:
[1] Woo, E. H. *et al.*: *Arch. Pharmacal Res.* **1989**, 12, 223.
[2] Chang, I. S. *et al.*: *Planta Med.* **1989**, 55, 544.

[C.K. Sung]

236.   *Cyathula officinalis* **Kuan**   (Amaranthaceae)

Chuan-niu-xi (C), Chuan-ngau-sut (H)

Root (CP)
Local Drug Name: Chuan-niu-xi (C), Chuan-ngau-sut (H), Sen-go-shitsu (J).
Processing: 1) Eliminate foreign matter and root stock, wash clean, soften thoroughly, cut
                into thin slices, and dry (C).
             2) Stir-fry the slices with wine to dryness (C).
Method of Administration: Oral (decoction: C, H, J).
Folk Medicinal Uses:
             1) Amenorrhea with mass formation in the lower abdomen (C, H, J).
             2) Retention of afterbirth (C).
             3) Arthralgia (C, H, J).
             4) Hematuria (C, H, J).
             5) Traumatic injuries (C, H).
             6) Rheumatism (H).
Contraindication : Pregnancy (C).

Scientific Research:
Chemistry
    1) Steroids: isocyasierone, 5-epicyasterone, sengosterone, cyasterone, amarasterone A,
       amarasterone B, capitasterone, poststerone, ecdysterone (crusterdysome),
       precyasterone [1–4], inokosterone [5].
    2) Alkaloid: betaine [6].
Pharmacology
    1) Effect on womb [7].

Literature:
[1] Hikino, H. *et al.*: *Tetrahedron* **1968**, 24, 4895.
[2] Hikino, H. *et al.*: *Chem. Pharm. Bull.* **1970**, 18, 1078; **1970**, 19, 433.
[3] Hikino, H. *et al.*: *Phytochemistry* **1971**, 10, 3173.
[4] Takemoto, T. *et al.*: *Tetrahedron Letters* **1968**, 4929, 4953.
[5] Liu, S. S. et al: *"Zhongyao Yanjiu Weixian Zhaiyao"* **1975-1979**, 221.
[6] Nanjing College of Pharmacy: *"Zhongcaoyao Xue"* **1976**, 2, 191.
[7] Zhang, Y. D. *et al.*: *Yaoli Yanjiu Baogao* **1935**, 1,157.

[J.X. Guo]

237.   *Cinnamomum camphora* **Sieb.**   (Lauraceae)

Zhang (C), Cheung-shue (H), Kusunoki (J), Nok-na-mu (K)

Camphor   (CP, JP)
  Local Drug Name: Zhang-lao (C), Jang-noe (K).
  Processing: Steam distilation of the wood (C, J, K).
  Method of Administration: Oral (powder or medicine wine; C); Topical (ointment, tincture:
                            C, H, J, K).
  Folk Medicinal Uses:
                  1) Neuralgia (J, K).
                  2) Congelation (J, K).
                  3) Traumatic injury (J, K).
                  4) Insect bite (J, K).
                  5) Bruise (J, K).
                  6) Swelling caused by gastritis (K).
                  7) Skin-irritation (C, H).
                  8) Vomiting and diarrhea due to cold-dampness (C).
                  9) Gastralgia and abdominalgia (C).
                  10) Toothache (C).
                  11) Scabies (C).

Stem
  Local Drug Name: Shoboku (J), Jang-mok (K).
  Processing: Dry in shade (K).
  Method of Administration: Oral (decoction: K).
  Folk Medicinal Uses:
                  1) Erysipelas (K).

Root, Wood
  Local Drug Name: Zhang-shu-gen, Zhang-shu (C), Cheung-shue (H).
  Processing: Dry in shade (C, H).
  Method of Administration: Oral (decoction: C, H).
  Folk Medicinal Uses:
                  1) Common cold, headache (C, H).
                  2) Stomach ache and distention (C, H).
                  3) Rheumatic pain (C, H).
                  4) Traumatic injury (C, H).

Leaf
  Local Drug Name: Zhang-shu-ye (C), Cheung-shue-yip (H).
  Processing: Fresh (C, H).
  Method of Administration: Topical (decoction: C, H).
  Folk Medicinal Uses:
                  1) Chronic leg ulcer (C, H).
                  2) Ringworm (H).
                  3) Pruritus (C, H).
                  4) Centipede bites (H).

Fruit

Local Drug Name: Zhang-shu-guo (C), Cheung-shue-gwor (H).
Processing: Dry under the sun (C, H).
Method of Administration: Oral (decoction: C, H).
Folk Medicinal Uses:

1) Stomachache, gastroenteritis (C, H).

Scientific Research:

Chemistry

1) Monoterpenes: *d*-camphor [1]. Campherenone, campherenol [6], linalool monoxide [8], 9-oxonerolidol [13].
2) Sesquiterpenes: S-guajazulene, Se-guajazulene, cadina-9,11(12)-diene, *d*-nerolidol, humulene, selinene, α-hlangene, β-elemene, α-santalene, β-santalene, γ-guaiene, γ-cadinene, calamenene, calacorone, caryophyllene, myristicin, elemol, guaiol, α-cadinol, β-eudesmol, juniper-camphor [5, 7, 12] .
3) Flavonoids: proanthocyanidin A-1, A-4 and A-5 [2].
4) Alkaloids: laurolitsine and reticuline [9].

Pharmacology

1) Local irritant effect (camphor).
2) Bacteriocidal effect (camphor).
3) Central nervous system stimulant effect (camphor).
4) Respiratory stimulant effect (camphor).
5) Angiotonic effect (camphor).
6) Cardioinhibitory effect (camphor) and cardiac stimulatory effect (oxocamphor) [3–4].

Literature:

[1] Freudenberg, K. *et al.*: *Ann.* **1954**, 587, 213; **1955**, 594, 76.
[2] Nonaka, G. *et al.*: *Chem. Pharm. Bull.* **1987**, 35, 149.
[3] Yamaguchi, H.: "*Rinsho no Yakuri*" 1952, 317.
[4] Asahina, Y. *et al.*: *Ber.* 1933, 66, **1975**.
[5] Hayashi, S. *et al.*: *Kashi.* **1960**, 81, 1136.
[6] Hikino, H. *et al.*: *Chem. Pharm. Bull.* **1968**, 16, 832; **1971**, 19, 87; *Tetrahedron Lett.*, **1967**, 5069.
[7] Araki, M. *et al.*: *Kashi* **1966**, 87, 63.
[8] Nagashima, K. *et al.*: *Shionogi Kenkyusho Kiyo* 1957, 22, 91.
[9] Tomita, M. *et al.*: *Yakugaku Zasshi* **1964**, 84, 365.
[10] Hirai, M. *et al.*: *Bull. Chem. Soc.Japan* **1967**, 40, 1003.
[11] Hayashi, S. *et al.*: *Bull. Chem. Soc. Japan* **1968**, 41, 234;
[12] Hayashi, S. *et al. Bull. Chem. Soc. Japan* **1968**, 41, 1465.
[13] Hirai, M. *et al.*: *Chem. Lett.* **1972**, 1213.

[T. Kimura]

238.   *Lindera strychnifolia* **(Sieb. et Zucc.) F. Vill.**   (Lauraceae)
(*Benzoin strychnifolium* (Sieb. et Zucc.) O. Kuntze)

Wu-yao (C), Woo-yuek (H), Tendai-uyaku (J)

Related plant: *L. aggregata* (Sims) Kosterm.: Wu-yao (C).

Root
Local Drug Name: Wu-yao (C), Woo-yuek (H), U-yaku (J), O-yak (K).
Processing: Slice and dry (C, J).
Method of Administration: Oral (decoction: C, H, J).
Folk Medicinal Uses:
  1) Gastrointestinal disorder (H, J).
  2) Headache (J).
  3) Distending pain in the chest and abdomen accompanied by dyspnea (C).
  4) Frequent urination (C, H, J).
  5) Hernia (C, H).
  6) Dysmenorrhea (C).

Scientific Research:
Chemistry
  1) Monoterpenes: α-pinene, β-pinene, camphene, limonene, ocimene, myrcene, *p*-cymene, borneol (linderol), bornyl acetate [5].
  2) Sesquiterpenes: Linderan, lindra acid [1–2], linderene[1–2, 6], isolinderene [3], α-humulene, β-humulene, [4–5], ylangene, β-elemene, β-selinene, γ-cadinene [5], linderazulene, ujacazulene [7], linderalactone [8, 11], isolinderalactone [8, 10], neolinderalactone [9, 11], linderane [11–12], neolinderane, pseudolinderane, linderadiene [12], linderoxide, isogermafurene [13], caryophyllene [14].
  3) Steroids: Campesterol, stigmasterol and β-sitosterol [14].
  4) Alkaloids: Laurolitsine[15], boldine, (+)-reticuline [16].
Pharmacology
  1) Inhibitory effect on β-hexosaminidase release from rat basophilic leukemia cells [17].

Literature:
[1] Kondo, H. *et al.*: *Yakugaku Zasshi* **1926**, 526, 1047; **1939**, 59, 504.
[2] Takeda, K. *et al.*: *Yakugaku Zasshi* **1944**, 64, 32.
[3] Suzuki, H. : *Yakugaku Zasshi* **1930**, 50, 714.
[4] Benesova, V. *et al.*: *Coll. Czech. Chem. Comm.* **1961**, 26, 1832.
[5] Motl, O. *et al.*: *Coll. Czech. Chem. Comm.* **1962**, 27, 987.
[6] Takeda, K. *et al.*: *Tetrahed. Lett.* **1964**, 277; **1966**, 1159; 2991; *J. Chem. Soc.* **1969**, 1920.
[7] Takeda, K. *et al.*: *J. Chem. Soc.* **1964**, 2591; 3577.
[8] Takeda, K. *et al.*: *J. Chem. Soc.* **1964**, 4578.
[9] Takeda, K. *et al.*: *J. Chem. Soc.* **1969**, 2786.
[10] Takeda, K. etal.: *Chem. Comm.* **1968**, 378.
[11] Takeda, K. etal.: *Chem. Comm.* **1968**, 637; **1969**, 1491.
[12] Takeda, K. etal.: *Chem. Comm.* **1968**, 1168.
[13] Ishii, H. *et al.*: *Tetrahedron* **1968**, 24, 625.
[14] Tomita, M. *et al.*: *Phytochem.* **1969**, 8, 2249.
[15] Tomita, M. *et al.*: *Yakugaku Zasshi* **1969**, 89, 737.
[16] Kozuka, M. *et al.*: *J. Natural Prod.* **1984**, 47, 1063.
[17] Kataoka, M. *et al.*: *Natural Medicines* **1996**, 50, 344.

[T. Kimura]

239.   *Anemone raddeana* Regel   (Ranunculaceae)

Duo-bei-yin-lian-hua (C), Oku-no-azuma-ichige (J), Ggweong-wui-ba, Ram-ggot (K)

Rhizome (CP)
Local Drug Name: Liang-tou-jian (C), Leung-tau-jim (H), Ryo-to-sen (J), Juk-jeol-hyang-
              bu (K).
Processing: Eliminate rootlet, wash clean, and dry (C, K).
Method of Administration: Oral (decoction: C, H, K); Topical (decoction: C; paste: K).
Folk Medicinal Uses:
              1) Rheumatoid arthritis (C, H, K).
              2) Carbuncle with ulceration (C, H).

Scientific Research:
Chemistry
    1) Lactone: ranunculin [1].
    2) Saponins and sapogenins: diosgenin, oleanolic acid, oleanolic acid 3-(O-α-L-arabino-
       pyranoside) [2], raddeanin A–D [3], oleanolic acid 3-O-β-D-glucopyranosyl-
       (1→2)-α-L-arabinopyranoside [4], raddeanin E–F [5], 3-O-α-L-rhamnopyranosyl-
       (1→2)-O-β-D-glucopyranosyl-(1→2)-α-L-arabino-pyranosyloleanolic acid 28-O-
       α-L-rhamnopyranosyl-(1→4)-O-β-D-glucopyranosyl-(1→6)-β-D-glucopyrano-
       side, 3-O-α-L-rhamnopyranosyl-(1→2)-O-β-D-glucopyranosyl-(1→2)-α-L-
       arabino-pyranosyl-27-hydroxyoleanolic acid 28-O-α-L-rhamnopyranosyl-(1→4)-
       O-β-D-glucopyranosyl-(1→6)-β-D-glucopyranoside [6–7].
Pharmacology
    1) Antitumor effect [3, 8].

Literature:
 [1] Liu, D. Y.: *Zhongcaoyao* **1983**, 14, 532.
 [2] Wu, F. G. *et al.*: *Gaodeng Xuexiao Huaxue Xuebao* **1983**, 4, 595.
 [3] Wu, F. G. *et al.*: *Lanzhou Daxue Xuebao, Ziran Kexueban* **1983**, 19(4), 188.
 [4] Wu, F. G. *et al.*: *Huaxue Xuebao* **1984**, 42, 253.
 [5] Wu, F. G. *et al.*: *Lanzhou Daxue Xuebao, Ziran Kexueban* **1984**, 20(2), 164.
 [6] Wu, F. G. *et al.*: *Chem. Pharm. Bull.* **1989**, 37, 2445.
 [7] Wu, F. G. *et al.*: *Chem. Pharm. Bull.* **1989**, 37, 3435.
 [8] Liu, L. S. *et al.* : *Zhongguo Yaoli Xuebao* **1985**, 6, 192.
 [9] Wu, F. G. *et al.*: *Huaxue Xuebao* **1984**, 42, 1266.
[10] Wu, F. G. *et al.*: *Huaxue Xuebao* **1985**, 43, 692.

[J.X. Guo]

240.   *Clematis armandii* Franch.   (Ranunculaceae)

Xiao-mu-tong (C), Muk-tung (H)

Related plant: *C. montana* Buch.-Ham.: Xiu-qiu-teng (C).

Stem (CP)

Local Drug Name: Chuan-mu-tong(C), Muk-tung (H).

Processing: Remove the coarse bark, and dry in the sun; or cut into thin slices when fresh, and dry in the sun (C).

Method of Administration: Oral (decoction: C).

Folk Medicinal Uses:

> 1) Edema, stranguria oliguria (C, H).
> 2) Arthralgia (C, H).
> 3) Amenorrhea (C).
> 4) Lack of lactation (C).

Scientific Research:

Chemistry

> 1) Saponins: hederagenin-3-*O*-β-ribopyranosyl-(1→3)-α-rhamnopyranosyl-(1→2)-α-arabinopyranoside-28-*O*-α-L-rhamnopyranosyl-(1→4)-β-D-glucopyranosyl-(1→6)-β-D-glucopyranoside, hederagenin-3-*O*-β-ribopyranosyl-(1→3)-α-rhamnopyranosyl-(1→2)-α-arabinopyranoside [1], clemontanoside B [2], clemontanoside C [3].
> 2) Flavanone glycoside: 5,4'-dihydroxy-3'-methoxyflavanone-7-(6"-*O*-β-L-rhamnopyranosyl)-β-D-glucopyranoside [4].

Literature:

[1] Bahuguna, R. P.: *Int. J. Crude Drug Res.* **1990**, 28, 125.
[2] Jangwan, J. S.: *Int. J. Crude Drug Res.* **1990**, 28, 39.
[3] Thapligal, R. P.: *Phytochemistry* **1993**, 33, 671.
[4] Chen, Y. F. *et al.*: *Tetrahedron* **1993**, 49, 5169.

[J.X. Guo]

241.   *Clematis chinensis* **Osbeck**   (Ranunculaceae)

Wei-ling-xian (C), Wai-ling-sin (H)

Related plants: *C. hexapetala* Pall.: Mian-tuan-tie-xian-lian (C); *C. manshurica* Rupr.: Dong-bei-tie-xian-lian (C), Eu-a-eri (K); *C. terniflora* DC.: Sen-nin-so (J).

Root (CP)

Local Drug Name: Wei-ling-xian (C), Wai-ling-sin (H), I-rei-sen (J), Wi-ryeong-seon (K).

Processing: Eliminate foreign matter, wash clean, soften thoroughly, cut into sections, and dry (C, K).

Method of Administration: Oral (decoction: C, H, J, K).

Folk Medicinal Uses:

> 1) Rheumatic or rheumatoid arthralgia (C, H, J, K).
> 2) Fish bone stuck in the throat (C, H).
> 3) Leukorrhea (K).
> 4) Tooth caries (K).
> 5) Sputum (K).

Scientific Research:

Chemistry

1) Triterpenoid saponins: clematoside A, A', B, C [1–2], prosapogenin CP_2, CP_6, CP_7, CP_8 [3], CP_1, CP_3, CP_4, CP_5 [4], CP_{2b}, CP_{3b}, CP_9, CP_{10} [5], CP_0, CP_{2a}, CP_{3a} [6], oleanolic acid 3-O-β-D-glucopyranosyl-(1→4)-β-D-xylopyranosyl-(1→3)-α-L-rhamnopyranosyl-(1→2)-α-L-arabinopyranoside, hederagenin 3-O-β-D-glucopyranosyl-(1→4)-β-D-xylopyranosyl-(1→3)-α-L-rhamnopyranosyl-(1→2)-α-L-arabinopyranoside, oleanolic acid 3-O-β-D-glucopyranosyl-(1→4)-β-D-glucopyranosyl-(1→4)-β-D-xylopyranosyl-(1→3)-α-L-xylopyranosyl-(1→2)-α-L-arabinopyranoside, hederagenin 3-O-β-D-glucopyranosyl-(1→4)-β-D-glucopyranosyl-(1→4)-β-D-xylopyranosyl-(1→3)-α-L-rhamnopyranosyl-(1→2)-α-L-arabinopyranoside [7].
2) Lactones: protoanemonin [8], anemonin [9].
3) Alkaloids [9].
4) Steroid: sitosterol [9].
5) Organic acids: α,β-myristic acid, linoleic acid [9].
6) Macrocyclic compound: clemochinenoside A [10].

Pharmacology

1) Antihistaminic effect [8].
2) Stimulative effect [8].
3) Bacteriostatic effect [8, 11].
4) Antihepertensive effect [12].
5) Effect on heart [12].

Literature:

[1] Chirva, V. Y. *et al.*: *Khim. Biokhim. Uglevodov, Mater. Vses. Konf., 4th* **1967**, 98.
[2] Agarwal, S. K. *et al.*: *Phytochemistry* **1974**, 13, 2623.
[3] Kizu, H. *et al.*: *Chem. Pharm. Bull.* **1979**, 27, 2388.
[4] Kizu, H. *et al.*: *Chem. Pharm. Bull.* **1980**, 28, 2827.
[5] Kizu, H. *et al.*: *Chem. Pharm. Bull.* **1980**, 28, 3555.
[6] Kizu, H. *et al.*: *Chem. Pharm. Bull.* **1982**, 30, 3340.
[7] Kizu, H. *et al.*: *Chem. Pharm. Bull.* **1982**, 30, 859.
[8] Nanjing College of Pharmacy: *"Zhongcaoyao Xue"*, **1976**, Vol. 2, 237, 258.
[9] Tang, T. H. *et al.*: *Guo Li Shandong Daxue Huaxuexi Shiyanshi Baogao* **1934**, (3,4), 19.
[10] Song, C. Q. *et al.*: *Chin. Chem. Lett.* **1992**, 3, 119.
[11] Cao, R. L. *et al.*: *Zhonghua Pifuke Zazhi* **1957**, (4), 286.
[12] Pi, X. P.: *Qingdao Yixueyuan Xuebao* **1957**, (1), 9.

[J.X. Guo]

242.   *Coptis japonica* (Thunb.) Makino var. *dissecta* Nakai
(Ranunculaceae)

Seriba-oren (J)

Related Plant: *Coptis japonica* (Thunb.) Makino: Kikuba-oren (J), Wae-hwang-ryeon (K); *C. chinensis* Franch. Hwang-ryeon (K) ; *C. deltoidea* C. Y. Cheng et Hsiao: Sam-gak-yeop-hwang-ryeon (K).

Rhizome (JP)

Local Drug Name: Oren (J), Hwang-ryeon (K).

Processing: Cut off fibrous roots and dry and burns with fire (J, K).

Method of Administration: Oral (decoction: J, K).

Folk Medicinal Uses:

1) Diarrhea and dysentery (J, K).
2) Bloody flux (K).
3) Vomiting (J, K).
4) Eye diseases (J, K).
5) Gastritis (J, K).
6) Boil of oral cavity (K).
7) Dyspepsia and anorexia (J, K).
8) Eczema and skin diseases (J).
9) Food intoxication (J).

Scientific Research:

Chemistry

1) Alkaloids: Berberine, palmatine, jatrorrhizine [1], coptisine, worenine [2], magnoflorine [3].
2) Phenyl propanoids: Ferulic acid [4].

Pharmacology

1) Gastric secretion increasing effect (water extract, decoction) [5].
2) Pancreas protease precursor activation effect (water extract) [6].
3) Gastric movement (water extract) [7].
4) Antispasmodic effect (35% ethanol extract) [8].
5) Antiulcer effect (water extract) [9].
6) Antiinflammatory effect (methanol extract, berberine) [10, 16].
7) Antibacterial effect (50% ethanol extract, berberine, coptisine) [11, 13].
8) Antihypertensive effect (berberine) [12, 14].
9) Antipyretic effect (berberine) [15].
10) Choleretic effect (berberine) [17].
11) Blood sugar lowering effect (berberine) [18].
12) Blood cholesterol lowering effect (berberine) [19].
13) Anti-tumor-promoter effect (berberine) [20].
14) Central nervous system depressing effect (berberine) [21].
15) Hepatonic effect (35% ethanol extract) [22].
16) Acetylcholine suppressing effect (berberine) [23].
17) Inhibitory effect on catecholamine biosynthesis [24].
18) Antispasmodic effect [25].

Literature:

[1] Tani, C. *et al.*: *Yakugaku Zasshi* **1957**, 77, 805.

[2] Kitazato, Z.: *Yakugaku Zasshi* **1927**, 47, 315.

[3] Tomita, M. *et al.*: *Yakugaku Zasshi* **1956**, 76, 1425.

[4] Ito, H. *et al.*: *Yakugaku Zasshi* **1954**, 74, 812; Yahara, S. *et al.*: *Chem. Pharm. Bull.* **1985**, 33, 527.

[5] Sato, I.: *Kyotofuritsu Ikadaigaku Zasshi*, **1936**, 16, 443; Ikuta, M.: *Osaka Igakkai Zasshi*, 1940, 39, 2072; **1941**, 40, 711, 727.

[6] Uchiyama, T. *et al.*: *Wakan Iyaku Gakkaishi*, **1989**, 6, 201.

[7] Suga, S.: *Osaka Igakkai Zasshi*, **1942**, 41, 649.

[8] Haginiwa, T. *et al.*: *Yakugaku Zasshi* **1962**, 82, 726.

[9] Takase, H. *et al.*: *Jap. J. Pharmacol.* **1989**, 49, 301.

[10] Otsuka, K. *et al.*: *Yakugaku Zasshi* **1981**, 101, 883.

[11] Chang, N. C.: *Proc. Soc. Exptl. Biol. Med.*, **1948**, 69, 141; Yamahara, J. *et al.*: *Shoyakugaku Zasshi* **1972**, 26, 84; Sawada, T. *et al.*: *Shoyakugaku Zasshi* **1971**, 25, 74.

[12] Aonuma, S. *et al.*: *Yakugaku Zasshi* **1957**, 77, 1303.

[13] Ukita, T. *et al.*: *Penishirin*, **1949**, 2, 534; Amin, A. H. *et al.*: *Can.J. Microbiol.*, **1969**, 15, 1067; Sun, D. *et al.*: *Antimicrob. Agents Chemother.*, **1988**, 32, 1274, 1370; Higaki, S. *et al.*: *Wakan Iyaku Gakkaishi*, **1987**, 4, 458; Lahiri, S. C. *et al.*: *J. Indian Med. Assoc.*, **1967**, 48, 1; Dutta, N. K. *et al.*: *Br. J. Pharmacol.*, **1972**, 44, 153; Sabir, M. *et al.*: *Indian J. Med. Res.* **1977**, 65, 305.

[14] Suzuki, S.: *Tohoku J. Exptl. Med.,* **1939**, 36, 134.

[15] Sabir, M. *et al.*: *Indian J. Physiol. Pharmacol.*, **1978**, 22, 9.

[16] Fujimura, H. *et al.*: *Yakugaku Zasshi* **1970**, 90, 782.

[17] Oshiba, S. *et al.*: *Nihon Univ. J. Med.*, **1974**, 16, 69.

[18] Chen, Q. M. *et al.*: *Yaoxue Xuebao*, **1986**, 21, 401; **1987**, 22, 161.

[19] Vad, B. G. *et al.*: *Indian J. Pharm.*, **1971**, 33, 23.

[20] Nishino, H. *et al.*: *Onchology*, **1986**, 43, 131.

[21] Shanbhag, S. M. *et al.*: *Japan. J. Pharmacol.,* **1970**, 20, 482.

[22] Yang, L. L. *et al.*: *Wakan Iyaku Gakkaishi*, **1990**, 7, 28.

[23] Uchizumi, S. *et al.*: *Nippon Yakurigaku Zasshi*, **1957**, 53, 63; Shimamoto, T. *et al.*: *Nippon Yakurigaku Zasshi* **1957**, 53, 75.

[24] Lee, M.K. *et al.*: *Planta Med.* **1996**, 62, 31.

[25] Boegge, S.C. *et al.*: *Planta Med.* **1996**, 62, 173.

[T. Kimura]

243.   *Pulsatilla koreana* **Nakai ex Mari**   (Ranunculaceae)

Chao-xian-bai-tou-weng (C), Cho-sen-haku-to-o (J), Hal-mi-ggot (K)

Related plant: *Pulsatilla chinensis* (Bge.) Reg.: Bai-tou-weng (C).

Root
Local Drug Name: Chao-xian-bai-tou-weng (C), Baek-du-ong (K).
Processing: Dry under the sun (C, K).
Method of Administration: Oral (decoction: C, K).
Folk Medicinal Uses:

         1) Abdominal pain (K).

         2) Sputum (K).

         3) Dysentery (C, K).

         4) Toothache (K).

         5) Fever (K).

         6) Acute gastritis (K).

         7) Cough (K).

         8) Spasm (K).

9) Fracture of bone (K).
10) Bone pain (K).
11) Hemorrhoid (C).
12) Epistaxis (C).
13) Lochia (C).
Side Effects: Toxic.

Scientific Research:
Chemistry
1) Saponins [1].

Literature:
[1] Kang, S. S.: *Arch. Pharmacal Res.* **1989**, 12, 42.

[C.K. Sung]

244.   *Epimedium grandiflorum* **Morr.**   (Berberidaceae)
(*E. grandiflorum* Morr. var. *thunbergianum* Nakai)

Yum-yeung-fork (H), Ikari-so (J), Sam-ji-gu-yeop-cho (K)

Related plant: *E. sagittatum* (Sieb. et Zucc.) Maxim., Jian-ye-yin-yang-huo (C), Hozaki-
ikari-so (J); *E. brevicornum* Maxim., Yin-yang-huo (C); *E. pubescens*
Maxim., Ren-mao-yin-yang-huo (C); *E. koreanum* Nakai, Zhao-xian-yin-
yang-huo (C).

Whole herb
Local Drug Name: Yin-yang-huo (C), Yum-yeung-fork (H), In-yo-kaku (J), Eum-yang-
gwak (K).
Processing: Dry under the sun or in shade (C, J, K).
Method of Administration: Oral (Decoction: C, J, K).
Folk Medicinal Uses:
1) Neurasthenia (J, K).
2) Amnesia (J, K).
3) Impotence, seminal emission, weakness of the limbs (C, H, J, K).
4) Rheumatic or rheumatoid arthralgia (C, H).
5) Climacteric hypertensia (C).
6) Weakness (K).
7) Hemiplegia (H).
8) Lumbago (H).
9) Rheumatalgia (H).

Scientific Research:
Chemistry
1) Flavonoids: ikariin [1], des-O-methylicariin [2, 5], β-anhydroicaritn, des-O-methyl-β-
anhydroicaritn, norikariin [3], anhydroikaritin-3-rhamno-7-glucoside [4], icariside

B3 and E1 [8], icariside B10, A5, and A6 [9], ikarisoside B, C, D, E and F [10], epimenoside A, B, C, D and E [11].
2) Alkaloids: magnoflorine [5].
3) Alyphatic compounds: ginnol [6], ceryl alcohol [7].
4) Lignans: (–)-olivil, icarisoresinol, icarisoresinol 4'-β-D-glucopyranoside and (–)-olivil 4'-β-D-glucopyranoside [12].

Literature:
[1] Akai, S. *et al.*: *Yakugaku Zasshi* **1935**, 55, 537; 705; 719, 788.
[2] Akai, S. *et al.*: *Yakugaku Zasshi* **1935**, 55, 1139.
[3] Fujita, M. *et al.*: *Abstr., Annual Meeting of Jap. Soc. Pharmacognosy* **1970**.
[4] Takemoto, T. *et al.*: *Abstr., December Meeting of Jap. Soc. Pharm. Tohoku Branch* **1970**.
[5] Tomita, M. *et al.*: *Yakugaku Zasshi* **1957**, 77, 114; 212.
[6] Matsuura, S. *et al.*: *Shoyakugaku Zasshi* **1971**, 25, 122.
[7] Yuoh, T. C. *et al.*: *J. Chinese Chem. Soc.*, **1936**, 4, 312.
[8] Miyase, T. *et al.*: *Chem. Pharm. Bull.*, **1987**, 35, 1109; 3713; **1988**, 36, 2475.
[9] Wu, L. J. *et al.*: *Phytochemistry* **1991**, 30, 1727.
[10] Fukai, T. *et al.*: *Phytochemistry* **1988**, 27, 259.
[11] Takemoto, T. *et al.*: *Yakugaku Zasshi* **1975**, 95, 312; 321; 698.
[12] Tokuoka, Y. *et al.*: *Yakugaku Zasshi* **1975**, 95, 557.

[T. Kimura]

245.   *Cocculus trilobus* **(Thunb.) DC.**   (Menispermaceae)

Mu-fang-ji (C), Muk-fong-gay (H), Ao-tsuzura-fuji (J), Daeng-daeng-i-deong-gul (K).

Rhizome and **Root**
Local Drug Name: Mu-fang-ji (C), Muk-fong-gay (H), Moku-boi (J), Mok-bang-gi (K).
Processing: Slice and dry (C), dry under the sun (J, K).
Method of Administration: Oral (decoction: C, H, J, K); Topical (fresh: H).
Folk Medicinal Uses:

        1) Neuralgia (C, J, K).
        2) Rheumatism (C, J, K).
        3) Gout (J, K).
        4) Cystitis (J).
        5) Cystodynia (K).
        6) Edema (C, J, K).
        7) Hypertension (C, H).
        8) Snake-bite (C) (H: topical).
        9) Acute nephritis (C, H).
        10) Congestion of the brain (K).
        11) Costalgia (H).
        12) Gastric pain (H).
        13) Dysmenorrhea (H).
        14) Sore throat (H).
        15) Boils, pyodermas (H: topical).

Scientific Research:

Chemistry

　　1) Alkaloids: Trilobine, isotrilobine, magnoflorine, homotrilobine[1], trilobamine [2], normenisarine [3], cocculolidine [4, 6], coclobine [5], dihydrocrysovine [6], coccutrine, cocculine [6–7], aristolochic acid and aristolic acid [8] (probably based on misidentification of a species of *Aristolochia*).

Pharmacology

　　1) Effects against congestive edema [9].

　　2) Insect resistant effect (aristolochic acid, aristolic acid) [8].

Literature:

[1] Kondo, H. *et al.*: *Yakugaku Zasshi* **1924**, 44, 69; **1926**, 46, 461; 465; **1927**, 47, 265; Nakano, T.: *Chem. Bull. Japan*, **1956**, 4, 69; Tomita, M. *et al.*: *Yakugaku Zasshi* **1958**, 78, 194.

[2] Kondo, H. *et al.*: *Yakugaku Zasshi* **1931**, 51, 451; **1935**, 55, 646.

[3] Kondo, H. *et al.*: *Yakugaku Zasshi* **1935**, 55, 911.

[4] Wada, K. *et al.*: *Tetrahedron Lett.* **1966**, 5179.

[5] Ito, K. *et al.*: *Yakugaku Zasshi* **1969**, 89, 1163.

[6] Juichi, M. *et al.*: *Chem. Pharm. Bull.* **1977**, 25, 533; *Yakugaku Zasshi* **1978**, 98, 886.

[7] McPhail. A. *et al.*: *Tetrahedron Lett.* **1976**, 485.

[8] Watanabe, A. *et al.*: *Agr. Biol. Chem. Japan* **1988**, 52, 1079.

[9] Yamahara, J. *et al.*: *Chem. Pharm. Bull.*, **1979**, 27, 1464.

[T. Kimura]

246.　　　　　*Euryale ferox* **Salisb.**　(Nymphaeaceae)

Qian (C), See-sut (H), Oni-basu (J), Ga-si-yeon-ggot (K)

Seed (CP)

Local Drug Name: Qian-shi (C), See-sut (H), Ketsu-jitsu (J), Geom-sil (K).

Processing:　1) Eliminate foreign matter (C, K).

　　　　　　　2) Stir-fry with bran to pale yellow (C).

Method of Administration: Oral (decoction: C, H, J, K)

Folk Medicinal Uses:

　　　　　　　1) Nocturnal emission, spermatorrhea, enuresis, frequent urination (C, H, J, K).

　　　　　　　2) Chronic diarrhea due to hypofunction of the spleen (C, H, J).

　　　　　　　3) Turbid discharge mixed with urine, excessive leukorrhea (C, H).

　　　　　　　4) Articular pain (H).

　　　　　　　5) Incontinence of urine (H).

　　　　　　　6) Hangover (K).

Scientific Research:

Chemistry

　　1) Steryl glycosides: 24-methycholest-5-enyl-3β-*O*-pyranoglucoside, 24-ethylcholest-5-enyl-3β-*O*-pyranoglucoside, 24-ethylcholesta-5,22*E*-dienyl-3β-*O*-pyranoglucoside

[1], 24-ethylcholesta-5-en-3β-*O*-β-D-pyranoglucosyl palmitate, 24-ethylcholesta-5,22*E*-dien-3β-*O*-β-D-pyranoglucosyl palmitate [2].

2) Tocopherols: α-tocopherol, β-tocopherol, γ-tocopherol, δ-tocopherol [3].

3) Amino acids [4]; starch [5].

Pharmacology

1) Antioxidative effect [6].

2) Inhibit the activities of murine retroviral reverse transcriptase [7].

Literature:

[1] Zhao, H. R. *et al.*: *J. Lipid Res.* **1989**, 30, 1633.

[2] Zhao, H. R. *et al.*: *Phytochem. Anal.* **1992**, 3, 38.

[3] Yeh, J. S. *et al.*: *Donghai Xuebao* **1993**, 34, 1115.

[4] Nath, B. K. et al: *J. Food. Sci. Technol.* **1985**, 22, 293.

[5] Nath, B. K. *et al.*: *Starch/Staerke* **1985**, 37, 361.

[6] Su, J. P. *et al.*: *Agric. Biol. Chem.* **1986**, 50, 199.

[7] Ono, K. *et al.*: *Chem. Pharm. Bull.* **1989**, 37, 1810.

[J.X. Guo]

247.   *Nelumbo nucifera* **Gaertn.**   (Nymphaeaceae)

Lian (C), Lin (H), Hasu (J), Yeon-ggot (K)

Seed (CP)

Local Drug Name: Lian-zi (C), Lin-gee (H), Ren-shi, Ren-niku (J), Yeon-ja (K).

Processing: Dry under the sun (C).

Method of Administration: Oral (fresh, soup, decoction, powder: C, H, J, K).

Folk Medicinal Uses:

1) Malabsorption (C, H, J, K).

2) Diarrhea (C, H, J, K).

3) Spermatorrhea (C, H, J).

4) Leukorrhea (C, J).

5) Uterine bleeding (J).

6) Palpitation (C).

7) Insomnia (C).

Contraindications: Constipation.

Fruit

Local Drug Name: Shi-lian-zi (C), Sak-lin-gee (H), Ren-jitsu (J), Seok-yeon-ja (K).

Method of Administration: Oral (decoction, C, H, J, K).

Folk Medicinal Uses:

1) Malabsorption (C, J, K).

2) Diarrhea (C, J, K).

3) Spermatorrhea (C, H).

4) Leukorrhea (C, H, J).

5) Vomiting (C).

6) Menstrual disorder (J).

Contraindications: Constipation.

Embryo (CP)
Local Drug Name: Lian-zi-xin (C), Lin-gee-sum (H), Ren-shin (J), Yeon-ja-sim (K).
Processing: Remove from seeds, dry under the sun.
Method of Administration: Oral (decoction: C, H, J, K).
Folk Medicinal Uses:
> 1) Febrile disease (C, H, K).
> 2) Thirst (C, H, K).
> 3) Palpitation (C, H).
> 4) Insomnia (C, H).
> 5) Hypertension (C, H, K).
> 6) General weakness (J).
> 7) Delirium due to heat (C).
> 8) Hemoptysis due to heat in blood (C).

Seed coat
Local Drug Name: Lian-yi (C), Ren-i (J), Yeon-eui (K).
Processing: remove from seeds.
Method of Administration: Oral (decoction: C).
Folk Medicinal Uses:
> 1) Hemorrhage (C).

Flower
Local Drug Name: Lian-hua (C), Lin-far (H), Ren-ka (J), Yeon-hwa (K).
Processing: Dry under the sun.
Method of Administration: Oral (decoction or powder: C, H, J, K).
Folk Medicinal Uses:
> 1) Traumatic injury (C, H, K).
> 2) Hematemesis (C, H, J, K).
> 3) Impetigo (C, H).
> 4) Internal hemorrhage (J).
> 5) Hemorrhoids (J).
> 6) Eczema (J).

Receptacle (CP)
Local Drug Name: Lian-fang (C), Lin-fong (H), Ren-bo (J), Yeon-bang (K).
Processing: Dry under the sun, or carbonize.
Method of Administration: Oral (decoction: C, H).
Folk Medicinal Uses:
> 1) Massive uterine bleeding (C, H).
> 2) Lochia postpartum (C, H).
> 3) Lower abdominal pain from stagnant blood (C, H).
> 4) Melena (C, H).
> 5) Hematuria (C, H).
> 6) Hemorrhoid bleeding (C).
> 7) Impetigo (C).

Stamen (CP)
Local Drug Name: Lian-xu (C), Lin-soe (H), Ren-shu (J), Yeon-su (K).
Processing: Remove from flowers and dry under the sun.
Method of Administration: Oral (decoction: C, H, J).

Folk Medicinal Uses:
>   1) Spermatorrhea (C, H, J).
>   2) Leukorrhea (C, H, J).
>   3) Enuresis (C, H).
>   4) Hematemesis (C).
>   5) Hematuria (C).
>   6) Dysentery (C).
>   7) Frequent urination (C).

Contraindications: Oliguria.

Leaf (CP)

Local Drug Name: He-ye (C), Hor-yip (H), Ka-yo (J), Ha-yeop (K).
Processing: Dry under the sun, or carbonize.
Method of Administration: Oral (decoction: C, H, J).
Folk Medicinal Uses:
>   1) Heat stroke (C, H).
>   2) Enteritis (C, H).
>   3) Hematemesis (H, J).
>   4) Hemorrhinia (H, J).
>   5) Leukorrhea (C).
>   6) Diarrhea (C, J).
>   7) Melena (C, J).
>   8) Spermatorrhea (C).
>   9) Edema (J).
>   10) Food intoxication (J).
>   11) Epistaxis (C).

Contraindications: Debility.

Rhizome and rhizome node (CP)

Local Drug Name: Ou-jie (C), Lin-ngau, Ngau-git (H), Gu, Gu-setsu (J), U (K).
Processing: Dry under the sun, or carbonize.
Method of Administration: Oral (decoction: C, H, J, K).
Folk Medicinal Uses:
>   1) Febrile disease (C, H, K).
>   2) Thirst (C, H, K).
>   3) Hemorrhinia (C, H, J).
>   4) Hemoptysis (C, H).
>   5) Hematemesis (C, H, J).
>   6) Melena (C, H, J).
>   7) Hematuria (C, H).
>   8) Abnormal uterine bleeding (C).

Scientific Research

Chemistry
1) Plumule contains liensinine, isoliensinine, neferine, nuciferine, pronuciferine, lotusine, methylcorypalline, demethylcoclaurine, galuteolin, hyperin, rutin; S-*N*-methyl isococlaurine, *dl*-armepavine) [1, 15, 20].
2) Receptacle contains nelumbine, quercetin [16], *N*-nornuciferine, oxoushinsunine, *N*-noramepavine, nuciferine [23].
3) Flower contains quercetin, luteolin, isoquercitrin, kaempferol.

51

4) Stamen contains quercetin, isoquercitrin, luteolin.

5) Seed contains starch [18], raffinose, oxoushinsunine, N-norarmepavine, polysaccharide [21], β-sitosterol, β-sitosterol fatty ester, glucose, palmitic acid [25].

6) Leaf contains roemerine, nuciferine, nornuciferine, armepavine, pronuciferine, anonaine, liriodenine, quercetin, *N*-methylcoclaurine, isoquercitrin, nelumboside, *cis*-3-hexenol, diphenylamine, α-longifolene, hexanol, benzene [22], dehydronuciferine, dehydro-anonaine, *N*-methylisococlaurine, dehydroroemerine [24], quercitrin-3-glucoside, isoquercitrin [26], *cis*-3-hexenol, hexanol, benzene, diphenylamine, α-longifolene [22].

7) Petiole contains roemerine, nornuciferine.

8) Rhizome contains asparagine.

9) Asimilobine, lirinidine [2].

10) Elements in pericarp: Na, Mg, Al, Si, P,S, Cl, K, Ca, Mn, Fe [17].

11) Flower scent contains 1,4-dimethoxybenzene, 1,8-cineole, terpinen-4-ol, linalool [19].

Pharmacology

1) Serotonergic receptor anatgonistic effect (asimilobine and lirinidine) [2].

2) Antiarrhythmic effects (neferine [3–8]; liensinine and methylliensinine) [9–11].

3) Hypotensive effect (liensinine) [13–14].

4) Calcium-antagonistic effect (liensinine, neferine, S-*N*-methyl isococlaurine) [3–8, 11, 15].

5) Antihemorrhagic effect (quercetin) [16].

6) Cytotoxic effect [23].

7) Blood-coagulation effect [26].

8) ATPase-inhibitory effect [27].

9) Potentiation of sodium pentobarbitone sleep [28].

10) Effect on alteration in general behaviour pattern [28].

Literature

[1] Xu, L. X. *et al.*: *Yaowu Fenxi Zazhi* **1991**, 11, 349.

[2] Shoji, N. *et al.*: *J. Nat. Prod.* **1987**, 50, 773.

[3] Li, G. R. *et al.*: *Zhongguo Yaoli Xuebao* **1989**, 10, 328.

[4] Li, G. R. *et al.*: *Zhongguo Yaoli Xuebao* **1989**, 10, 406.

[5] Li, G. R. *et al.*: *Zhongguo Yaoli Xuebao* **1990**, 11, 158.

[6] Li, G. R. *et al.*: *Zhongcaoyao* **1988**, 19, 217.

[7] Li, G. R. *et al.*: *Zhongguo Yaoli Xuebao* **1988**, 9, 139.

[8] Li, G. R. *et al.*: *Chin. J. Pharmacol. Toxicol.* **1987**, 1, 268.

[9] Wang, J. L. *et al.*: *Yaoxue Xuebao* **1992**, 27, 881.

[10] Xia, G. J. *et al.*: *Acta Univ. Med. Tongji* **1986**, 15, 200.

[11] Wang, J. L. *et al.*: *Yaoxue Xuebao* **1993**, 28, 812.

[12] Wang, J. L. *et al.*: *Acta Univ. Med. Tongji* **1992**, 21, 317.

[13] Chen, W. Z. *et al.*: *Yueh Hsueh Hsueh Pao* **1962**, 9, 271.

[14] Chen, W. Z. *et al.*: *Yueh Hsueh Hsueh Pao* **1962**, 9, 277.

[15] Pan, J. X. *et al.*: *J. Beijing Med. Univ.* **1989**, 21, 401.

[16] Ishida, H. *et al.*: *Chem. Pharm. Bull.* **1988**, 36, 4585.

[17] Jiang, Z. J. *et al.*: *Beijing Shifan Daxue Xuebao, Ziran Kexueban* **1991**, 27, 471.

[18] Suzuki, A. *et al.*: *Cereal Chem.* **1992**, 69, 309.

[19] Omata, A. *et al.*: *J. Essent. Oil Res.* **1991**, 3, 221.

[20] Wang, J. L. *et al.*: *Zhongguo Zhongyao Zazhi* **1991**, 16, 673.

[21] Das, S. *et al.*: *Carbohydr. Res.* **1992**, 224, 331.

[22] Fu, S. Y. *et al.*: *Beijing Daxue Xuebao, Ziran Kexueban* **1992**, 28, 699.

[23] Yang, T. H. *et al.*: *J. Chin. Chem. Soc. (Taipei)* **1972**, 19, 143.
[24] Kunitomo, J. *et al.*: *Phytochemistry* **1973**, 12, 699.
[25] Dhar, D. N. *et al.*: *Curr. Sci.* **1972**, 41, 59.
[26] Thuan, B. T. *et al.*: *Tap Chi Duoc Hoc* **1980**, (6), 19.
[27] Thang, N. X. *et al.*: *Rev. Pharm.* **1983**, 82.
[28] Mukherjee, P.K. *et al.*: *J. Ethnopharm.* **1996**, 54, 63.

[P.P.H. But]

248. *Aristolochia fangchi* Y.C. Wu ex L.D. Chow et S.M. Hwang
(Aristolochiaceae)

Guang-fang-ji (C), Gwong-fong-gay (H), Gwang-bang-gi (K)

Root (CP)
Local Drug Name: Guang-fang-ji (C), Fong-gay (H), Ko-bo-i (J), Bang-gi (K).
Processing: Eliminate foreign matter and rough bark, wash clean, cut into thick slices, dry under the sun (C).
Method of Administration: Oral (decoction: C, H, J, K).
Folk Medicinal Uses:
        1) Edema (C, H, J, K).
        2) Beriberi (C, H, J, K).
        3) Tinea (C, H).
        4) Eczema (C, H, K).
        5) Articular rheumatism (J).
Contraindications: Yin-deficiency without wet-heat.
Side effects: Excessive or prolonged use may lead to kidney damage labelled as Chinese herbs nephropathy [1-6, 19] and urothelial malignancy [7].

Scientific Research
Chemistry
    1) Aristolochic acid , aristololactam, allantoin, magnoflorine, *p*-coumaric acid, syringic acid, palmitic acid, aristolochic acid IV methyl ether methyl ester, aristolactic acid IV methylether, β-sitosterol, moupinamide, *N*-(*p*-hydroxyphenethyl)-*p*-coumaramide [8–9].
Pharmacology
    1) Inhibitory effect on acetylcholine esterase [10].
    2) Carcinogenic and genotoxic effects of aristolochic acid [11–17].
    3) Fertility regulatory effect (aristolochic acid) [18].

Literature
[1] Vanherweghem, J.L. *et al.*: *Lancet* **1993**, 341, 387.
[2] Jadoul, M. *et al.*: *Lancet* **1993**, 341, 892.
[3] But, P.P.H.: *Lancet* **1993**, 341, 637.
[4] Vanhaelen, M. *et al.*: *Lancet* **1994**, 343, 174.

[5] De Smet, P.A.G.M.: In: De Smet, P.A.G.M. *et al.*(eds.) *Adverse Effects of Herbal Drugs*. Springer-Verlag, Berlin, **1992**, 79.

[6] Cosyns, J.P. *et al.*: *Kidney Intl.* **1994**, 45, 1680.

[7] Cosyns, J.P. *et al.*: *Lancet.* **1994**, 344, 188.

[8] Xu, L.Z. *et al.*: *Zhongyao Tongbao* **1984**, 9, 206.

[9] Chou, L.T. *et al.*: *Yao Hsueh T'ung Pao* **1981**, 16(2), 51.

[10] Yamaguchi, T. *et al.*: *Jpn. Kokai Tokkyo Koho JP* **1992**, 04,159,225 [92,159,225] .

[11] Mengs, U. *et al.*: *Arch. Toxicol.* **1982**, 51, 107.

[12] Mengs, U. *et al.*: *Arch. Toxicol.* **1983**, 52, 209.

[13] Mengs, U.: *Arch. Toxicol.* **1987**, 59, 328.

[14] Mengs, U. *et al.*: *Planta Med.* **1988**, 502.

[15] Mengs, U.: *Arch. Toxicol.* **1988**, 61, 504.

[16] Mengs, U.: *Med. Sci. Res.* **1990**, 18, 855.

[17] Mengs, U.: *Arch. Toxicol.* **1993**, 67, 307.

[18] Wang, W.H. *et al.*: *Yao Hsueh Hsueh Pao* **1984**, 19, 405.

[19] Vanherweghem, J.L.: *Bull. Mem. Acad. R. Med. Belg.* **1994**, 149, 128.

[P.P.H. But]

249. *Asarum heterotropoides* Fr. var. *mandshuricum* (Maxim.) Kitag.
(Aristolochiaceae)
[=*Asiasarum heterotropoides* F. Maekawa var. *mandshuricum* F. Maekawa]

Bei-xi-xin (C), Sight-sun (H), Keirin-saishin (J), Jok-do-ri-pul (K)

Related plants: *A.sieboldii* Miq. var. *seoulense* Nakai: Han-cheng-xi-xin (C); *A.sieboldii* Miq. (*Asiasarum sieboldii* F. Maekawa): Hua-xi-xin (C), Usuba-saishin (J), Min-jok-do-ri-pul (K).

Herb (CP)

Local Drug Name: Xi-xin (C), Sight-sun (H), Se-sin (K).

Processing: Eliminate foreign matter, dry in shade (C, K).

Method of Administration: Oral (decoction: C, H, J, K); Topical (decoction: C; powder: H, K).

Folk Medicinal Uses:

1) Common cold, headache, toothache (C, H, J, K).

2) Sinusitis with nasal obstruction (C, H, J, K).

3) Rheumatic arthralgia (C, H, J, K).

4) Cough and dyspnea due to retention of phlegm and fluid (C, H, J, K).

5) Fur (K).

Contraindication: Incompatible with rhizome of *Veratrum* species (C).

Scientific Research:

Chemistry

1) Volatile oils: eucarvone, α-pinene, β-pinene, 1,8-cineole, croweacin, safrole, elemicin, methyleugenol, asaricin [1], kakuol, *n*-pentadecane, 3,5-dimethoxytoluene [2],

limonene, linalool, 3,4,5-trimethoxytoluene, 2,3,5-trimethoxytoluene, 2,3,4-trime-
thoxy-1-propenyl-benzene [3], estragole, camphene [4] α-terpineol, myristicine, α-
thujene, myrcene, terpin-4-ol, [5], 1,2,4-trimethoxy-5-allylbenzene [6], *dl*-car-3-
ene-2,5-dione [7], borneol, transasarone.
2) Alkaloids and nitrogen compound: *dl*-demethylcoclaurine (higenamine) [8], (2*E*,4*E*)-
   N-isobutyl-2,4- decadienamide (pellitorine), (2*E*,4*E*,8*Z*,10*E*)-*N*-isobutyl-2,4,8,10-
   dodecatetraenamide, (2*E*,4*E*,8*Z*,10*Z*)-*N*-isobutyl-2,4,8,10-dodecatetraenamide [9].
3) Steroids: sitosterol, campesterol, stimasterol [10].
4) Organic acid: palmitic acid [11].
5) Others: sesamine [9], *l*-asarinin, *l*-epiasarinin [12].
Pharmacology
1) Insecticidal effect [6].
2) Local anesthesia [13].
3) Antipyretic effect [14].
4) Analgesic effect [14].
5) Hair tonic effect [15].
6) Effect on cardiovascular system [13, 16].
7) Antibacterial effect [17].
8) Inhibitory effect on central nervous system [18].
9) Antiinflammatory effect [19].
10) Inhibitory effect on Δ^5-desaturase [12].

Literature:

[1] Saiki, Y. *et al.*: *Yakugaku Zasshi* **1967**, 87, 1529.
[2] Saiki, Y. *et al.*: *Yakugaku Zasshi* **1970**, 90, 103.
[3] Mori, N. *et al.*: *Shoyakugaku Zasshi* **1977**, 31, 175.
[4] Tian, Z. *et al.*: *Yaoxue Tongbao* **1981**, 2, 53.
[5] Shen, Z.X. *et al.*: *Yaowu Fenxi Zazhi* **1982**, 6, 335.
[6] Miyazawa, M. *et al.*: *Chem. Express* **1992**, 7, 69.
[7] Endo, J. *et al.*: *Yakugaku Zasshi* **1978**, 98, 789.
[8] Kosuge, T. *et al.*: *Kanpo Kenkyu* **1978**, 11, 429.
[9] Ichiro, Y. *et al.*: *Chem. Pharm. Bull.* **1981**, 29, 564.
[10] Nakamura, T. *et al.*: *Dai 9ji Shokubutsu Jikken Bunruigaku Toronkai Koenroku* **1979**.
[11] Kaku, T. *et al.*: *Yakugaku Zazhi* **1931**, 51, 8.
[12] Shimizu, S. *et al.*: *Phytochemistry* **1992**, 31, 757.
[13] He, Y. J.: *Qingdao Yixueyuan Xuebao* **1959**, (2), 20.
[14] Ishihara, T.: *Igaku Chao Zasshi* **1960**, 153, 338.
[15] Yayama, K.: *Jpn. Kokai Tokkyo Koho* 79, 145, 228 (cl. A61k7/06), 13 Nov **1979**, Appl.
    78/51, 309, 30 Apr **1978**.
[16] Chen, Z.Z. *et al.*: *Yaoxue Xuebao* **1981**, 16, 721.
[17] Ohmoto, T. *et al.*: *Shoyakugaku Zasshi* **1981**, 35, 71.
[18] Jiang, Y. *et al.*: *Yaoxue Xuebao* **1982**, 17, 87.
[19] Qu, S.Y. *et al.*: *Yaoxue Xuebao* **1982**, 17, 12.

[J.X. Guo]

250. *Camellia japonica* **L.** (Theaceae)

Shan-cha (C), Sarn-char (H), Tsubaki(J), Dong-baek-na-mu(K)

Oil (JP, KP)
Local Drug Name: Tsubaki-abura (J), Dong-baek-yu (K).
Processing: Dry under the sun, grind, steam and compress (J, K).
Method of Administration: Oral (K).
Folk Medicinal Uses:
>   1) Dandruff (K).
>   2) Measles (K).
>   3) Wound (K).
>   4) Common cold (K).
>   5) Ringworm (K).
>   6) Tonsillitis (K).

Leaf
Local Drug Name: Tsubaki-no-ha (J), Dong-baek-yeop (K).
Processing: use in fresh (J).
Method of Administration: Oral (decoction: J); Topical (J).
Folk Medicinal Uses:
>   1) Contusion (J).
>   2) Nocturia (J).
>   3) Insect bite (J).

Flower
Local Drug Name: Shan-cha-hua (C), Sarn-char-far (H).
Processing: Dry under the sun (C, H).
Method of Administration: Oral (decoction: C, H), Topical (paste: C; powder: H).
Folk Medicinal Uses:
>   1) Hematemesis (C, H).
>   2) Epistaxis (H).
>   3) Bleeding hemorrhoids (C, H).
>   4) Scalds (C, H).
>   5) Burns (H).
>   6) Cracked nipples (H).
>   7) Boils (H).
>   8) Pyodermas (H).

Scientific Research:
Chemistry
1) Saponins: camellidin I, II [1, 11].
2) Flavonols: quercetin, kaempferol, sexangularetin [12], flavan-3-ol, catechin, (–)-epi-catechin [24].
3) Phenols: *p*-hydroxybenzoic acid, protocatechuic acid, gallic acid [12], eugenol [20].
4) Sterols [21]: α-spinasterol, stigmast-7-en-3β-ol, stigmasteryl-D-glucoside, β-sitoster-yl-D-glucoside [12], 5α-stigmasta-7,22-dien-3β-ol, 5α-stigmast-7-en-3β-ol [24].
5) Triterpenes [16]: 3β-hydroxy-28-norolean-17-en-16-on-12,13-epoxide [12], maragenin II, camellenodiol [14], β-amyrin [21, 24], lupeol [24].
6) Anthocyans [19, 23]: cyanidin 3-*O*-b-D-(6-*O*-*p*-coumaroylglucoside [5], cyanidin 3-galactoside, cyanidin 3-glucoside [6, 15].
7) Purine bases: theobromine [22].
8) Tannins: camelliin A [2], B [2–3], gemin D [7, 13].
9) Fatty acids: palmitic acid, oleic acid [21].

10) Enzymes: fructokinase, hexokinase [9].
11) Sugars: raffinose, pectin [24].
12) Miscellaneous: theanine [10], ascorbic acid [18].
Pharmacology
  1) Antifungal effect [1, 11].
  2) Antitumor effect (camelliin B) [3].
  3) Skin-lightening effect [4].
  4) Dental caries prevention effect [8].
  5) L-Ascorbic acid oxidase inhibition effect [17].

Literature:
 [1] Nagata, T. et al.: Agric. Biol. Chem. **1985**, 49, 1181.
 [2] Yoshida, T. et al.: Chem. Pharm. Bull. **1990**, 38, 2681.
 [3] Yoshida, T. et al.: Chem. Pharm. Bull. **1989**, 37, 3174.
 [4] Mori, K. and Shinomiya, T.: Jpn. Kokai Tokkyo Koho JP **63,303,910**, 12 Dec. **1988**,
     Appl. 87/139,379, 03 Jun. **1987**, 6 pp.
 [5] Saito, N. et al.: Phytochemistry **1987**, 26, 2761.
 [6] Sakata, Y. et al.: Engei Gakkai Zasshi **1986**, 55, 82.
 [7] Yoshida, T. et al.: Phytochemistry **1985**, 24, 1041.
 [8] Sakai, T. et al.: Shoyakugaku Zasshi **1985**, 39, 165.
 [9] Nakamura, N. et al.: Physiol. Plant. **1991**, 81, 215.
[10] Tsushida, T. et al.: Agric. Biol Chem. **1984**, 48, 2861.
[11] Hamaya, E. et al.: Nippon Shokubutsu Byori Gakkaiho **1984**, 50, 628.
[12] Nakajima, H. et al.: Yakugaku Zasshi **1984**, 104, 157.
[13] Yoshida, T. et al.: Chem. Pharm. Bull. **1982**, 30, 4245.
[14] Itokawa, H. et al.: Phytochemistry **1981**, 20, 2539.
[15] Sakata, Y. et al.: Mem. Fac. Agric. Kagoshima Univ. **1981**, 17, 79.
[16] Itoh, T. et al.: Lipids **1980**, 15, 407.
[17] Takahashi, K. et al.: Mukogawa Joshi Daigaku Kiyo, Shokumotsu-hen **1980**, 28, F5.
[18] Sakamura, F.: Kaseigaku Zasshi **1975**, 26, 256.
[19] Ishikura, N.: Bot. Mag. **1975**, 88, 41.
[20] Fujita, Y. et al.: Osaka Kogyo Gijutsu Shikensho Kiho, **1974**, 25, 198.
[21] Endo, S. et al.: Tokyo Gakugei Daigaku Kiyo, Dai-4-Bu **1974**, 26, 107.
[22] Bohine, P. et al.: Farm. Vestn.(Ljubljana) **1972**, 23, 219
[23] Thompson, R., S. et al.: J. Chem. Soc., Perkin Trans. I **1972**, 1387.
[24] Suau Suarez, R.: Acta Cient. Compostelana, **1971**, 8, 185.

                                                [C.K. Sung]

251.   *Camellia sinensis* **(L.) O. Kuntze** (Theaceae)
                    [=*Thea sinensis* L.]

Cha (C), Char (H), Cha (J), Cha-na-mu (K)

Leaf
  Local Drug Name: Cha (C), Char-yip (H), Cha-yo (J), Da-yeop (K).
  Processing: Stir-fry (C); steam and dry in heated air (J, K).

Method of Administration: Oral (infusion: C, H, J, K); Topical (paste: C).
Folk Medicinal Uses:

    1) Diarrhea, dysentery, enteritis (C, H, J, K).
    2) Stomatitis (J, K).
    3) Sore throat (J, K).
    4) Edema (C, H).
    5) Hypnopathia (C).
    6) Dysuria (C).
    7) Scald (C).
    8) Indigestion (H).
    9) Common cold (H).
    10) Oliguria (H).
    11) Alcohol intoxication (H).
    12) Drowsiness (H).
    13) Anasarca (K).
    14) Headache (K).
    15) Enuresis (K).
    16) Panaritium (K).

Scientific Research:
Chemistry
    1) Alkaloids: caffeine, theophylline, theobromine[1]
    2) Flavonoids: quercitrin, quercetin [1], camelliaside C [5].
    3) Tannins: *l*-epigallocatechol, *dl*-gallocatechol, *l*-epicatechol, *l*-epigallocatechol gallate, *l*-epicatechol gallate, *dl*-catechol [8].
    4) Aromatic compounds: 5,7-dihydroxycoumarin, (−)-epiafzelechin, phloroglucinol, pyrogallol [2], *l*-quinic acid, shikimic acid [7].
    5) Steroids: α-spinasterol (theosterin) [3].
    6) Aliphatic compound: [9].
Pharmacology
    1) Central nervous system stimulant effect [4].
    2) Cardiotonic effect [4].
    3) Diuretic effect [4].
    4) Analgesic effect [4].
    5) Gastric secretion increasing effect [4].
    6) Inhibitory effects on arachidonate 5-lipoxygenase [5].
    7) Antioxidant effect [6].

Literature:
[1] Iwasaki, : *Yakugaku Zasshi* **1896**, 144, 119.
[2] Myers, M. etal.: *Chem. & Ind.* **1959**, 950.
[3] Sakato, Y. *et al.*: *Nogeishi.* **1959**, 33, 374; **1942**, 18, 524.
[4] Burg, A. W. *et al.*: *Toxicol. Appl. Pharmacol.* **1974**, 28, 162.
[5] Sekine, T. *et al.*: *Chem. Pharm. Bull.* **1993**, 41, 1185.
[6] Lea, C. H. *et al.*: *Chem. & Ind.* **1957**, 1073.
[7] Zaprometov, M. N.: *Biokhimiya* **1961**, 26, 373.
[8] Dzhemukhadze, K. M. *et al.*: *Doklady Acad. Nuk S.S.S.R.* **1961**, 136, 1471.
[9] Hatanaka, A. *et al.*: *Agr. Biol. Chem. Japan* **1961**, 25, 7.

[T. Kimura]

252.   *Chelidonium majus* **L.**   (Papaveraceae)
[=*C. sinense* DC]

Bai-qu-cai (C), Kusano-o (J), Ae-gi-ddong-pul (K)

Herb
Local Drug Name: Bai-qu-cai (C), Haku-kutsu-sai (J), Baek-gul-chae (K).
Processing: Dry under the sun (C, K) or use in fresh (C).
Method of Administration: Oral (decoction: C, K); Topical (paste: C; decoction, fresh juice:
J).
Folk Medicinal Uses:
> 1) Insect bite (C, J).
> 2) Gastric ulcer (C, K).
> 3) Scabies (J, K).
> 4) Abdominal pain (C).
> 5) Gastritis (C).
> 6) Enteritis (C).
> 7) Dysentery (C).
> 8) Jaundice (C).
> 9) Chronic bronchitis (C).
> 10) Pertussis (C).
> 11) Eczema (J).
> 12) Bruise (J).
> 13) Stomach cancer (K).
> 14) Hepatopathy (K).
> 15) Dislocation (K).
> 16) Neuralgia (K).
> 17) Psoriasis (K).
> 18) Dermatitis (K).

Side Effects: Poisonous, hypesthesia.

Scientific Research:
Chemistry
> 1) Alkaloids [1]: sanguinarine [2, 8, 11–12], magnoflorine, oxysanguinarine, dihydro-sanguinarine, dihydrochelerythrine, dihydrochelilutine, dihydrochelirubine, N-demethyl-9,10-dihydro-sanguinarine, (–)-stylopine α-methohydroxide, coptisine, (–)-stylopine methohydroxide [4], chelidonine [4, 6, 8, 14], allocryptopine, protopine [4, 16], corysamine [4], berberine [4, 8], homochelidonine, scoulerine [5], chelerythrine [5, 11–12], colchamine [6], chelidonine-thotepa, amitosine [7], DL-stylopine, 6-methoxydihydro-chelerythrine, 6-methoxydihydro- sanguinarine, 8-oxocoptisine, L-canadine [17], (–)-turkiyenine [18], tetrahydrocoptisine [20], celidoniol [21].
> 2) Coumarins [3].
> 3) Pigments: neoxanthin, violxanthin, zeaxanthin, lutein, β-cryptoxanthin, α-crypto-xanthine, β-carotene, chlorophyll-a, chlorophyll-b [9].
> 4) Lectins [13].

Pharmacology
> 1) Antiviral effect (total alkaloid, colchamine, chelidonine) [6–7, 15].
> 2) Antitumor effect (chelidonine) [8, 10, 14, 22].

3) Antifungal effect (chelerythrine) [11].
4) Antimitotic effect (chelidonine) [14].
5) Antiallergic effect (chelidonine) [14].
6) Spasmolytic effect (chelidonine) [14].
7) Hypotensive effect (chelidonine) [14].
8) Analgesic effect (chelidonine) [14].
9) Antitussive effect (chelidonine) [14].
10) Anti-AIDS effect (thiophosphate derivative of total alkaloid) [19].
11) Affinity for $GABA_A$ receptor [23].
12) Inhibitory effect on keratinocytes [24].

Literature:

[1] Matile, P.: *Nova Acta Leopold.* **1976**, Suppl. **7**, 139.
[2] Takao, N. *et al.*: *Chem. Pharm. Bull.* **1976**, 24, 2859.
[3] Florya, V. N. *et al.*: *Tezisy Dokl. Soobshch. Konf. Molodykh Uch. Mold., 9th,* **1974**, 147
[4] Slavik, J. *et al.*: *Collec. Czech. Chem. Commun.* **1977**, 42, 2686.
[5] Nyomarkay, K. M. *et al.*: *Ann. Univ. Sci. Budap. Rolando Eotvos Nominatae, Sect. Biol.* **1977**, 18-19, 113.
[6] Lozyuk, L. V.: *Mikrobiol. Zh.(Kiev)* **1977**, 39, 343.
[7] Lozyuk, L. V.: *Mikrobiol. Zh.(Kiev)* **1978**, 40, 92.
[8] Hladon, B. *et al.*: *Ann. Pharm.(Poznan)* **1978**, 13, 61.
[9] Neamtu, G. *et al.*: *Stud. Cercet. Biochim.* **1979**, 22, 175.
[10] Petlichnaya, L. *et al.*: *Farm. Zh.(Kiev)* **1982**, (6), 68-69.
[11] Hejtmankova, N. *et al.*: *Fitoterapia* **1984**, 55, 291.
[12] Walterova, D. *et al.*: *Planta Med.* **1984**, 50, 149.
[13] Peumans, W. J. *et al.*: *Plant Physiol.* **1985**, 78, 379.
[14] Jusiak, L. *et al.*: Pol. PL 128,822, 15 Mar. **1986**, Appl. 217,458, 28 Jul. 1979; 2 pp.
[15] Kery, A. *et al.*: *Acta Pharm. Hung.* **1987**, 57, 19.
[16] Jusiak, L. and Rompala, A.: Pol. PL 144,246, 31 May **1988**, Appl. 250,271, 30 Oct. **1984**; 3 pp.
[17] Zhou, J. *et al.*: *Zhongcaoyao* **1989**, 20, 146.
[18] Kadan, G. *et al.*: J. Nat. Prod. **1990**, 53, 531.
[19] Nowisky, W.: U. S. US 4,970,212, 13 Nov. **1990**, US Appl. 379,415, 18 May **1982**; 25 pp.
[20] Gulubov, A. Z. *et al.*: *Nauch. Tr. Vissh. Pedagog. Inst., Plovdiv, Mat., Fiz., Khim., Biol.* **1970**, 8, 135.
[21] Scoane, E. *et al.*: *An. Quim.* **1969**, 65, 303.
[22] Sokoloff, B.: *Oncology* **1968**, 22, 49.
[23] Haberlein, H. *et al.*: *Planta Med.* **1996**, 62, 227.
[24] Vavreckova, C. *et al.*: *Planta Med.* **1996**, 62, 491.

[C.K. Sung]

253. *Corydalis decumbens* (Thunb.) Pers. (Papaveraceae)

Fu-sheng-zi-jing (C), Har-tin-moe (H), Jirobo-engosaku (J), Jom-hyeon-ho-saek (K)

Rhizome (CP)
Local Drug Name: Xia-tian-wu (C), Har-tin-mo (H), En-go-saku (J), Ha-cheon mu (K).
Processing: Dry under the sun (C, J).
Method of Administration: Oral (powder: C, decoction: J, H).
Folk Medicinal Uses:
  1) Rheumatic arthritis (C, H, J, K).
  2) Hypertension (H, J, K).
  3) Hemiplegia, sequelae of poliomyelitis (C).
  4) Sciatica (C, H).
  5) Traumatic injury (C, H).

Scientific Research:
Chemistry
  1) Alkaloids: Tetrahydropalmatine [1], protopine, bulbocapine, adulmidine [2], ecumbenine-C [3], jatrorrhizine [4], decumbesine, epi- -decumbesine [5], (–)-corydecumbine [7].
Pharmacology
  1) Effects on isolated cat cilialy muscle and guinea pig ileum (protopine) [6].

Literature:
[1] Osada, : *Yakugaku Zasshi* **1927**, 47, 99; 100; 102; 104.
[2] Naruto, S. et al: *Phytochemistry* **1972**, 11, 2462.
[3] Zhang, J. S. *et al.*: *Huaxue Xuebao* **1988**, 46, 595.
[4] Liao, J. *et al.*: *J. Chromatogr.* **1994**, 669, 225, 236.
[5] Zhang, J. S. *et al.*: *J. Nat. Prod.*, **1988**, 51, 1241.
[6] Chu, T. Y. *et al.*: *Chung Tsao Yao* **1980**, 11, 341.
[7] Basnet, P., *et al.*: *Heterocycles* **1993**, 36, 2205.

[T. Kimura]

254.　　　　　*Papaver somniferum* L.　(Papaveraceae)

Ying-su (C), Ngunk-suk (H), Keshi (J), Yan-gwi-bi (K)

Related plant: *Papaver setigerum* DC.: Atsumi-geshi (J).

Latex (JP)
Local Drug Name: A-hen (J), A-pyeon (K).
Processing: Latex of the unripe fruit. Adjust content of morphine at 10% (J).
Method of Administration: Oral (powder or tincture: J).
Folk Medicinal Uses:
  1) Diarrhea (J, K).
  2) Pain (J, K).
Side effects: Narcotic. Drug dependency on repeated medication.

Pericarp (CP)
Local Drug Name: Ying-su-qiao (C), Ngunk-suk-hok (H), Ou-zoku-koku (J).

Processing: 1) Break to pieces, cut into slices (C).
               2) Stir-fry with vinegar or honey (C).
Method of Administration: Oral (decoction: C).
Folk Medicinal Uses:
               1) Chronic cough (C, H).
               2) Chronic diarrhea with prolapse of the rectum (C).
               3) Epigastric and abdominal pain (C, H).
Side effects: Narcotic.

Scientific Research:
Chemistry
    1) Alkaloids: morphine [1], codeine, thebaine, papaverine, noscapine (narcotine),
        narceine, neopine [2], narcotoline[6–7], 2,2'-dimorphine (pseudomorphine) [8].
    2) Chromones: meconic acid.
    3) Steroid: β-sitosterol [9].
Pharmacology
    1) Analgesic (morphine).
    2) Sedative (morphine).
    3) Obstipation (alkaloids) [3-5].

Literature:
[1] Gulland, J. M. et al: *J. Chem. Soc.* **1925**, 123, 980.
[2] Kabay, J.: *Brit. Pat.* 406,107; *Ger. Pat.* 524,964.
[3] Kromer, W. *et al.*: *Life Sci.* **1989**, 44, 579.
[4] Coupar, I. M.: *Br. J. Pharmacol.* **1978**, 63, 57.
[5] Beubler, E. *et al.*: *Naunyn-Scmiedeberg's Arch. Pharmacol.* **1979**, 306, 113.
[6] Pfeifer, S.: *Arch. d. Pharm.* **1957**, 290, 209, and 261.
[7] Miram, R., *et al.*: *Naturwiss.* **1958**, 45, 573.
[8] Bentley, K. W. *et al.*: *Chem. & Ind.* **1957**, 398.
[9] Takemoto, T. *et al.*: *Yakugaku Kenkyu* **1957**, 29, 880.

                                               [T. Kimura]

255.   *Orostachys japonicus* **A. Berger**   (Crassulaceae)
                      (*O. erubescens* Ohwi)

Wa-hua (C), Tsumerenge (J), Ba-wi-sol (K)

Herb
Local Drug Name: Wa-song (C, K).
Processing: Dry under the sun (C, K).
Method of Administration: Oral (decoction: C, K), topical (paste of fresh herb or powder:
               C).
Folk Medicinal Uses:
               1) Hematochezia (C).
               2) Hematemesis (C).
               3) Gingivitis (K).

4) Coagulation metritis (K).
5) Dried mouth pain (K).
6) Hemorrhoid (K).

Scientific Research:
Chemistry
1) Triterpenes: taraxerone [1], seco-A-triterpene mix., glutinone, friedelin, β-amyrin, glutinol, epi-fridelanol, 1-hexatriacontanol [3].
2) Steroids: stigmast-4-ene-3-one, ergost-4-ene-3-one [1], sterol mixture, steryl glucoside mixture [3].
3) Fatty acids [3].
Pharmacology
1) Cytotoxic effect to murine and human cacer cells [2].
2) Pyruvate-orthophosphate dikinase acitivity [4].

Literature:
[1] Park. H. J. *et al.*: *Saenghak Hakhoechi* **1994**, 25(1), 20.
[2] Lee, Ihn Rhan, et al: *Saenghak Hakhoechi* **1992**, 23(3), 132.
[3] Park, H. J. *et al.*: *Saenghak Hakhoechi* **1991**, 22(2), 78.
[4] Sanada, Y. *et al.*: *Z. Pflanzenphysiol.* **1982**, 105(2), 189.

[C.K. Sung]

256.   *Sedum erythrostichum* **Miquel** (Crassulaceae)

Jing-tian (C), Benkeiso (J), Ggweong-eu-bi-reum (K)

Herb
Local Drug Name: Jing-tian (C), Kei-ten (J), Gyeong-cheon (K).
Processing: Dry under the sun (C, J, K) or use in fresh (C).
Method of Administration: Oral (decoction: C, J, K); Topical (decoction: C).
Folk Medicinal Uses:
1) Trauma (J, K).
2) Mastitis (C, K).
3) Dermatopathy (J, K).
4) Laryngitis (C).
5) Urticaria (C).
6) Hematemesis (C).
7) Infantile erysipelas (C).
8) Carbuncle (C).
9) Swelling (J).
10) Abcess (J).
11) Abdominal pain (K).
12) Lymphadenitis (K).
13) Neuralgia (K).
14) Lymphoma (K).
15) Furuncle (C).

Scientific Research:
Chemistry
   1) Sedoheptulose [1].

Literature:
[1] Yamada, S.: *Fukushima J. Med.* **1959**, 6, 253.

[C.K. Sung]

257.   *Dichroa febrifuga* **Lour.** (Saxifragaceae)

Chang-shan (C), Sheung-sarn (H), Jo-zan-ajisai (J)

Root (CP)
Local Drug Name: Chang-shan (C), Sheung-sarn (H), Jo-zan (J).
Processing: 1) Eliminate foreign matter, grade according to size, soak in water, soften
                thoroughly, cut into thin slices, and dry in the sun (C).
          2) Stir-fry slices until the colour darkened (C).
Method of Administration: Oral (decoction: C, H, J).
Folk Medicinal Uses:
               1) Malaria (C, H, J).
               2) Productive cough (H).
               3) Food poisoning (H).
               4) Febrile diseases (J).
Contraindication: Pregnancy (C).
Side Effect: Vomiting (C).

Scientific Research:
Chemistry
   1) Alkaloids: dichroine A, dichroine B [1–3], α,β,γ-dichroine, 4-quinazolone [4],
      dichroidine [2].
   2) Coumarin: umbelliferone [5].
   3) Trace elements: Cu, Pb [6].
Pharmacology
   1) Antimalarial effect [7].
   2) Antiamebic effect [8].
   3) Antileptospiral effect [9].
   4) Antiviral effect [10].
   5) Febrifuge effect [11].
   6) Emetic action [12].
   7) Effect on cardiovascular system [13].

Literature:
[1] Zhang, C. S. *et al.*: *Science* **1946**, 103, 59.
[2] Fu, Y. F. *et al.*: *Sc. Technol. China* **1948**, 1(3), 56.
[3] Koepfli, J. B. *et al.*: *J. Amer. Chem. Soc.* **1950**, 72, 3323.
[4] Zhao, C. H. *et al.*: *J. Amer. Chem. Soc.* **1948**, 70, 1765.
[5] Yanagida, S. *et al.*: *Shanghai Ziran Kexue Yanjiusuo Huibao* **1942**, 12(1). 94.

[6] Qin, J. F. *et al.*: *Zhongcaoyao* **1983**, 14(11), 492.

[7] Zhang, C. S. *et al.*: *Zhonghua Yixue Zazhi* **1947**, 33(5), 177.

[8] Zhang, T. M. *et al.*: *Wuhan Yixueyuan Xuebao* **1958**, (1), 11.

[9] Sicuan Institute of Chinese Materia Medica: *Zhongcaoyao Yanjiu Ziliao* **1971**, (6) , 32.

[10] Wang, S. Y. *et al.*: *Kexue Tongbao* **1958**, (3), 90; (5), 155.

[11] Sun, S. X.: *Zhonghua Yixue Zazhi* **1956**, 42(10), 964.

[12] Jiang, W. D.: *Shengli Xuebao* **1961**, 24(3), 180.

[13] Zhang, C. S.: *Shengli Xuebao* **1956**, 20(1), 30.

[J.X. Guo]

258.   *Saxifraga stolonifera* **Meerb**   (Saxifragaceae)

Hu-er-cao (C), Foo-yee-cho (H), Yukinoshita (J), Ba-wi-chwi (K)

Herb
Local Drug Name: Hu-er-cao (C), Foo-yee-cho (H), Ko-ji-so (J), Ho-i-cho (K).
Processing: Dry under the sun (C, K) or use in fresh (C, K).
Method of Administration: Oral (decoction: C, H, J, K); Topical (paste: C, fresh juice: J, K).
Folk Medicinal Uses:
        1) Otitis media (C, H, J, K, topical).
        2) Eczema (H, J, K).
        3) Frost-bite (H, K).
        4) Fever in child (C).
        5) Cough and wheezing (C).
        6) Intertrigo (H, topical).
        7) Sputum from lung abscess (H).
        8) Furunculosis (C, H, topical).
        9) Bleeding wound (H, topical).
        10) Swelling (J).
        11) Abcess (J).
        12) Meningitis (K).
        13) Vomiting (K).
        14) Diarrhea (K).
        15) Fever (K).
        16) Neuralgia (K).

Scientific Research:
 Chemistry
    1) Flavonol glycosides [1].
    2) Phenol glycosides: bergenin, arbutin [2–3].
    3) Coumarins; isocoumarins [4].
    4) Miscellaneous: catechol, K(−)-quinate, γ-aminobutyric acid [5].
    5) Oils [6].

Literature:
[1] Morita, N. *et al.*: *Chem. Pharm. Bull.* **1974**, 22, 1487.

[2] Taneyama, M. *et al.*: *Bot. Mag.* **1979**, 92, 69.
[3] Taneyama, M. *et al.*: *Bot. Mag.* **1978**, 91, 109.
[4] Nitto Electric Instrial Co., Ltd.: *Jpn. Kokai Tokkyo Koho* JP **60,53,150**, 26 Mar. **1985**, Appl. 83/160,057, 31 Aug. **1983**; 4 pp.
[5] Aoki, T. *et al.*: *J. Sci. Hiroshima Univ. Ser. A. Phys. Chem.* **1984**, 48, 81.
[6] Kameoka, H. *et al.*: *Yukagaku* **1976**, 25, 490.

[C.K. Sung]

259.   *Geum japonicum* Thunb.   (Rosaceae)

Ri-ben-shui-yang-mei (C), Daikonso (J), Baem-mu (K)

Related plant: *Geum japonicum* Thunb. var. *chinense* Bolle.: Nan-shui-yang-mei (C).

Whole herb
Local Drug Name: Nan-bu-zheng (C), Sui-yo-bai (J), Su-yang-mae (K).
Processing: Dry under the sun or in the shade (C, J, K). Fresh (C).
Method of Administration: Oral (decoction: C, J, K); Topical (paste or fresh: C).
Folk Medicinal Uses:
       1) Edema with nephropathy (J).
       2) Nocturia (J, K).
       3) Diabetes (J).
       4) Hypertension (C).
       5) Headache (C).
       6) Menoxenia (C).
       7) Pain of lower abdomen (C).
       8) Infantile convulsion (C).
       9) Lumbago due to pathogenic wind-dampness (C).
       10) Carbuncle (C).
       11) Abscess (K).
       12) Spermatorrhea (K).
       13) Traumatic injury (C).

Scientific Research:
Chemistry
    1) Tannins: geponin [1].
    2) Phenylpropanoids: gein, geoside [2].
Pharmacology
    1) Antiviral effect (geponin) [1].

Literature:
[1] Xu, H.X., *et al.*:`Heterocycles` **1994**, 38, 167.
[2] Takahashi, M. *et al.*:*J. Pharm. Soc. Japan* **1955**, 75, 1567.

[T. Kimura]

260.   *Prunus japonica* **Thunb.**   (Rosaceae)

Yu-li (C), Niwa-ume (J), Cham-ok-mae-hwa (K)

Related plant: *Prunus nakai* L.: Chosen-niwa-ume (J); *P. humilis* Bunge.: Ou-li (C), Ko-niwa-zakura (J); *P. pedunculata* Maxim.: Chang-bing-bian-tao (C).

Seed (CP)
Local Drug Name: Yu-li-ren (C), Yuk-lay-yun (H), Iku-ri-nin (J), Uk-ri-in (K).
Processing: Dry under the sun (C, J).
Method of Administration: Oral (decoction: C, H, J, K).
Folk Medicinal Uses:
        1) Edema (H, J, K).
        2) Weakness and edema of the legs with oliguria (C).
        3) Constipation (H, J, K).
        4) Stagnancy of undigested food with abdominal distension and
           constipation (C).

Scientific Research:
Chemistry
    1) Flavonoids: afzelin, kaempferitrin, multiflorin A (prunuside) [1], multiflorin B [2].
    2) Triterpenoids: ursolic acid [2].
    3) Phenolic compounds: vanillic acid, protocatechuic acid [2].
Pharmacology
    1) Purgative [2].

Literature:
[1] Oshio, H. *et al.*: *Yakugaku Zasshi* **1975**, 95, 484.
[2] Takagi, S. *et al.*: *Yakugaku Zasshi* **1979**, 99, 439.

[T. Kimura]

261.   *Prunus mume* **Sieb. et Zucc.**   (Rosaceae)

Mei (C), Mui (H), Ume (J), Mae-sil-na-mu (K)

Fruit (CP)
Local Drug Name: Wu-mei (C), Woo-mui (H), U-bai (J), O-mae (K).
Processing: 1) Unripe fruit, dry over the gentle charcoal fire for 3–4 days (C, J, K).
          2) Discard kernel (C).
Method of Administration: Oral (decoction: C, H, J, K); Topical (ash: H).
Folk Medicinal Uses:
        1) Fever (J, K).
        2) Cough and sputum (C, H, J, K).
        3) Vomiting, nausea (J, K).
        4) Chronic dysentery and diarrhea (C, H, J, K).
        5) Thirst in consumptive diseases (C, H).

6) Colic and vomiting caused by ascaris (C).

7) Biliary ascariasis (C, H).

8) Stomachache (K).

9) Gastric spasm (K).

10) Cholecystitis (H).

11) Granulomas (H, topical).

12) Nasal polyps (H, topical).

13) Corns (H, topical).

Flower (CP)

Local Drug Name: Mei-hua (C).

Processing: Dry at low temperature (C).

Method of Administration: Oral (decoction: C).

Folk Medicinal Uses:

1) Depression with fidgetness (C).

2) Epigastric pain due to stagnation of qi of the liver and stomach (C).

3) Globus hystericus (C).

4) Scrofula, ulcers (C).

Scientific Research:

Chemistry

1) Organic acids: Citric acid, malic acid, succinic acid, tartaric acid.

2) Glycosides: Amygdalin.

3) Flavonoids: Mumenin (kaempferid-7-glucoside), naringenin, prunin, (+)-catechin,
(−)-epicatechin, leucoanthocyanidin [1].

4) Polysaccharide: P-1 [2].

Pharmacology

1) Inhibitory effect on β-hexosaminidase release from rat basophilic leukemia cells [3].

Literature:

[1] Hasegawa, M.: *J. Org. Chem.* **1959**, 24, 408.

[2] Dogasaki, C. *et al.*: *Biol. Pharm. Bull.* **1995**, 18, 377.

[3] Kataoka, M. *et al.*: *Natural Medicines* **1996**, 50, 344.

[T. Kimura]

262.   *Rubus coreanus* **Miquel** (Rosaceae)

Cha-tian-pao (C), Tokkuri-ichigo (J), Bok-bun-ja-ddal-gi (K)

Fruit

Local Drug Name: Fu-pan-zi (C), Bok-bun-ja (K).

Processing: Dry under the sun (C, K).

Method of Administration: Oral (decoction: C, K).

Folk Medicinal Uses:

1) Impotence (C).

2) Spermatorrhea (C).

3) Enuresis (C).

4) Leukorrhea (C).
5) Weakness (K).
6) Stomachache (K).
7) Ophthalmia (K).
8) Gonorrhoea (K).

Root
Local Drug Name: To-sei-kon (J), Bok-bun-ja-geun (K).
Processing: Dry under the sun (J, K).
Method of Administration: Oral (decoction: J, K).
Folk Medicinal Uses:
1) Hematemesis (J, K).
2) Menstrual disorder (J, K).
3) Bruise (J).

Scientific Research:
Chemistry
1) Triterpenes: 23-hydroxytormentic acid, rosamultin, niga-ichigosides F1, F2 [1], coreanoside F1 [2], 28b-D-glucopyranosyl 2α,3β,19α,23-tetrahydroxyurs-12-en-28-oate [3].
2) Steroids: β-sitosterol glucoside [1].

Literature:
[1] Kim, Y. H. et al.: Arch. Pharmacal Res. **1993**, 16, 109.
[2] Ohtani, K. et al.: Phytochemistry **1990**, 29, 3275.
[3] Kim, E. et al.: Saengyak Hakhoechi **1987**, 18, 188.

[C.K. Sung]

263.   *Abrus cantoniensis* **Hance**   (Leguminosae)

Guang-zhou-xiang-si-zi (C), Gight-gwut-cho (H)

Whole Plant (CP)
Local Drug Name: Ji-gu-cao (C), Gight-gwut-cho (H), Kei-kotsu-so (J).
Processing: Eliminate foreign matter and legumes, and cut into sections (C).
Method of Administration: Oral (decoction: C, H, J).
Folk Medicinal Uses:
1) Jaundice with hypochondriac distress and epigastric distension and pain (C, H, J).
2) Acute and chronic hepatitis (C, H).
3) Mastitis (C).
4) Cirrhosis with ascites (H).
5) Gastric pain (H).
6) Urinary tract infection (H).
7) Dysuria (H).
8) Rheumatic arthralgia (H).
9) Traumatic injury (H).

69

10) Cervical lymphadenitis (H).

11) Snake bites (H).

Scientific Research:

Chemistry

1) Alkaloids: abrine, choline [1], barbeline, barbinidine, barbinine, browniine, 14-dehydro-browniine, delcosine, delelatine, delpheline, 6-dehydrodeltamine, dictyocarpine, 14-acetyl-dictyo-carpine, glaucenine, glaucerine, methyl-lycaconitine, 14-deacetyl-nudicauline [2].

2) Triterpenes: abrisapogenol A, abrisapogenol C, glycyrrhetinic acid [3], cantoniensis-triol, soyasapogenol A [4], sophoradiol, soyasapogenol B [5], glabrolide [2], soyasaponin I [6].

3) Anthraquinones: chrysophanic acid, physcion [7].

4) Saponins: abrisaponins A, Ca, D_1, D_3, F, L, SB, So_1 and So_2, soyasaponins I and A_3, kaikasaponin III, dehydrosoyasaponin I, sophoraflavoside II, kudzusaponin A_3, robinioside E, subproside I, wistariasaponin B_2, subproside V, phaseoside IV, saponin 2 [11–12].

Pharmacology

1) Calcium channel bloker [8].

2) Cholecystokinin receptor binding effect [8].

3) HMG-CO-A reductase inhibition [8].

4) Platelet activating factor binding inhibition [8].

5) Glutamate-pyruvate-transaminase inhibition [9].

6) Antihepatotoxic effect [6].

7) Antiinflammatory effect [10].

Literature:

[1] Yu, D. Q. *et al.*: *Yaoxue Xuebao* **1974**, 9, 424.

[2] Pelletier, S. W. *et al.*: *Phytochemistry* **1989**, 28, 1521.

[3] Sakai, Y. *et al.*: *Chem. Pharm. Bull.* **1990**, 38, 824.

[4] Chiang, T. C. *et al.*: *Planta Med.* **1980**, 39, 225.

[5] Chiang, T. C. *et al.*: *Planta Med.* **1982**, 46, 52.

[6] Takeshita, T. *et al.*: *J. Pharmacobio. Dyn.* **1990**, 13(3), 54.

[7] Wong, S. M. *et al.*: *Planta Med.* **1982**, 46, 191.

[8] Han, G. Q. *et al.*: *Int. J. Chinese Med.* **1991**, 16(1), 1.

[9] Kiso, Y. *et al.*: *Shoyakugaku Zasshi* **1982**, 36, 238.

[10] Remy, R. *et al.*: *C. R. Acad. Sci., Paris, Ser. D* **1967**, 264, 2426.

[11] Miyao, H. *et al.*: *Chem. Pharm. Bull.* **1996**, 44, 1222.

[12] Miyao, H. *et al.*: *Chem. Pharm. Bull.* **1996**, 44, 1228.

[J.X. Guo]

264.   *Canavalia gladiata* **(Jacq.) DC.**   (Leguminosae)

Dao-dou (C), Nata-mame (J), Jak-du-kong (K)

Seed (CP)

Local Drug Name: Dao-dou (C), Hatu-to-zu (J), Do-du (K).

Processing: Eliminate foreign matter, break to pieces before use (C, K).

Method of Administration: Oral (decoction: C, J, K).
Folk Medicinal Uses:
> 1) Hiccup and vomiting of deficiency-cold type (C, K).
>
> 2) Cough and sputum with weakness (J).

Scientific Researches:
Chemistry
1) Amiono acids, proteins and enzymes: urease, canavaline, canavanine [1], concanavalin A (Con A) [2], arginase [3], D-α-amino-n-butyric acid [4], lysine, phenylalanine, glutamic acid [5], endo-β-N-acetylgluco-samminidase [6], histidine, arginine, tryptophan, threonine, cystine, valine, methionine, isoleucine, leucine, tyrosine [7].
2) Fatty acids: palmitic acid, stearic acid, oleic acid, linolenic acid, eicosadienoic acid, linoleic acid [7].
3) Amines: canavalmine (1,13-diamino-5,9-diazatridecane) [8], guaniddinooxypropy-lamine [9], aminopropyl canavalmine, aminobutylcanavalmine [10], N^4-methyl-thermospermine [11].
4) Oliosaccharides: glucose, fructose, sucrose, D-3-O-Me chiro-inositol [12].
Pharmacology
1) Hemagglutinating effect [13].
2) Mitogenic effect [13].
3) Anticancer effect [14].
4) Protease inhibiting effect [15].

Literatures:
[1] Konoshima, M. *et al.*: *Hirokawa Yakuyo Shokubutsu Daijiten* **1963**, 255.
[2] Surolia, A. *et al.*: *Indian J. Biochem. Biophys.* **1973**, 10(3), 145.
[3] Tomiya, T. *et al.*: *Seikagaku* **1973**, 45(4), 194.
[4] Ogawa, T. *et al.*: *Agric. Biol. Chem.* **1976**, 40(8), 1661.
[5] Penteado, Marilene de Vuono Camargo *et al.*: *Rev. Farm. Bioquim. Univ. Sao Paulo* **1983**, 19(2), 126.
[6] Iwase, H. *et al.*: *Jpn. Kokai Tokyo Koho* JP 62 44, 180 [87 44, 180] (C1, C12N9/42), 26 Feb **1987**, Appl. 85/183, 859, 23 Aug **1985**.
[7] Spoladore, D. S. *et al.*: *Bragantia* **1987**, 46(1), 133.
[8] Fujihara, S. *et al.*: *Biochem. Biophys. Res. Commun.* **1982**, 107, 403.
[9] Hamana, K. *et al.*: *Biochem. Biophys. Res. Commun.* **1985**, 129, 46.
[10] Matsuzak, S. *et al.*: *Phytochemistry* **1990**, 29, 1311.
[11] Hamana, K. *et al.*: *Phytochemistry* **1992**, 31, 1410.
[12] Teixeira, M. A. *et al.*: *Quim. Nova* **1990**, 13, 263.
[13] Yadav, M.: *Proc. Malays. Biochem. Soc. Conf.* **1977**, 4, 39.
[14] Lu, L. *et al.*: *Zhejiang Yike Daxue Xuebao* **1983**, 12(1), 7.
[15] Kumari, N. N. et al: *J. Food Sci. Technol.* **1991**, 28(2), 105.

[J.X. Guo]

265.   *Cassia nomame* (Sieb.) Kitag.   (Leguminosae)
[=*C. mimosoides* L. ssp. *nomame* Ohashi]

Dou-cha-jue-ming (C), Sarn-bin-dau (H), Kawara-ketsumei (J), Cha-pul (K)

Whole herb
Local Drug Name: Shan-ye-bian-dou (C), Sarn-bin-dau (H), San-pen-zu (J), San-pyon-du
    (K).
Processing: Dry under the sun (C, J, K).
Method of Administration: Oral (tea or decoction: C, H, J, K).
Folk Medicinal Uses:
  1) Gastrointestinal disorder (J).
  2) Constipation (C, H, J, K).
  3) Chronic nephritis (C).
  4) Nephritic edema (H).
  5) Cough (C, H).
  6) Jaundice (H).
  7) Sputum (H).
  8) Infantile malnutrition (H).
  9) Stomachache (K).
  10) Cardiac disorder (K).
  11) Meteorism (K).

[T. Kimura]

266.   *Cassia obtusifolia* **L.**   (Leguminosae)

Jue-ming (C), Kuet-ming (H), Ebisugusa (J), Gyeol-myeong-cha (K)

Related Plant: *Cassia tora* L.: Xiao-jue-ming (C), Kuet-ming (H), Hosomi-ebisugusa (J).

Seed (CP, JP)
Local Drug Name: Jue-ming-zi (C), Kuet-ming-gee (H), Ketsu-mei-shi (J), Gyeol-
                myeong-ja (K).
Processing: 1) Dry under the sun (C, J, K), break into pieces before use (C).
            2) Stir-fry until slightly scented, break into pieces before use (C).
Method of Administration: Oral (decoction: C, H, J, K).
Folk Medicinal Uses:
  1) Gastrointestinal disorder (J, K).
  2) Constipation (C, H, J, K).
  3) Glaucoma, nyctalopia (H, J).
  4) Photophobia and lacrimation (C).
  5) Conjunctivitis (C, H, K).
  6) Headache, dizziness, blurred vision (C).
  7) Hypertension (H).
  8) Hepatitis (H).
Scientific Research:
Chemistry
  1) Anthraquinones: emodin, obtusifolin, obtusin, chryso-obtusin, aurantio-obtusin and
     their glycosides [1].
  2) Naphthopyrones: rubrofusarin, norrubrofusarin [2].
Pharmacology
  1) Secretion of gastric juice (extract) [3].

2) Antibacterial (emodin, toralactone, isotoralactone) [4].

3) Inhibition of cyclic AMP phospho-diesterase effect (emodin, obtusin) [5].

4) Inhibition of platelet coagulation (gluco-obtusifolin, gluco-chryso-obtusin, gluco-aurantio-obtusin) [6].

5) Hepatotonic (cassiaside, rubrofusarin-6-β-gentiobioside) [7].

6) Weak inhibitory effect on aldose reductase [8].

Literature:

[1] Takido, M.: *Chem. Pharm. Bull.* **1958**, 6, 398; **1960**, 8, 246; Kitanaka, S. *et al.*: *Chem. Pharm. Bull.* **1984**, 32, 860; **1985**, 33, 1274; Wong, S. M., *et al.*: *Phytochemistry* **1988**, 28, 211.

[2] Kimura, Y., *et al.*: *Yakugaku Zasshi* **1966**, 86, 1087; Shibata, S., *et al.*: *Chem. Pharm. Bull.*, **1969**, 17, 454; **1969**, 17, 458; Kitanaka, S. *et al.*: *Chem. Pharm. Bull.*, **1988**, 36, 3980.

[3] Sato, I.: *Kyotofuritsu Ikadaigaku Zasshi* **1936**, 16, 443.

[4] Kitanaka, S., *et al.*: *Yakugaku Zasshi* **1986**, 106, 302.

[5] Nikaido, T., *et al.*: *Chem. Pharm. Bull.*, **1984**, 32, 3075.

[6] Yun-Choi, H. S., *et al.*: *J. Nat. Prod.*, **1990**, 53, 630; **1990**, 53, 638.

[7] Wong, S.-M., *et al.*: *Planta Med.* **1989**, 55, 276.

[8] Matsuda, H. *et al.*: *Biol. Pharm. Bull.* **1995**, 18, 463.

[T. Kimura]

267.   *Gleditsia japonica* **Miq.**   (Leguminosae)
                  [=*G. horrida* (Thunb.) Makino]

Shan-zao-jiao (C), Saikachi (J)

Related plant: *Gleditsia sinensis* Lam.: Zao-jia (C), To-saikachi (J), Jo-gak-ja-na-mu (K).

Fruit

Local Drug Name: Shan-zao-jiao (C), So-kyo (J), Jo-hyeop (K).

Processing: Dry under the sun (C, J, K).

Method of Administration: Oral (decoction: C, J, K).

Folk Medicinal Uses:

        1) Bronchitis (J).

        2) Swelling (J, K).

        3) Skin diseases (J).

        4) Apoplexy (C).

        5) Cough (C).

        6) Epilepsy (C).

        7) Nasal disease (K).

        8) Bone stuck in the throat (K).

Side effect: Hemolytic poisoning.

Scientific Research:

Chemistry

   1) Saponins: gleditsia saponin A, B, C, D, E, F, G, H, I, J, K [1–5].

2) Flavonoids: fisetin, fustin, mollisacacidin (gledistin) [8–9].
Pharmacology
   1) Hemolytic effect, diuretic and Antiinflammatory effects (saponins) [6].
   2) Anti-tumor promotion by TPA in the mouse papilloma [7].

Literature:

[1] Hashimoto, Y. *et al.*: *Phytochemistry* **1975**, 14, 1467.
[2] Okada, Y. *et al.*: Planta Med. **1980**, 40, 185.
[3] Konoshima, T. *et al.*: *Phytochemistry* **1980**, 20, 139.
[4] Konoshima, T. *et al.*: *Chem. Pharm. Bull.* **1980**, 27, 3437.
[5] Konoshima, T. *et al.*: *Chem. Pharm. Bull.* **1987**, 35, 1982.
[6] Yamahara, J. *et al.*: *Yakugaku Zasshi* **1975**, 95, 1179.
[7] Tokuda, H. *et al.*: *Onchology* **1991**, 48, 77.
[8] Mitsuno, M. *et al.*: *Yakugaku Zasshi* **1957**, 77, 557.
[9] Mitsuno, M. *et al.*: *Yakugaku Zasshi* **1957**, 77, 1280.

[T. Kimura]

268.   *Gleditsia sinensis* **Lam.** (Leguminosae)
[=*G. officinalis* Hemsl.]

Zao-jia (C), Joe-garp (H), To-saikachi (J), Jo-gak-ja-na-mu (K)

Related plant: *Gleditsia japonica* Miq.: Shan-zhao-jiao (C), Saikachi (J).

Fruit (CP)
  Local Drug Name: Zhu-ya-zao (C), Joe-garp (H), So-kyo (J), Jo-hyeop (K).
  Processing: Dry under the sun, break into pieces before use (C).
  Method of Administration: Oral (decoction: H, J, K; pill or powder: C); Suppository
                    (powder: J); Topical (powder for blowing into nostrils to
                    induce sneezing, or paste: C).
  Folk Medicinal Uses:
          1) Bronchitis (J).
          2) Swelling (J, K).
          3) Skin diseases (H, J).
          4) Restorative inducing a sneeze (J).
          5) Enterostenosis (J).
          6) Loss of consciousness in stroke and epilepsy (C).
          7) Sore throat, dispnea and cough with sputum difficult to spit out (C).
          8) Constipation (C).
          9) Subcutaneaous pyogenic infections (C).
         10) Nasal disease (K).

Seed
  Local Drug Name: So-kyo-shi (J), Jo-hyeop-ja (K).
  Processing: Dry under the sun.
  Method of Administration: Oral (decoction: J).

Folk Medicinal Uses:
>   1) Constipation (J, K).
>   2) Diarrhea (J).
>   3) Melena (J).
Contraindications: Pregnancy.

Thorn (CP)

Local Drug Name: Zao-jiao-ci (C), Joe-gok-chi (H), So-kaku-shi (J), Jo-gak-ja (K).
Processing: Eliminate tips and dry under the sun (J). Cut into thick slices and dry (C). Steam
>   with vinegar (C).
Method of Administration: Oral (decoction: C, H, J); Topical (powder: J).
Folk Medicinal Uses:
>   1) Swelling (H, J, K).
>   2) Suppuration (H, J, K).
>   3) Carbuncle and boil (C).
>   4) Scabies and leprosy (C).
>   5) Bone stuck in the throat (K).

Scientific Research:
Chemistry
>   1) Saponins: Gymnocladus saponin A, B, C, D, D1, E, F1, F2, G [1-4].
>   2) Monoterpenoid glucocsides: (6S)-2-*trans*-6-α-L-arabinopyranosyloxy-2,6-dimethyl-
>   2,7-octadienoic acid, (6S)-2-*trans*-2,6-dimethyl-6-[3-O-(β-D-glucopyranosyl)-4-
>   O-(2-methylbutyroyl)-α-L-arabinopyrano-syloxy]-2,7-octadienoic acid [5].
Pharmacology
>   1) Anti-tumor-promoter effect (saponins) [6].

Literature:
[1] Konoshima, *et al.*: *Chem. Pharm. Bull.* **1984**, 32, 4833.
[2] Konoshima, *et al.*: *Chem. Pharm. Bull.* **1985**, 33, 4732.
[3] Konoshima, *et al.*: *Chem. Pharm. Bull.* **1987**, 35, 1982.
[4] Konoshima, *et al.*: *Chem. Pharm. Bull.* **1987**, 35, 46.
[5] Konoshima, *et al.*: *Chem. Pharm. Bull.* **1984**, 32, 2617.
[6] Tokuda, H. *et al.*: *Cancer Letters* **1988**, 40, 309.

>   [T. Kimura]

269.   *Psoralea corylifolia* L. (Leguminosae)

>   Bu-gu-chi (C), Boe-gwut-gee (H), Oranda-biyu (J), Pa-go-ji (K)
Fruit (CP)
Local Drug Name: Bu-gu-chi (C), Boe-gwut-gee (H), Ho-kotsu-shi (J), Bo-gol-ji (K).
Processing: Dry under the sun (C, K), stir-fry with salt-water until slightly inflated (C).
Method of Administration: Oral (decoction: C, J, K); Topical (tincture: C).
Folk Medicinal Uses:
>   1) Psoriasis (H, J, K).
>   2) Vitiligo (C, H, K).
>   3) Weakness (J, K).

4) Alopecia (J, K).

5) Impotence, seminal emission (C).

6) Enuresis, frequent urination (C).

7) Aching of the loins and knees with cold sensation (C).

8) Asthma in deficiency syndromes of the kidney (C).

9) Diarrhea occurring before dawn daily (C).

10) Impotence (H).

11) Lumbago (H).

12) Spermatorrhea (H).

Contraindications: Yin-deficiency.

Scientific Research:

Chemistry

1) Isoflavones: neobavaisoflavone [1, 6], corylin [5], corylinal methylether, neobavaisoflavone-7-*O*-Me ether [12], psoralenol [13].

2) Monoterpenes: bakuchiol [2, 8, 18, 20].

3) Coumarins: psoralen [3, 19], isopsoralen [3, 4], angelicin [9, 19].

4) Chromenes: bavachromene [6].

5) Chalcones: 5'-formyl-2',4-dihydroxy-4'-methoxychalcone [7, 10], corylifolinin [14], isoneobavachalcone [15], bavachromanol [17].

6) Coumesterols: corylidin [11, 15], psoralidin 2',3'-oxide diacetate [16].

7) Flavanones: corylifolin [14].

8) Steroids: β-sitosterol D-glucoside [11].

Pharmacology

1) Inotropic effect (psoralen).

2) Antimicrobial effect (bakuchiol) [8].

3) Photosensitizing effect [9].

4) Coronary vasodilation effect (corylifolinin) [14].

5) Antitumor effect (corylifolinin) [14].

6) Enhancing effect on bone calcification [21].

Literature:

[1] Bajwa, B. S. *et al.*: *Curr. Sci.* **1972**, 41, 882.

[2] Mehta, G. *et al.*: *Tetrahedron* **1973**, 29, 1119.

[3] Desai, R. V. *et al.*: *Indian* 84,828, 14 Sep. **1974**, Appl. 84,828, 29 Oct. **1962**; 3 pp.

[4] Franco Indian Pharmaceutical Private Ltd.: Fr. 1,605,327, 02 Aug. **1974**, Indian Appl. 117,079, 03 Aug. **1968**, 7 pp.

[5] Jain, A. *et al.*: *Indian J. Chem.* **1974**, 12, 659.

[6] Bajwa, B. S. *et al.*: *Indian J. Chem.* **1974**, 12, 15.

[7] Gupta, S. R. *et al.*: *Indian J. Chem.* **1975**, 13, 632.

[8] Kaul, R.: *Arzneim.-Forsch.* **1976**, 26, 486.

[9] Innocenti, G. *et al.*: *Planta Med.* **1977**, 31, 151.

[10] Gupta, S. R. *et al.*: *Phytochemistry* **1977**, 16, 1995.

[11] Gupta, G. K. *et al.*: *Phytochemistry* **1977**, 16, 403.

[12] Gupta, G. K. *et al.*: *Phytochemistry* **1978**, 17, 164

[13] Suri, J. L. *et al.*: *Phytochemistry* **1978**, 17, 2046.

[14] Zhu, D.-Y. *et al.*: *Yao Hsueh Hsueh Pao* **1979**, 14, 605.

[15] Gupta, B. K. *et al.*: *Phytochemistry* **1980**, 19, 2034.

[16] Gupta, B. K. *et al.*: *Phytochemistry* **1980**, 19, 2232

[17] Suri, J. L. *et al.*: *Phytochemistry* **1980**, 19, 336.

[18] Banerji, A. *et al.*: *Int. Conf. Chem. Biotechnol. Biol. Act. Nat. Prod.* 1st, **1981**, 3, 349.
[19] Chang H.-J. *et al.*: *Shan-hsi Hsin I Yao* **1981**, 10, 55.
[20] Banerji, A. *et al.*: *Phytochemistry* **1945**, 22.
[21] Miura, H. *et al.*: *Planta Med.* **1996**, 62, 150.

[C.K. Sung]

270.   *Vigna angularis* **(Willd.) Ohwi et Ohashi** (Leguminosae)
    [=*Phaseolus angularis* Wight, *Azukia angularis* (Willd.) Ohwi]

Chi-xiao-dou (C), Hung-dou (H), Azuki (J), Pat (K)

Related Plants: *Phaseolus calcaratus* Roxb. [*Vigna umbellata* (Thunb.) Ohwi et Ohashi]:
    Chi-xiao-dou (C), Tsuru-azuki (J).

Seed (CP)
    Local Drug Name: Chi-xiao-dou (C), Hung-dou (H), Seki-sho-zu (J), Jeok-so-du (K).
    Processing: Dry under the sun (C, K).
    Method of Administration: Oral (decoction: C, H, J, K); Topical (paste: C).
    Folk Medicinal Uses:
                1) Edema (C, H, J, K).
                2) Boil (C, H, K).
                3) Beri-beri (H, K).
                4) Urticaria (J, K).
                5) Nephritis (H, K).
                6) Jaundice with dark urine (C).
                7) Acute rheumatic arthritis (C).
                8) Carbuncles, appendicitis (C).
                9) Coloration on the face (K).
                10) Hemorrhage (K).
                11) Alcoholism (K).
                12) Hypotension (K).
                13) Erysipelas (K).

Scientific Research:
 Chemistry
    1) Polysaccharides: acidic arabinogalactan (F2A, F2B) [1], α-glucan [3].
    2) Odor constituents: alkyl alcohol (hexanol), furfural, benzaldehyde, furfuryl alcohol,
        pyridine, 4-vinylphenol [4].
    3) Triterpenes: acetyloleanolic acid, oleanolic acid, β-amyrin, lupeol, cyclobranol, 24-
        methylenecyclo-artanol [5].
    4) Sterol derivs: stigmasterol, sitosterol, isofucosterol, cholesterol, campesterol,
        avenasterol, 7-stigmastenol, citrostadienol, gramisterol, 4-desmethylsterol,
        acylsterol, 4,4-dimethylsterol, 4-monomethylsterol [5].
    5) Enzymes: nitrite reductase [6], plant starch granule-degrading enzyme [13].
    6) Protease inhibitors: Subtilisin inhibitor [7], Bowman-Birk protease inhibitor [8], adzuki
        proteinase inhibitors I-A, I-A' [9], II [12, 14, 15].

7) Lipids: ceramide, cerebroside [10].

8) Proteins: 7S protein-I (major storage protein) [11].

9) Pipecolic acid [16].

Pharmacology

1) Serine proteinase inhibitory effect [8].

2) α-Amylase inhibitory effect [2].

Literature:

[1] Wei, B. *et al.*: *Oyo Toshitsu Kagaku* **1994**, 41, 157.

[2] Ishimoto, M.: *Baiosaiensu to Indasutori*, **1994**, 52, 645.

[3] Wei, B. *et al.*: *Denpun Kagaku* **1993**, 40, 299.

[4] Tokitomo, Y.: *Mem. Fac. Lib. Arts Educ., Part 2 (Yamanashi Univ.)* **1985**, 36, 117.

[5] Ito, S. *et al.*: *Nippon Nogei Kagaku Kaishi* **1985**, 59, 895.

[6] Ishiyama, Y. *et al.*: *Plant Sci. Lett.* **1985**, 37, 251.

[7] Yoshikawa, M. *et al.*: *Agric. Biol. Chem.* **1985**, 49, 367.

[8] Tanaka, Y. *et al.*: *J. Biochem.(Tokyo)* **1983**, 94, 611.

[9] Kiyohara, T. *et al.*: *J. Biochem.(Tokyo)* **1981**, 90, 721.

[10] Ohnishi, M. *et al.*: *Agric. Biol. Chem.* **1981**, 45, 1283

[11] Sakakibara, M. *et al.*: *Agric. Biol. Chem* **1979**, 43, 1951.

[12] Yoshikawa, M. *et al.*: *Agric. Biol. Chem.* **1978**, 42, 1753.

[13] Hizukuri, S. *et al.*: *Kagoshima Digaku Nogakubu Gakujutsu Hokoku* **1978**, 28, 131.

[14] Yoshikawa, M. *et al.*: *Agric. Biol. Chem.* **1977**, 41, 2235.

[15] Yoshida, C. *et al.*: *J. Biochem.(Tokyo)* **1975**, 78, 935.

[16] Hatanaka, S.: *Sci. Pap. Coll. Gen. Educ., Univ. Tokyo* **1967**, 17, 219.

[C.K. Sung]

271. *Croton crassifolius* **Geisel.** (Euphorbiaceae)

Ji-gu-xiang (C), Gight-gwut-heung (H)

Root

Local Drug Name: Ji-gu-xiang (C), Gight-gwut-heung (H).

Processing: Dry under the sun (C).

Method of Administration: Oral (decoction: C, H).

Folk Medicinal Uses:

       1) Gastric ulcer, duodenal ulcer (C, H).

       2) Gastrointestinal disorder (H).

       3) Abdominal discomfort (H).

       4) Rheumatoid arthritis (C, H).

       5) Lambago (H).

       6) Traumatic injury (H).

       7) Hernial pain (H).

       8) Dysmenorrhea (H).

       9) Soar throat (C).

      10) Snake bite (H).

Contraindications: Pregnancy.

Scientific Research
Chemistry
    1) Amino acid, organic acid [1].

Literature
[1] Yin, W. Q. *et al.*: In: Wu, Z. Y. (Eds.) *Xinhua Bencao Gangyao,* Shanghai Science and Technology Press, Shanghai, **1991**, 2, 211.

[P.P.H. But]

272.   *Croton lachnocarpus* **Bentham**   (Euphorbiaceae)

Mao-guo-ba-dou (C), Siu-yip-sheung-ngan-lung (H)

Root and leaf
Local Drug Name: Xiao-ye-shuang-yan-long (C), Siu-yip-sheung-ngan-lung (H).
Processing: Eliminate foreign matter, wash clean, cut into slices, dry in the sun, or use when fresh (C).
Method of Administration: Oral (decoction or soak in wine: C, H,); Topical (paste of fresh leaf: C, H).
Folk Medicinal Uses:
        1) Rheumatioid arthritis (C, H).
        2) Swelling pain of trauma (C, H).
        3) Snake bites (C, H).
        4) Pruritus, pyodermas (C, H).
        5) Ringworm (H).

Scientific Research
Chemistry
    1) Alkaloid, triterpene [1].

Literature
[1] Yin, W. Q. *et al.*: In: Wu, Z. Y. (Eds.) *Xinhua Bencao Gangyao,* Shanghai Science and Technology Press, Shanghai, **1991**, 2, 211.

[P.P.H. But]

273.   *Croton tiglium* **L.**   (Euphorbiaceae)

Ba-dou (C), Bar-dou (H), Hazu (J), Pa-du-na-mu (K)

Root
Local Drug Name: Ba-dou-gen (C), Bar-dou-gun (H).
Processing: Dry under the sun.
Method of Administration: Topical (decoction: H).

Folk Medicinal Uses:
>   1) Rheumatic arthritis (H).
>   2) Hematoma (H).
>   3) Snake bite (H).

Side effects: Poisonous.

Fruit (CP)

Local Drug Name: Ba-dou (C), Bar-dou (H), Ha-zu (J), Pa-du (K).
Processing: Dry under the sun; remove the pericarp and use the kernel.
Method of Administration: Oral (powder: C, H, J, K); Topical (powder or paste: C, H).
Folk Medicinal Uses:
>   1) Malignant ulcer (C, H).
>   2) Scabies (C).
>   3) Warts (C).
>   4) Chest and abdominal distention (H).
>   5) Diphtheria (H).
>   6) Malaria (H).
>   7) Intestinal obstruction (H).
>   8) Constipation (C, J).
>   9) Abdominal dropsy (K).
>   10) Colic pain (K).

Contraindication: Pregnancy.
Side effects: Poisonous. Intoxication symptoms resemble acute gastroenteritis.

Scientific Research

Chemistry
>   1) Steroid: β-sitosterol [1].
>   2) Phorbol [17], phorbol-12,13-diesters, phorbol-12,13,20-triesters [2, 6, 19–20], crotonic acid, tiglic acid.
>   3) Protein: crotins I-II [7], lectin [9].

Pharmacology
>   1) Cocarcinogenic and cancer-inducing effect [2–5, 15–16].
>   2) Antileukemic effect [6].
>   3) Inhibitory effect on protein synthesis by a reticulocyte lyase [7–8].
>   4) Hemolytic effect [9, 12–13].
>   5) Enhancing effect on Epstein-Barr virus (EBV)-associated early and viral capsid antigens in EBV genome-carrying human lymphoblastoid cell lines [10].
>   6) Hemagglutinating effect [13–14].
>   7) Inhibitory effect on thymidine-incorporation in thymus [20].

Literature

[1] Mukherjee, J.: *Indian J. Appl. Chem.* **1969**, 32, 211.
[2] Sivak, A. *et al.*: *Cancer Res.* **1969**, 29, 624.
[3] Van Duuren, B. L. *et al.*: *Cancer Res.* **1968**, 28, 2349.
[4] Van Duuren, B. L. *et al.*: *J. Med. Chem.* **1963**, 6, 616.
[5] Van Duuren, B. L. *et al.*: *Cancer Res.* **1965**, 25, 1871.
[6] Kupchan, S. M. *et al.*: *Science* **1976**, 191, 571.
[7] Stirpe, F. *et al.*: *Biochem. J.* **1976**, 156, 1.
[8] Sperti, S. *et al.*: *Biochem. J.* **1976**, 156, 7.

[9] Banerjee, K. K. *et al.*: *Arch. Biochem. Biophys.* **1981**, 212, 740.

[10] Ito, Y. *et al.*: *Cancer Lett.* **1981**, 12, 175.

[11] Ito, Y. *et al.*: *Cancer Lett.* **1981**, 13, 29.

[12] Banerjee, K. K. *et al.*: *J. Biosci.* **1983**, 5(suppl. 1), 121.

[13] Banerjee, K. K. *et al.*: *FEBS Letti.* **1983**, 162, 248.

[14] Fuh, L. F. *et al.*: *Sheng Wu K'o Hsueh* **1982**, 19, 45.

[15] Chen, M. H. *et al.*: *Xibao Shengwuxue Zazhi* **1985**, 7, 110.

[16] Arroya, E.R. *et al.*: *J. Med. Chem.* **1965**, 8, 672.

[17] Hecker, E. *et al.*: *Tetradedron Lett.* **1967**, (33), 3165.

[18] Farnsworth, N. R. *et al.*: *Lloydia* **1969**, 32, 1.

[19] Pieters, L.A. *et al.*: *Planta Med.* **1986**, 465.

[20] Hellman, B. *et al.*: *Planta Med.* **1986**, (4), 294.

[P.P.H. But]

274. *Euphorbia humifusa* **Willd.** (Euphorbiaceae)

Di-jin (C), Ddang-bin-dae (K)

Related plant: *E. maculata* L.: Ban-di-jin (C), Keun-ddang-bin-dae (K).

Herb (CP)

Local Drug Name: Di-jin-cao (C), Ji-kin-so (J), Ji-geum-cho (K).

Processing: Eliminate foreign matter, spray with water, soften briefly, cut into sections, and dry in the sun (C, K).

Method of Administration: Oral (decoction: C, K); Topical (decoction: C, K).

Folk Medicinal Uses:

> 1) Dysentery, colitis (C, K).
> 2) Hemoptysis, hematuria, hematochezia (C, K).
> 3) Abnormal uterine bleeding (C, K).
> 4) Boils, carbuncles (C).

Scientific Research:

Chemistry

> 1) Flavonoids: two kaempferide glycosides, quercetin glycoside [1], isoquercitrin-2"-gallate [2], quercetin [3].
> 2) Triterpenes: β-amyrin acetate, lupenyl acetate, 3β-acetoxy-3*O*-norlupan-2*O*-one, α-amyrenonol, gult-5-en-3β-yl acetate, ursa-9(11):12-dien-3β-ol [4].
> 3) Coumarins: scopoletin, umbelliferone, ayapin [5].
> 4) Tannins: gallic acid [3], pyrogallol, pyrocatechol [6], eumaculin A, eusupinin A [7].
> 5) Others: inactive inositol [3], palmitic aicd [5].

Pharmacology

> 1) Antibacterial effect (scopoletin, umbelliferone) [5].
> 2) Hemostatic effect [8].
> 3) Inhibitory effect on xanthine oxidase [2].

Literature:

[1] Li, R. Z. *et al.*: *Beijing Yixueyuan Xuebao* **1983**, 15(1), 72.

[2] Hatano, T. *et al.*: *Planta Med.* **1991**, 57, 83.

[3] Fujii, K. *et al.*: *Yakugaku Zasshi* **1937**, 75, 140.

[4] Matsunaga, S. *et al.*: *Phytochemistry* **1988**, 27, 535.

[5] Kashihara, M. *et al.*: *Shoyakugaku Zasshi* **1986**, 40, 427.

[6] Tsunematsu, T. *et al.*: *Yakugaku Zashi* **1958**, 78, 289.

[7] Agata, I. *et al.*: *Chem. Pharm. Bull.* **1991**, 39, 881.

[8] Shaoxin Chinese Pharmaceutical Factory: *Zhongcaoyao Tongxun* **1970**, (4), 40.

[J.X. Guo]

275. *Euphorbia kansui* T.N. Liou ex T.P. Wang (Euphorbiaceae)

Gan-sui (C), Gum-shui (H), Gam-su (K)

Root (CP)
Local Drug Name: Gan-sui (C), Gum-shui (H), Kan-sui (J), Gam-su (K).
Processing: 1) Eliminate foreign matter, wash clean, and dry in the sun (C, K).
             2) Stir-fry with vinegar to dryness (C).
Method of Administration: Oral (powder or pills: C, H, J, K).
Folk Medicinal Uses:
            1) Anasarca (C, H, J, K).
            2) Hydrothorax or ascites with dyspnea (C).
            3) Constipation (C, H, J, K).
            4) Oliguria (C, J, K).
Contraindications: Pregnancy. Incompatible with licorice (C).

Scientific Research:
Chemistry
    1) Diterpenes: a derivative of 13-oxyingenol, two derivatives of 20-deoxyingenol [1],
        kansuinine A, kansuinine B [2], kansuiphorin A, kansuiphorin B [3], kansuiphorin
        C, kansuiphorin D [4], two derivatives of ingenol [5].
    2) Steroids: γ-euphorbol (euphadienol, α-euphol) [6], kanzuiol (tirucallol) [7], α-
        euphor-bol (euphorbadienol) [8].
    3) Carbohydrates: sucrose, *d*-glucose [9], starch [10].
    4) Organic acids: citric acid, oxalic acid [9], palmitic acid [10].
    5) Vitamine: vitamin B_1 [11].
    6) Tannins [9].
    7) Resin [10].
Pharmacology
    1) Abortion-inducing effect (euphol) [12–14].
    2) Urinative effect [15].
    3) Antitumor effect (kansuiphorin C, kansuiphorin D) [4].
    4) Antileukemic effect (kansuiphorin A, kansuiphorin B) [3].
    5) Immune complex binding to macrophages enhancing effect [5].

Literature:
[1] Daisuke, U. *et al.*: *Tetrahedron Lett.* **1974**, (29), 2527.

[2] Daisuke, U. *et al.*: *Tetrahedron Lett.* **1975**, (21), 1697.

[3] Wu, J. S. *et al.*: *J. Nat. Prod.* **1991**, 54, 823.

[4] Pan, D. J. *et al.*: *Phytochemistry* **1991**, 30, 1018.

[5] Matsumoto, T. *et al.*: *Planta Med.* **1992**, 58, 255.

[6] Murakami, S. *et al.*: *Yakugaku Zasshi* **1955**, 75, 1169.

[7] Murakami, S. *et al.*: *Yakugaku Zasshi* **1955**, 75, 1171.

[8] Inagaki, M. *et al.*: *Yakugaku Zasshi* **1955**, 75, 1571.

[9] Yanagida, S. *et al.*: *Yakugaku Zasshi* **1944**, 64, 9.

[10] Yanagida, S. *et al.*: *Yakugaku Zasshi* **1943**, 63, 408.

[11] Yang, E. F. *et al.*: *Chin. J. Physiol.* **1940**, 15(1), 9.

[12] Chen, X. S. *et al.*: *Yaoxue Tongbao* **1982**, 17(6), 43.

[13] Lu, Y. F. *et al.*: *Jilin Yixue* **1983**, 4(1), 33.

[14] Yu, T. W. *et al.*: *Zhongxiyi Jiehe Zazhi* **1984**, 4, 201.

[15] Kanfuchun Hospital: *Xin Yixue* **1972**, (11), 55.

[J.X. Guo]

276.   *Euphorbia lathyris* L.   (Euphorbiaceae)

Xu-sui-zi (C), Horutoso (J), Sok-su-ja (K)

Seed (CP)

Local Drug Name: Qian-jin-zi (C), Zoku-zui-shi (J), Sok-su-ja (K).

Processing: 1) Eliminate foreign matter, sift and wash clean, dry in the sun. Break to pieces before use (C, K).

2) Rub off the seed coat, wrap in a piece of paper, bake until the fatty oil is expelled entirely, discard paper, cool, or pulverize the seed, wrap in a piece of paper and bake by gentle heat, remove the fatty oil by pressing, then pulverize to fine powder (C).

Method of Administration: Oral (pills or powder: C, J, K); Topical (paste: C, K; decoction: J).

Folk Medicinal Uses:

1) Edema or retained fluid with abdominal distension (C, J, K).

2) Oliguria and constipation (C, J, K).

3) Amenorrhea due to blood stasis (C).

4) External use for ringworm and verruous vegetations (C).

5) Freckle (K).

Contraindications: Contraindicated in pregnancy or debility with loose bowels (C).

Scientific Research:

Chemistry

1) Diterpenes: ingenol 3-hexadecanoate, ingenol 3-tetradeca-2,4,6,8,10-pentanoate [1], ingenol 20-hexadecanoate, lathyrol diacetate benzoate, lathyrol diacetate nicotinate, 7-hydroxy lathyrol, 6,20-epoxy lathyrol [2], 6,20-epoxylathyrol-phenylacetate-diacetate [3], epoxylathyrol [4], ester L_3 [5], ester L_{7a}, ester L_{7b} [6], ester L_8, ester L_9 [7].

2) Coumarins: aesculin, euphorbetin (bisaesculetin) [8], isoeuphorbetin [9], daphnetin [10].

3) Flavonoids: 4',5,7-trihydroxyflavone-3-mono-β-D-glucuronide, 3',4',5,7-tetrahydro-xyflavone-3-mono-β-D-glucuronide [11].

4) Triterpenes: lanosterol, cycloartenol, 24-methylene cycloartenol [12], butyrospermol [13].

5) Steroids: campesterol, stigmasterol, β-sitosterol, Δ^7-stigmasterol [12].

6) Aliphatic acids: palmitic acid, oleic acid, linoleic acid, linolenic acid [14], palmitoleic acid, lauric acid, dodecanoic plus tridecanoic acid, myristic acid, pentadecanoic, heptadecanoic acid, heptadecanoic plus octadecanoic acid, stearic acid, arachidic acid, behenic acid, lignoceric acid [12].

7) Enzyme: sucrose phosphatase [15].

Pharmacology

1) Antitumor activity (ingenol-3-hexadecanoate) [16].

2) Therapy schistosomiasis [17].

3) Toxic reaction [18].

Literatures:

[1] Adolf, W. *et al.*: *Z. Krebsforsch. Klin. Onkol.* **1975**, 84, 325.

[2] Adolf, W. *et al.*: *Experientia* **1971**, 27, 1393.

[3] Adolf, W. *et al.*: *Tetrahedron Lett.* **1970**, (26), 2241.

[4] Toshihiro, S. *et al.*: *Yakugaku Zasshi* **1973**, 93, 1052.

[5] Toshihiro, S. *et al.*: *Yakugaku Zasshi* **1975**, 95, 760.

[6] Adolf, W. *et al.*: *Phytochemistry* **1984**, 23, 1461.

[7] Itokawa, H. *et al.*: *Phytochemstry* **1990**, 29, 2025.

[8] Dutta, P.K. *et al.*: *Tetrahedron Lett.* **1972**, (7), 601.

[9] Dutta, P.K. *et al.*: *Indian J. Chem.* **1973**, 11, 831.

[10] Jaretzky, R. *et al.*: *Pharm. Zentrathalle* **1942**, 83, 517.

[11] Dumkow, K. *et al.*: *Z. Naturforsch.* **1969**, 24B, 358.

[12] Conti, L. *et al.*: *Chim. Ind.* **1983**, 65, 753.

[13] Nishimura, H. *et al.*: *Enerugi Shigen* **1984**, 5, 176.

[14] Toshihibro, S. *et al.*: *Yakugaku Zasshi* **1975**, 95, 764.

[15] Hawker, J.S. *et al.*: *Phytochemistry* **1984**, 23, 245.

[16] Itokawa, H. *et al.*: *Planta Med.* **1989**, 55, 271.

[17] Cheng, S.Z. *et al.*: *Xin Zhongyiyao* **1956**, 7(7), 23.

[18] Xiao, R. Q.: *Zhonghua Erke Zazhi* **1982**, 20, 119.

[J.X. Guo]

277. *Jatropha curcas* **L.** (Euphorbiaceae)

Ma-feng-shu (C), Mar-fung-shue (H), Ban-u-kon (J)

Bark and leaf

Local Drug Name: Ma-feng-shu (C), Mar-fung-shue (H), San-na (J).

Processing: Use when fresh.

Method of Administration: Topical (paste: C, H).

Folk Medicinal Uses:

       1) Traumatic injury (C, H).

       2) Wound bleeding (C, H).

3) Sprains (C, H).
4) Pruritus (C, H).
5) Eczema (H).
6) Tinea pedis (H).
7) Kerion (H).
8) Leprosy (C, H).
9) Trichomonal vaginitis (H).
10) Dyspepsia (J).
11) Toothache (J).

Side effects: Poisonous.

Scientific Research

Chemistry
1) Glycoside: [1]
2) Sterol: stigmasterol, β-sitosterol, β-sitosterol-β-D-glucoside, 7-keto-β-sitosterol, campesterol, 1-triacontanol stigmast-5-en-3β,7α-diol, stigmast-5-en-3β,7β-diol, [1–2].
3) Flavonoids: vitexin, isovitexin, apigenin [3].
4) Fatty acid: palmitic acid, oleic acid, linoleic acid [4].
5) Protein and peptide: [5], curcin [6], curcacycline A [9].

Pharmacology
1) Inhibitory effect on protein formation by a reticulocyte lyase [5].
2) Cytoprotective effect against HIV in cultured human lymphoblastoid CEM-SS cells [7].
3) Inhibitory effect on P-388 lymphocytic leukemia [2].
4) Inhibitory effect on human complement [9].
5) Inhibitory effect on proliferation of human T-cells [9].

Literature

[1] Khafagy, S. M. *et al.*: *Planta Med.* **1977**, 31, 274.
[2] Hufford, C. D. *et al.*: *Lloydia* **1978**, 41, 161.
[3] Sankara Subramanian, S *et al.*: *Phytochemistry* **1971**, 10, 2548.
[4] Siddiqui, I.A. *et al.*: *J. Oil Technol. Ass. India* **1973**, 5, 8.
[5] Stirpe, F. *et al.*: *Biochem. J.* **1976**, 156, 1.
[6] Yin, W. Q. *et al.*: In: Wu, Z.Y. (Eds.) *Xinhua Bencao Gangyao,* Shanghai Science and Technology Press, Shanghai, **1991**, 2, 225.
[7] Muanza, D. N. *et al.*: *Int. J. Pharmacognosy* **1995**, 33, 98.
[8] Hirota, M. *et al.*: *Cancer Res.* **1988**, 48, 5800.
[9] van den Berg, A. J. *et al.*: *FEBS Lett.* **1995**, 358, 215.

[P.P.H. But]

278.　　*Knoxia valerianoides* **Thorel et Pitard.**　(Euphorbiaceae)

Hong-da-ji (C), Die-gik (H), Ko-ga-dai-geki (J)

Root (CP)

Local Drug Name: Hong-da-ji (C), Die-gik (H), Ko-ga-dai-geki (J).

Processing: Eliminate foreign matter, cut into sections, dry under the sun (C).

Method of Administration: Oral (decoction: C, H, J).
Folk Medicinal Uses:
> 1) Edema (C, H, J).
> 2) Scrofula (C, H, J).
> 3) Carbuncles (C, H).
> 4) Hydrothorax and ascites (C, H).
> 5) Constipation (C).
> 6) Oliguria (C).
> 7) Sores (C).

Scientific Research
Chemistry
> 1) Anthraquinone: knoxiadin, 3-hydroxymorindone, damnacanthal, rubiadin, syringic acid [1], 2-ethoxymethylknoxiavaledin, 2-formylknoxiavaledin, 2-hydroxymethylknoxia-valedin [2].

Literature
[1] Wang, X. F. *et al.*: *Yaoxue Xuebao* **1985**, 20, 615.
[2] Zhou, Z. *et al.*: *Phytochemistry* **1994**, 36, 765.

[P.P.H. But]

279.　　*Mallotus japonicus* **Muell.-Arg.**　　(Euphorbiaceae)

Akamegashiwa (J), Ye-deok-na-mu (K)

Bark
Local Drug Name: Aka-me-gashiwa (J), Ya-o-deung (K).
Processing: Dry under the sun (J, K).
Method of Administration: Oral (decoction: J, K); Topical (bath: J, K).
Folk Medicinal Uses:
> 1) Gastrointestinal disorder (J).
> 2) Gastric ulcer (J, K).
> 3) Duodenal ulcer (J, K).
> 4) Gallstone (J).
> 5) Prickly heat (J, K).
> 6) Neuralgia (K).

Scientific Research:
Chemistry
> 1) Phloroglucins: isomallotolerin, isomallotochromanol , butyrylmallotochromanol, isobutyrylmallotochromanol, mallotojaponol [1].
> 2) Tannins: five hydrolyzable tannins [2–3], malloprenol, malloprenol linolenate [5], ellagic acid [6].
> 3) Glycosides: 3-O-α-L-rhamnopyranoside and 3-O-β-D-glucopyranosyl-(1→4)-α-L-rhamnopyranoside of corotoxigenin, mallogenin, coroglaucigenin, panogenin [4].
> 4) Flavonoids: quercetin and rutin [6].

86

5) Anthocyanins [7].

Pharmacology

    1) Cytotoxic (butyrylmallotochromanol, isobutyrylmallotochromanol, mallotojaponol)
       [1].

Literature:

[1] Arisawa, M. *et al.*: *Chem. Pharm. Bull.*, **1990**, 38, 698; *J. Nat. Prod.*, **1990**, 53, 638.

[2] Nonaka, G. *et al.*: *Chem. Pharm. Bull.*, **1989**, 37, 2063.

[3] Saijo, R. *et al.*: *Phytochemistry* **1989**, 28, 2443; **1990**, 29, 267; 279.

[4] Okabe, H. *et al.*: *Chem. Pharm. Bull.*, **1976**, 24, 108.

[5] Abe, J. *et al.*: *Japan Pat.* 72 29,965.

[6] Yanagida, K. *et al.*: *Osaka Kogyo-Daigaku Kiyo (Riko)* **1969**, 14, 47.

[7] Yoshitama, K. *et al.*: *Shokubutsugaku Zasshi* **1972**, 85, 303.

[T. Kimura]

280.   *Ricinus communis* **L.**   (Euphorbiaceae)

Bi-ma (C), Bay-mar (H), Togoma (J), A-ju-gga-ri (K)

Seed (CP)

  Local Drug Name: Bi-ma-zi (C), Bay-mar-gee (H), Hi-ma-shi (J), Pi-ma-ja (K).

  Processing: Dry under the sun (C, J, K).

  Method of Administration: Topical (paste or ointment: C, H, J); Oral (pill: C, J, K).

  Folk Medicinal Uses:

        1) Abscess, scrofula (C, J).

        2) Carbuncle (C).

        3) Boil and skin infection (C).

        4) Prolapse of rectum or uterus (H).

        5) Sore throat (C).

        6) Dystocia, retained placenta (H; apply to Yungchuan point).

        7) Facial nerve palsy (H).

        8) Lymphadenitis (K).

        9) Toothache (K).

      10) Ear-ache (K).

      11) Tympanitis (K).

      12) Constipation (C).

  Side effects: Nausea, vomiting, abdominal pain, diarrhea, shock, respiratory arrest, death
        (C).

Seed oil (CP, JP)

  Local Drug Name: Bi-ma-you (C), Himashi-yu (J), Pi-ma-ja-yu (K).

  Processing: Compression of the seed, and decolorization and deodorization (C, J).

  Method of Administration: Oral (C, J, K).

  Folk Medicinal Uses:

        1) Constipation (J, K).

        2) Food intoxication (J, K).

3) Acute gastritis (K).

4) Abdominal pain (K).

Contraindications: Constipation, appendictis, peritonitis, pregnancy, habitual abortion. Incompatible with fat-soluble anthelmintics (C, J).

Side effects: Diarrhea, abortion, intestinal injury [1].

Scientific Research:

Chemistry

1) Fatty oil: ricinolein (glyceride of ricinoleic acid).

2) Flavonoids: 2"-O-*p*-coumaroylprunin [7].

3) Proteins: ricin.

Pharmacology

1) Purgative (ricinoleic acid) [2].

2) Action potential change in cat colon (oil, sodium ricinoleate) [3].

3) Lowering annular smooth muscle effect (oil) [4].

4) Depressing bowel contraction (sodium ricinoleate) [5].

5) Inhibition of bowel absorption of water and inorganic ions (sodium ricinoleate) [6].

6) Antimicrobial (ricinoleic acid) [7].

Literature:

[1] Gaginella, T. S. *et al.*: *J. Pharmacol. Exptl. Therap.* **1977**, 201, 259.

[2] Iwao, I. *et al.*: *Jap. J. Pharmacol.*, **1962**, 12, 137; Watson, W. C. *et al.*: *Biochem. Pharmacol.*, **1962**, 11, 229; Watson, W. C. et al: *J. Pharm. Pharmacol.*, **1963**, 15, 183.

[3] Christensen, J. *et al.*: *Gastroenterology,* **1972**, 62, 1159; **1972**, 63, 1011.

[4] Stewart, J. J. *et al.*: *J. Pharmacol. Exptl. Therap.*, **1975**, 192, 458.

[5] Stewart, J. J. *et al.*: *J. Pharmacol. Exptl. Therap.*, **1975**, 195, 347.

[6] Ammon, H. V. *et al.*: *J. Clin. Invest.*, **1974**, 53, 374; Ammon, H. V. *et al.*: *Gastroenterology* **1973**, 65, 744; Gadacz, T. R. *et al.*: *Am. J. Dig. Dis.* **1976**, 21, 859; Ammon, H. V. *et al.*: *J. Clin. Invest.*, **1974**, 53, 205; Gaginella, T. S. *et al.*: *J. Pharmacol. Exptl. Therap.*, **1975**, 195, 355; Bright-Asare, P. *et al.*: *Gastroenterology*, **1973**, 64, 81.

[7] Novak, A. F. *et al.*: *J. Am. Oil Chemisits Soc.*, **1961**, 38, 321; Utkina, N. K., *et al.*: *Chem. Nat. Compd.* **1993**, 29, 291.

[T. Kimura]

281.   *Acronychia pedunculata* **(L.) Miq.**   (Rutaceae)
[=*A. laurifolia* Bl.]

Jiang-zhen-xiang (C), Gong-chun-heung (H)

Root

Local Drug Name: Jiang-zhen-xiang (C), Gong-chun-heung (H)

Processing: Eliminate foreign matter, wash clean, dry under the sun or in shade.

Method of Administration: Oral (decoction: C, H)

Folk Medicinal Uses:

1) Rheumatalgia (C, H).

2) Traumatic injury (C, H).

3) Gastric pain (C, H).
4) Hernial pain (C, H).
5) Cough, wheezing (C).
6) Bronchitis (C).
7) Influenza (C).

Fruit
Local Drug Name: Shan-you-gan-guo (C), Gong-chun-heung-gwor (H).
Processing: Scald with boiling water, then dry.
Method of Administration: Oral (decoction, C, H).
Folk Medicinal Uses:
>   1) Anorexia (C, H).
>   2) Indigestion (C, H).

Leaf
Local Drug Name: Shan-you-gan-ye (C), Gong-chun-heung-yip (H).
Method of Administration: Oral (decoction: C, H); Topical (fresh: C, H).
Folk Medicinal Uses:
>   1) Common cold and cough (C, H).
>   2) Traumatic injury (C, H).

Scientific Research:
Chemistry
1) Monoterpenes: α-pinene, limonene [1].
2) Alkaloids: evolitrine, kokusaginine [2], skimmianine, dictamine [3].
3) Triterpenoids: β-amyrin [3], bauerenol [4–5].
4) Arylketones: acrovestone [3–6], demethylacrovestone [7], acronylin, 6-demethyl-acronylin [8–9], 1-[2',4'-dihydroxy-3',5'-di-(3"-methylbut-2"-enyl)-6'-methoxy]-phenylethanone [3].
5) Coumarin: bergapten [3].
6) Potassium oxalate [2].
Pharmacology
1) Cytotoxic effect against A-549, P-388 and L-1210 cells (acrovestone) [6].
2) Estrogenic effect.

Literature
[1] Arthur, H. R. et al.: J. Chem. Soc. 1961, 3551.
[2] De Silva, L. B. et al.: Phytochemistry 1979, 18, 1255.
[3] Kumar, V. et al.: Phytochemistry 1989, 28, 1278.
[4] Arthur, H. R. et al.: Phytochemistry 1966, 5, 379.
[5] Zhou F. X. et al.: Zhongguo Zhongyao Zazhi 1989, 14(2), 94.
[6] Wu, T. S. et al.: J. Nat. Prod. 1989, 52, 1284.
[7] De Silva, L. B. et al.: Phytochemistry 1991, 30, 1709.
[8] Biswas, G. K. et al.: Chem. Ind. 1970, 654.
[9] Banerji, J. et al.: Indian J. Chem. 1974, 11, 693.

[P.P.H. But]

282.   *Atalantia buxifolia* **(Poir.) Oliv.**   (Rutaceae)
[*=Severinia buxifolia* (Poir.) Tenore]

Jiu-bing-le (C), Dung-fung-gwut (H)

Root and leaf
Local Drug Name: Dong-feng-ju (C), Dung-fung-gwut (H).
Method of Administration: Oral (decoction: C, H).
Folk Medicinal Uses:
                    1) Common cold and cough (C, H).
                    2) Bronchitis (C, H).
                    3) Malarial disease (C, H).
                    4) Epigastric pain, abdominal pain (C, H).
                    5) Rheumatic arthritis (C, H).
                    6) Lumbago (C, H).
                    7) Traumatic injury (C, H).
                    8) Snake bite (C).
                    9) Headache (C).
                    10) Gastric pain (C).

Scientific Research
  Chemistry
    1) Alkaloid: atalafoline [1], atalafoline B [2], N-methylatalaphylline, N-methylseverifoline,
       atalaphylline, severifoline, 5-hydroxy-N-methylseverifoline [3], severibuxine,
       atalantin [4].
    2) Coumarin: 6-methyl-7-geranyloxycoumarin [4].
    3) Triterpenoid: severinolide, cycloseverinolide [4]
  Pharmacology
    1) Antiasthmatic effect [1].
    2) Antifeedant effect [4].
    3) Antimicrobial effect [4].
    4) Cytotoxic effect [4].

Literature
[1] Qin, D. K.: *Yaoxue Xuebao* **1986**, 21, 683.
[2] Gu, G. M.: *Yaoxue Xuebao* **1987**, 22, 886.
[3] Wu, T. S. *et al.*: *Phytochemistry* **1982**, 21, 1771.
[4] Wu, T.S. *et al.*: *Progress in Drug Development from Medicinal Plants*. Proceedings of
    UNESCO Regional Symposium on Drug Development from Medicinal Plants. Oct.
    25-27, 1996, Hangzhou, China, **1996**, 238.

[P.P.H. But]

283.   *Citrus maxima* **(L. Burman) Merrill**   (Rutaceae)
[*=C. grandis* (L.) Osbeck]

You (C), Yau (H), Buntan (J), Wang-gyul-na-mu (K)

Flower
  Local Drug Name: You-hua (C), Yau-far (H),Yu-hwa (K).
  Method of Administration: Oral (decoction: C, H).
  Folk Medicinal Uses:
                    1) Sputum (C).
                    2) Epigastric pain (C).

Fruit
  Local Drug Name: You (C), Yau (H), Yu (K).
  Method of Administration: Oral (decoction: C, K).
  Folk Medicinal Uses:
                    1) Anorexia (K).
                    2) Drunkenness (C, K).
                    3) Productive cough (C).
                    4) Indigestion (C).

Seed
  Local Drug Name: You-he (C), Yau-wut (H), Yu-haek (K).
  Method of Administration: Oral or topical (decoction or tincture: J).
  Folk Medicinal Uses:
                    1) Hernia (C).

Root
  Local Drug Name: You-gen (C), Yu-geun (K).
  Method of Administration: Topical (decoction: C).
  Folk Medicinal Uses:
                    1) Epigastric pain (C).
                    2) Hernial pain (C).
                    3) Cough (C).

Pericarp
  Local Drug Name: You-pi (C), Yau-pay (H), Yu-pi (K).
  Method of Administration: Oral (decoction: C, H, K).
  Folk Medicinal Uses:
                    1) Asthma (C, H, K).
                    2) Gastric pain (C, H, K).
                    3) Abdominal distention (C, H, K).
                    4) Indigestion (C, H, K).
                    5) Productive cough (C, H).
                    6) Hernial pain (H).

Leaf
  Local Drug Name: You-ye (H), Yau-yip (H), Yu-yeop (K).
  Method of Administration: Oral (decoction: C, H, K); Topical (H).
  Folk Medicinal Uses:
                    1) Mastitis (H).
                    2) Tonsillitis (H).
                    3) Abdominal distention (C, H, K).
                    4) Indigestion (C, H, K).
                    5) Hernia (C).

91

6) Epigastirc distention (C, H).
Contraindication: Pregnancy.

Scientific Research
Chemistry
1) Obacunone, obaculactone, limonin, deacetylnomilin, naringin, poncirin, neohesperidon, naringenin-4'-glucoside-7-neohesperiodside, methylanthranilate, geraniol, linalool, citral [1–2].
Pharmacology
1) Antiinflammatory effect.

Literature

[1] Albach, R.F. *et al.*: *Phytochemistry* **1969**, 8, 127.
[2] Huang, M.S. *et al.*: *Zhongcoayao* **1984**, 15, 203.

[P.P.H. But]

284. *Citrus maxima* (L. Burman) Merrill cv. Tomentosa (Rutaceae)
[=*C. grandis* (L.) Osbeck cv. Tomentosa]

Hua-zhou-you (C), Far-gwut-hung (H)

Pericarp (CP)
Local Drug Name: Hua-ju-hong (C), Far-gwut-hung (H).
Processing: Remove from fruit and dry under the sun or by heat, then slightly wetted with water and flattened (C).
Method of Administration: Oral (decoction: C, H).
Folk Medicinal Uses:
1) Indigestion (C, H).
2) Sputum (C, H).
3) Cough (C, H).
4) Hiccup (C, H).
5) Drunkenness (C).

Scientific Research
Chemistry
1) Naringen, rhoifolin [1–2].
Pharmacology
1) Antiinflammatory effect (naringin) [3].

Literature

[1] Ge, F. H. *et al.*: *Zhongyaocai* **1989**, 12(9), 35.
[2] Huang, M. S. *et al.*: *Zhongcaoyao* **1984**, 15, 203.
[3] Nothover, B. J. *et al.*: *Brit. J. Pharmacol.* **1962**, 18, 340.

[P.P.H. But]

285.   *Citrus medica* L., *C. wilsonii* **Tanaka**   (Rutaceae)

Ju-yuan, Xiang-yuan (C), Heung-yuan (H), Maru-bushukan (J)

Fruit (CP)
Local Drug Name: Xiang-yuan (C), Heung-yuan (H), Bu-shu-kan (J).
Processing: Break into pieces, dry in shade (C).
Method of Administration: Oral or topical (decoction: C, H, J).
Folk Medicinal Uses:
>   1) Gastrointestinal cancer (C, H).
>   2) Qi-stagnation in liver (C).
>   3) Epigastric pain and distention (C, H).
>   4) Hematemesis, hemoptysis, uterine bleeding (C, H, J).
>   5) Vomiting and belching (C, H).
>   6) Cough (C, H, J).
>   7) Asthma (C, J).
>   8) Soar throat (J).
>   9) Sputum (C).

Scientific Research
 Chemistry
>   1) Essential oil: *d*-limonene, geranial, neral, nerol, β-ocimen, (+)-carvone [1].
>   2) Lemittin, β-sitosterol, daucosterol, palmitic acid, succinic acid, citrusin [2].
 Pharmacology
>   1) Antifungal effect [3]

Literature
 [1] Wen, M. Z. *et al.*: *Zhiwu Xuebao* **1986**, 28, 511.
 [2] He, H.Y. *et al.*: *Zhongcaoyao* **1986**, 17, 530.
 [3] Dubey, N. K. *et al.*: *Tests Agrochem. Cultiv.* **1982**, 3, 58.

                                                                [P.P.H. But]

286.   *Citrus medica* **L. var.** *sarcodactylis* **(Noot.) Swingle**   (Rutaceae)

Fo-shou (C), Fut-sau (H)

Fruit (CP)
Local Drug Name: Fo-shou (C), Fut-sau (H).
Processing: Break into pieces, dry in shade.
Method of Administration: Oral (decoction: C, H,).
Folk Medicinal Uses:
>   1) Anorexia (C, H).
>   2) Epigastric pain and distention (C, H).
>   3) Vomiting and belching (C, H).
>   4) Cough (C, H, J).
>   5) Sputum (C, H, J).

Scientific Research
Chemistry
  1) Lemittin: *cis*-head-to-head-3,3',4,4'-lemittin dimer, *cis*-head-to-tail-3,3',4,4'-lemittin dimer [1].
  2) Flavone: 3,5,8-trihydroxy-4',7-dimethoxyflavone [2], 3,5,6-trihydroxy-4',7-dimethoxyfla-vone, 3,5,6-trihydroxy-3'4',7-trimethoxyflavone [2–3].
  3) Coumarin: 6,7-dimethoxycoumarin [2].
  4) Sterol: β-sitosterol, daucosterol [2].
  5) Acid: *p*-hydroxycinnamic acid, succinic acid, palmitic acid [2].
  6) Citropten, nomilin, limonin
Pharmacology
  1) Antagonistic effect on β-adrenergic receptor [4].
  2) Protectice effect against alcohol toxicity [4].

Literature
[1] He, H. Y. *et al.*: *Youji huaxue* **1987**, (3), 193.
[2] He, H. Y. *et al.*: *Zhongyao Tongbao* **1988**, 13, 352.
[3] He, H. Y. *et al.*: *Yaoxue Xuebao* **1985**, 20, 433.
[4] Wang, Y. M.. *et al.*: *Zhonacaoyao* **1982**, 13, 552..

[P.P.H. But]

287.   *Clausena lansium* **(Lour.) Skeels** (Rutaceae)
[=*C. wampi* Blanco]

Huang-pi (C), Wong-pay (H)

Leaf
Local Drug Name: Huang-pi-ye (C), Wong-pay-yip (H).
Processing: Eliminate foreign matter, dry or used fresh.
Method of Administration: Oral or topical (decoction: C, H).
Folk Medicinal Uses:
        1) Prevention of influenza, common cold and fever (H).
        2) Epidemic meningoencephalitis (C, H).
        3) Malaria (C, H).

Fruit
Local Drug Name: Huang-pi (C), Wong-pay (H).
Processing: Eliminate foreign matter, dry or used fresh (C).
Method of Administration: Oral or topical (decoction: C, H).
Folk Medicinal Uses:
        1) Indigestion (C, H).
        2) Productive cough (C, H).

Root
Local Drug Name: Huang-pi-gen (C), Wong-pay-gun (H).

Processing: Eliminate foreign matter, dry or used fresh (C).
Method of Administration: Oral or topical (decoction: C, H).
Folk Medicinal Uses:
　　　　　　　　1) Stomach ache, epigastric pain (C, H).
　　　　　　　　2) Hernial pain (C, H).
　　　　　　　　3) Dysmenorrhea (C, H).

Scientific Research
Chemistry
　　1) Coumarin: wampetin (dehydroindicolactone), imperatorin, 8-geranoxypsoralen,[2–4], indicolactone, anisolactone, 2",3"-epoxyanisolactone [5].
　　2) Ketone: (+)-oplopanone [4].
　　3) Carbzole alkaloid: 3-formyl-6-methoxycarbazole, methyl-6-methoxycarbazole-3-carboxylate, 3-formyl-1,6-dimethoxycarbazole, 3-formyl cabazole, methylcarbazole-3-carboxylate, murrayanine, indizoline, glycozoline [4], lansine [6].
　　4) Amide: lansamide-I [1, 6], lansiumamides A-C [6], clausenamide, neoclausenamide, cycloclausenamide [7, 10].
　　5) ∈-valerolactam [7], heptaphylline, β-sitosterol [1, 6].
Pharmacology
　　1) Hepatoprotective effect [7–9].
　　2) Smooth muscle relaxant effect [11].

Literature
[1] Prakash, D. et al.: Indian J. Chem. Sect. B. **1980**, 19B, 1075..
[2] Kong, Y.C. et al.: Fitoterapia **1983**, 54, 47.
[3] Khan, N. et al.: Phytochemistry **1983**, 22, 2624.
[4] Li, W. S. et al.: J. Chin. Chem. Soc. (Taipei) **1990**, 37, 571.
[5] Ding, Y. et al.: Zhongcaoyao **1990**, 21, 535.
[6] Lin, J.H.: Phytochemistry **1989**, 28, 621 .
[7] Yang, M.H. et al.: Yaoxue Xuebao **1987**, 22, 33.
[8] Yang, M.H. et al.: Ger. Offen. DE 3,700,703 **1987**, 6pp.
[9] Yang, M.H. et al.: Ger. Offen. DE 3,700,704 **1987**, 11pp.
[10] Yang, M.H. et al.: Phytochemistry **1988**, 27, 445.
[11] Kong, Y.C. et al.: Gen. Pharmac. **1986**, 17, 593.

[P.P.H. But]

288.　　*Dictamnus dasycarpus* **Turcz.** [=*D. albus* L.]　(Rutaceae)
　　　　　　　　D. angustifolius **G. Don.**

Bai-xian (C), Bark-sin (H), Hakusen (J), Baek-seon (K)

Root bark (CP)
Local Drug Name: Bai-xian-pi (C), Bark-sin-pay (H), Haku-sen-pi (J), Baek-seon-pi (K).
Processing: Eliminate foreign matter, cut into slices and dry (C).
Method of Administration: Oral (decoction: C, H, J, K); Topical (infusion or powder: C).

Folk Medicinal Uses:
    1) Eczema (C, H, J, K).
    2) Skin inflammation with yellowish watery discharge (C).
    3) Rubella (C).
    4) Tinea (C).
    5) Scabies (C, J).
    6) Rheumatalgia (C, J).
    7) Jaundice (C, H, J, K).
    8) Contusion (K).

Scientific Research
Chemistry
    1) Alkaloids: dictamine, skimmianine, γ-fagarine [2], *O*-ethylnordictamine, *O*-ethylnor-γ-fagarine, *O*-ethylnorskimmianine, isomaculosidine [4].
    2) Limonoids: limonin, fraxinellone, obacunone, limonin diosphenol, dictamdiol [7].
    3) Coumarins: psoralen, xanthotoxin, scopoletin, quercetin, isoquercetin [3], obacunonic acid [1].
    4) Sesquiterpene: dictamnol [6].
    5) Steroid: pregnenolone [6].
Pharmacology
    1) Mutagenic effect (dictamnine, γ-fagarine) [2].
    2) Vasorelaxant effect [5].

Literature
[1] Nikonov, G. K.: *Med. Prom. SSSR.* **1964**, 18, 15.
[2] Mizuta, M. *et al.*: *Mutat. Res.* **1985**, 144, 221..
[3] Komissarenko, N. F. *et al.*: *Khim. Prir. Soedin.* **1983**, (4), 529.
[4] Lin, T. P. *et al.*: *Hua Hsueh* **1986**, 44(3), 96.
[5] Yu, S. M. *et al.*: *Naunyn-Schmiedeberg's Arch. Pharmacol.* **1992**, 345, 349.
[6] Takeuchi, N. *et al.*: *Chem. Pharm. Bull.* **1993**, 41, 923.
[7] Hu, C. Q. *et al.*: *Zhiwu Xuebao* **1989**, 31, 453.

[P.P.H. But]

289.   *Fortunella margarita* **(Lour.) Swingle** (Rutaceae)

Jin-ju (C), Gum-gwut (H), Nagakinkan (J), Geum-gam (K)
Leaf
Local Drug Name: Jin-ju-ye (C), Geum-gyul-yeop (K).
Processing: Fresh or dry in shade.
Method of Administration: Oral (decoction: C).
Folk Medicinal Uses:
    1) Hiccup (C).
    2) Scrofula (C).

Root
Local Drug Name: Jin-Ju-gen (C), Geum-gyul-geun (K).
Processing: Dry in the sun.

Method of Administration: Oral (decoction: C, K).
Folk Medicinal Uses:
>   1) Stomachache (C, K).
>   2) Hernia (C).
>   3) Scrofula (C).
>   4) Prolapse of uterus (C).
>   5) Edema (C).

Fruit
Local Drug Name: Jin-Ju (C), Gum-gwut (H), Geum-gyul (K).
Processing: Use when fresh or after soaking in brine (C).
Method of Administration: Oral (infusion: C, H, K).
Folk Medicinal Uses:
>   1) Indigestion (C, H).
>   2) Soar throat (C, H).
>   3) Sputum (C, H).

Scientific Research
Chemistry
>   1) Vitamin C [1].
>   2) Glycoside: fortunellin [2].

Literature
[1] Hayashi, U.: *Rept. Osaka Municipal Research Inst. Domestic Sci.* **1940**, 17(1), 143.
[2] Matsuno, T.: *Yakugaku Zasshi* **1958**, 78, 1311.

[P.P.H. But]

290.   *Glycosmis citrifolia* **(Willd.) Lindl.** (Rutaceae)

Shan-shao-ju (C), Sarn-siu-gwut (H), Hana-shinbogi (J)

Root and leaf
Local Drug Name: Shan-shao-ju (C), Sarn-siu-gwut (H).
Processing: Dry in the sun.
Method of Administration: Oral or topical (decoction: C, H).
Folk Medicinal Uses:
>   1) Common cold (C, H).
>   2) Cough (C, H).
>   3) Indigestion (C, H).
>   4) Traumatic injury; fractures (C, H).
>   5) Gastric and duodenal ulcer (C, H).
>   6) Enteritis, dysentery (C, H).
>   7) Stomachache (H).
>   8) Hernia (C, H).
>   9) Frostbites (H).
>   10) Anorexia (C).

Contraindication: Pregnancy.

Scientific Research

Chemistry

  1) Alkaloid, flavonoid, amino acid [1].

Pharmacology

  1) Therapeutic effect on twisted ankle [2].

Literature

[1] Anonymous: *Nongcun Zhongcaoyao Zhiji Jizhu* **1971**, 234.

[2] Anonymous: *Xinyixue* **1975**, 6, 462.

[P.P.H. But]

291. *Melicope pteleifolia* (Champ. ex Benth.) T. Hartley (Rutaceae)
[=*Euodia lepta* (Spreng.) Merr.]

San-ya-ku (C), Sarm-ngar-foo (H)

Leaf and root

Local Drug Name: San-ya-ku (C), Sarm-ngar-foo (H).

Processing: Dry in shade.

Method of Administration: Oral or topical (decoction: C, H).

Folk Medicinal Uses:

        1) Pharyngitis, tonsillitis (C, H).

        2) Heat stroke, common cold, fever (C, H).

        3) Epidemic influenza, encephalitis (C, H).

        4) Pneumonitis, empyema (C, H).

        5) Hepatitis, jaundice (C, H).

        6) Rheumatalgia, sciatica, lumbago (C, H).

        7) Traumatic injury (C, H).

        8) Snake bites (C, H).

        9) Abscesses, wound infection, dermatitis (C, H).

        10) Hemorrhoids (H).

        11) Stomachache (C).

        12) Eczema (C, H).

Scientific Research

Chemistry

  1) Alkaloid: (–)-edulinine, (–)-ribalinine, (+)-isoplatydesmine [1].

  2) Chromenes: isoevodionol, methylevodinol, evodione, 6-(1-hydroxyethyl)-5,7-
     dimethoxy-2,2-dimethyl-2H-[1]-benzopyran, etc. [2].

Pharmacology

  1) Analgesic effect.

Literature

[1] Gunawardana, Y. A. G. P. *et al.*: *J. Sci. Soc. Thailand* **1987**, 13(2), 107.

[2] Li, G.L. *et al.*: *Progress in Drug Development from Medicinal Plants*. Proceedings of
    UNESCO Regional Symposium on Drug Development from Medicinal Plants. Oct.
    25-27, 1996, Hangzhou, China, **1996**, 200.

[P.P.H. But]

292.   *Brucea javanica* **(L.) Merr.**   (Simaroubaceae)

Ya-dan-zi (C), Ngar-darm-gee (H)

Fruit (CP)
Local Drug Name: Ya-dan-zi (C), Ngar-darm-gee (H), A-dan-shi (J).
Processing: Collect when mature, remove foreign matter, dry under the sun (C).
Method of Administration: Oral (whole kernel, C, H, J); Topical (C, H).
Folk Medicinal Uses:
> 1) Amebic dysentery (C, H, J).
> 2) Malaria (C, H, J).
> 3) Hemorrhoids (H).
> 4) Warts (C, H).
> 5) Corns (C, H).
> 6) Syphilis (C).
> 7) Gonorhea (C).

Contraindications: Pregnancy, gastrintestinal bleeding, liver disease, kidney disease.
Side effects: Vomiting, abdominal pain, diarrhea, dizziness, hypotension, drowsiness,
        paralysis, fibrillation, anaphylatic shock [1–2].

Scientific Research
Chemistry
> 1) Quassinoids: brusatol, bruceines, dehydrobruceines, bruceosides, yadanziosides,
>   yadanzigan, brusatol, javanicin [1, 6, 10–11, 16–19].
> 2) Bruceaketolic acid [10].
> 3) Cleomiscosin A.
> 4) Chrysophanol, chrysophanein, emodin, β-sitosterol, ethyl gallate [4, 8], quercetin-3-*O*-
>   β-D-galactoside, vanillic acid, luteolin-7-*O*-β-D-glucoside [7], daucosterol [11].
> 5) Alkaloids: 4-ethoxtcarbonyl-2-quinolone [7].
> 6) Triterpenoids: bruceajavinins A-B, dihydrobruceajavanin A [15].
> 7) Fatty acid [9].

Pharmacology
> 1) Antiamebic effect.
> 2) Antimalarial effect [10, 15].
> 3) Anthelmintic effect.
> 4) Antileukemic effect.
> 5) Cytotoxic effect [3].
> 6) Antitumor effect [10–12, 14].

Literature
[1] Zheng, G.Q. *et al.*: *Zhongyao Zazhi* **1986**, 11, 121.
[2] Zhang, Z.L. *et al.*: *Jilin Yiyao* **1985**, 6, 674.
[3] Fukamiya, N. *et al.*: *J. Nat. Prod.* **1992**, 55, 468.
[4] Yu, R.M. *et al.*: *Zhongcaoyao* **1988**, 19, 294.
[5] Zheng, G.Q. *et al.*: *Zhongyao Zazhi* **1986**, 11, 121.
[6] Zhang, J.S. *et al.*: *Huaxue Xuebao* **1983**, 41, 149.
[7] Yu, Y.N. *et al.*: *Yaoxue Xuebao* **1990**, 25, 382.
[8] Wang, S.X. *et al.*: *Shenyang Yaoxueyuan Xuebao* **1988**, 5, 196.
[9] Fukamiya, N. *et al.*: *Yaoxue Tongbao* **1990**, 42, 73.

[10] Lin, L.Z. *et al.*: *Huaxue Xuebao* **1982**, 40, 73.

[11] Xie, J.X. *et al.*: *Yaoxue Xuebao* **1981**, **16**, 53.

[12] Cheng, J.H. *et al.*: *Zhongchengyao* **1991**, 13, 21.

[13] Fan, Z.Z. *et al.*: *Zhongchengyao* **1989**, 11(6), 26.

[14] Su, S.Y. *et al.*: *Zhongxiye Jiehe Zazhi* **1985**, 5(2), 86.

[15] Kitagawa, I. *et al.*: *Chem. Pharm. Bull.* **1994**, 42, 1416.

[16] Lin, L.Z. *et al.*: *Phytochemistry* **1990**, 29, 2720.

[17] Fukamiya, N. *et al.*: *J. Nat. Prod.* **1992**, 55, 468.

[18] Gupta, J. *et al.*: *Hamdard Medicus* **1994**, 37(4), 40.

[19] Gupta, J. *et al.*: *Hamdard Medicus* **1996**, 39(1), 68.

[P.P.H. But]

293.   *Aesculus chinensis* **Bge.**   (Hippocastanaceae)

Qi-ye-shu (C)

Related plants: *A. chinensis* Bge. var. *chekingensis* (Hu et Fang) Fang: Zhe-jiang-qi-ye-shu (C), *A. wilsonii* Rehd.: Tian-shi-li (C), *A. turbinata* Blume: Tochinoki (J), Chil-yeop-su (K).

Seed (CP)

Local Drug Name: Suo-luo-zi (C), Sha-ra-shi (J), Sa-ra-ja (K).

Processing: Remove the outer coat and foreign matter. Break to pieces before use (C, K).

Method of Administration: Oral (decoction: C, K).

Folk Medicinal Uses:

1) Distress in the chest, distension in the abdomen, epigastric pain (C, J, K).

Scientific Research:

Chemistry

1) Alkane: eicosan-1-01 [1].

2) Steroid: dausosterol [1].

3) Carbohydrate: D-*d*-glucose [1].

4) Proteid: wilsonic acid [1].

5) Saponins [2].

6) Miscellaneous: *N*-butyl-β-D-fructopyranoside, 1-butosy-2-2-2-trichloro-ethanol [1].

Pharmacology

1) Antiinflammatory effect [3].

2) Anthydropic effect [4–5].

3) Enhancing effect on the secretion of corticosterone [6].

4) Hypoxia tolerance enhancing effect [2].

Literature:
[1] Qin, W. J. *et al.*: *Zhonghua Yaoxue Zazhi* **1992**, 27, 626.

[2] Dan, P. X. *et al.*: *Zhongchengyao Yanjiu* **1983**, (9), 24.

[3] Ogura: *Igaku Chuo Zasshi* **1976**, 330, 636.

[4] Zolta, O.T. *et al.*: *Arzneim. Forsch.* **1969**, 19, 287.

[5] Hampel, H. *et al.*: *Arzneim. Forsch.* **1970**, 20, 209.
[6] Susumu, H. *et al.*: *Chem. Pharm. Bull.* **1981**, 29, 490.

[J.X. Guo]

294.   *Ilex asprella* **(Hook.f. et Arn.) Champ. ex Bentham**   (Aquifoliaceae)

Mei-ye-dong-qing (C), Mui-yip-dung-ching (H)

Root
  Local Drug Name: Gang-mei-gen (C), Gong-mui-gun (H).
  Processing: Wash clean, cut into sections, dry in the sun (C).
  Method of Administration: Oral (decoction: C, H)
  Folk Medicinal Uses:
                1) Influenza, fever (C, H).
                2) Tonsillitis, pharyngitis (C, H).
                3) Bronchitis (C, H).
                4) Pertussis (C, H).
                5) Dysentery (C, H).
                6) Enteritis (C, H).
                7) Infectious hepatitis (C, H).
                8) Mushroom poisoning (C, H).

Leaf
  Local Drug Name: Gong-mui-yip (H).
  Method of Administration: Topical (paste: H).
  Folk Medicinal Uses:
                1) Traumatic injury (H).
                2) Pyodermas (H).

Scientific Research
  Chemistry
      1) Volatile oil [1].
      2) Triterpene: asprellic acids A-C [2].
  Pharmacology
      1) Cytotoxic effect [2].

Literature
  [1] Chen, C. T. *et al.*: *Bull. Inst. Chem., Acad. Sin.* **1976**, 23, 13.
  [2] Kashiwada, Y. *et al.*: *J. Nat. Prod.* **1993**, 56, 2077.

[P.P.H. But]

295.   *Ilex chinensis* **Sims.** (Aquifoliaceae)
                      [=*I. purpurea* Hassk]

Dong-qing (C), Nanamenoki (J)

Leaf, bark, root and seed
Local Drug Name: Dong-qing (C), To-sei-yo (J).
Processing: Dry under the sun (C).
Method of Administration: Oral (decoction: C, J); Topical (paste: C).
Folk Medicinal Uses:

    1) Dysentery (C).
    2) Upper respiratory infection (C).
    3) Bronchitis (C, J).
    4) Pyelonephritis (C).
    5) Pneumonia (J).
    6) Scalds (J).
    7) Traumatic injury (C, J).
    8) Burns, wound bleeding (C).

Scientific Research
Chemistry
  1) Ilexosides A-B [1], pedunculoside, protocatechuic acid, caffeic acid, syringin, rotundic acid, cyclohexanone peduculosyl-3,23-*O*-acetal [2].
Pharmacology
  1) Antibacterial effect [3-4].

Literature
[1] Inada, A. *et al.*: *Chem. Pharm. Bull.* **1987**, 35, 841.
[2] Zhao, H. R. *et al.*: *Zhongguo Zhongyao Zazhi* **1993**, 18, 226.
[3] Anonymous: *Zhongcaoyao Tongxun* **1971**, (3), 33.
[4] Anonymous: *Zhonghua Yixue Zazhi* **1973**, 53, 204.

[P.P.H. But]

296.   *Ilex cornuta* **Lindl.** (Aquifoliaceae)

Gou-gu (C), Gau-gwut (H), Ho-rang-ga-si-na-mu (K)

Leaf (CP)
Local Drug Name: Gou-gu-ye (C), Sup-die-gung-loe (H), Ku-kotsu-yo (J), Gu-gol-yeop (K).
Processing: Dry under the sun.
Method of Administration: Oral (decoction: C, H, J, K).
Folk Medicinal Uses:

    1) Headache (H, K).
    2) Pulmonary tuberculosis (H).
    3) Fever (H).
    4) Dizziness, hypertension (C, K).
    5) Hemoptysis (C, H).
    6) Traumatic injury, rheumatalgia (K).
    7) Vertigo (H, K).
    8) Inflammation (K).
    9) Arthritis (J).
Contraindication: Pregnancy.

Root

Local Drug Name: Gou-gu (C), Gung-loe-gun (H).

Processing: Dry under the sun.

Method of Administration: Oral (decoction: C, H).

Folk Medicinal Uses:

        1) Rheumatism, lumbago (C, H).

        2) Headache (C, H).

        3) Toothache (C, H).

        4) Hepatitis (C, H).

Contraindication: Pregnancy.

Scientific Research

Chemistry

1) Glycosides: pomolic acid 3β-O-α-L-2-acetoxyarabinopyranosyl-28-O-β-D-glucopyrano-side, 29-hydroxyoleanolic acid 3β-O-α-L-arabinopyranosyl-28-β-D-glucopyranoside [1], ilexide I (3β-O-[β-D-glucopyranosyl-(1→2)-α-L-arabino-yranosyl]pomolic acid) [2, 5], ilexide II [2], ziguglucosides 1-II, cornutaside A-D [4].

2) Glycolipid:cornuta-glycolipides A-B [3].

3) 3,4-dicaffeoylquinic acid, 3,5-dicaffeoylquinic acid, adenosine [3], lupeol, ursolic acid, daucosterol [4].

Pharmacology

1) Fertility regulating effect.

2) Increase coronary blood flow [1, 3].

3) PGI_2 -stimulatory effect [3].

4) Anti-platelet aggregation effect [3].

5) Antithrombotic effect [5].

6) Anticholesteremic effect [5].

Literature

[1] Qin, W. J. *et al.*: *Phytochemistry* **1986**, 25, 917.

[2] Nakanishi, T. *et al.*: *Phytochemistry* **1982**, 21, 1373.

[3] Qin, W. J. *et al.*: *Zhongcaoyao* **1988**, 19, 486.

[4] Qin, W. J. *et al.*: *Zhongcaoyao* **1988**, 19, 434.

[5] Otsuka Pharmaceutical Co., Ltd.: *Jpn. Kokai Tokkyo Koho JP 58,146,600* **1983**, 8pp.

                                                   [P.P.H. But]

297.   *Ilex latifolia* **Thunb.,** *I. kudingcha* **Tseng** (Aquifoliaceae)

Da-ye-dong-qing (C), Die-yip-dung-ching (H)

Leaf

Local Drug Name: Ku-ding-cha (C), Foo-ding-cha (H).

Processing: Dry under the sun.

Method of Administration: Oral (decoction: C, H).

Folk Medicinal Uses:

        1) Headache (C, H).

        2) Fever (H).

3) Dizziness, hypertension (C, H).
4) Hemoptysis (C, H).

Scientific Research
Chemistry
　1) Glycosides: latifolosides A-B [1].
　2) Arbutin [2].
Pharmacology
　1) Anti-implantation effect [3].
　2) Termination of early pregnancy [3].
　3) Uterotonic effect [4].

Literature
[1] Ochi, M. *et al.*: *Bull. Chem. Soc. Jpn.* **1975**, 48, 937.
[2] Miura, H. *et al.*: *Shoyakugaku Zasshi* **1985**, 39, 181.
[3] Xu, Y.X. *et al.*: *Xian Yixueyuan Xuebao* **1984**, (4), 379.
[4] Xu, Y.X. *et al.*: *Xian Yixueyuan Xuebao* **1985**, (6), 125.
[5] But, P. P. H. *et al.*: *Shoyakugaku Zasshi* **1985**, 39, 46.

[P.P.H. But]

298. 　　　　　*Ilex rotunda* **Thunb.** (Aquifoliaceae)

Tie-dong-qing (C), Tit-dung-ching (H), Meon-na-mu (K)

Stem bark
Local Drug Name: Jiu-bi-ying (C), Gou-bit-ying (H), Gu-pil-eung (K).
Method of Administration: Oral (decoction: C); Topical (paste: C, H).
Folk Medicinal Uses:
　　　　　1) Common cold (C, H).
　　　　　2) Hemorrhoid (C, H).
　　　　　3) Tonsillitis (C, H).
　　　　　4) Sore throat (C, H).
　　　　　5) Acute gastroenteritis (C, H).
　　　　　6) Acute pancreatitis (H).
　　　　　7) Gastric ulcer (H).
　　　　　8) Duodenal ulcer (H).
　　　　　9) Rheumatalgia (H).
　　　　　10) Hemorrhagic fever (H).
　　　　　11) Traumatic injury (H).
　　　　　12) Boils, pyodermas (H).
　　　　　13) Wound bleeding (H).
　　　　　14) Scald, burns (H).
　　　　　15) Neurodermatitis (H).

Scientific Research
Chemistry
　1) Rotundic acid [1], pedunculoside [2], ilexanin A (syringin) [3, 7], ursolic acid, rotungenic acid, rotundioic acid [5], rotundic acid isopropylidene [7], ilexolic acids A, B [8], sinapaldehyde, sinapaldehyde glucoside, ilexrotunin, syringaldehyde, 3-

acetyloleanolaic acid, rotundanonic acid, rotundanonic acid [7, 12], ilexosides XXIX-XXXII, XXXIII-XXXIX, XXXVIII-XL, XLI-XLV, XLVI-LI [6, 8–11],

rotungenoside, ziyu-glucoside I, suavissimoside F1 and chikusetsuaponin IVa [8]

2) Tannin: 1-caffeoylquinic acid, neochlorogenic acid, chlorogenic acid [4].

Pharmacology

1) Hemostatic effect [3].

Literature

[1] Oyama, T. *et al.*: *Tetrahedron Lett.* **1968**, (44), 4639.
[2] Hase, T. *et al.*: *Nippon Kagaku Kaishi* **1973**, (4), 778.
[3] Xie, P. S. *et al.*: *Yao Hsueh Hsueh Pao* **1980**, 15, 303.
[4] Nakatani, M. *et al.*: *Kagoshima Daigaku Rigakubu Kiyo, Sugaku, Butsurigaku, Kagaku* **1988**, (21), 127.
[5] Nakatani, M. *et al.*: *Phytochemistry* **1989**, 28, 1479.
[6] Nakatani, M. *et al.*: *Bull. Chem. Soc. Jpn.* **1989**, 62, 469.
[7] Wen, D. X. *et al.*: *Zhongcaoyao* **1991**, 22, 246.
[8] Amimoto, K. *et al.*: *Chem. Pharm. Bull.* **1992**, 40, 3138.
[9] Amimoto, K. *et al.*: *Phytochemistry* **1993**, 33, 1475.
[10] Amimoto, K. *et al.*: *Chem. Pharm. Bull.* **1993**, 41, 39.
[11] Amimoto, K. *et al.*: *Chem. Pharm. Bull.* **1993**, 41, 77.
[12] Wen, D.X. *et al.*: *Phytochem.* **1996**, 41, 657.

[P.P.H. But]

299.   *Rhamnus japonica* **Maxim.**   (Rhamnaceae)

Kuro-umemodoki (J)

Related plant: *Rhamnus davurica* Pall.: Shu-li (C), Gal-mae-na-mu (K).

Fruit

Local Drug Name: Shu-li-zi (C), So-ri-shi (J), Seo-ri-ja (K).
Processing: Dry under heated air (J, K).
Method of Administration: Oral (decoction: J, K).
Folk Medicinal Uses:

1) Edema (J, K).
2) Constipation (J, K).
3) Cough (K).

Scientific Research:

Chemistry

1) Sugars: bornesitol [1].

Literature:

[1] Plouvier, V.: *Compt. Rend.* **1958**, 247, 2190.

[T. Kimura]

300.   *Ampelopsis japonica* (**Thunb.**) **Makino**   (Vitaceae)

Bai-lian (C), Bark-lim (H), Byaku-ren (J), Ga-hoe-top (K)

Root (CP)
  Local Drug Name: Bai-lian (C), Bark-lim (H), Byaku-ren (J), Beak-ryeom (K).
  Processing: Eliminate foreign matter, wash clean, soften thoroughly, cut into thick slices,
        and dry (C, K).
  Method of Administrarion: Oral (decoction: C, K); Topical (powder: C; paste: K).
  Folk Medicinal Uses:
                1) Carbuncle (C, H, J, K).
                2) Deep-rooted boils (C).
                3) Scrofula (C, H).
                4) Scalds and burns (C, H, J, K).
  Contraindications: Incompatible with aconites and related herbs (C).

Scientific Research:
  Chemistry
    1) Iridoids [1].
  Pharmacology
    1) Antimycotic effect [2].
    2) Antiviral effect [3].
    3) Tyrosinase inhibitory effect [4].

Literature:
[1] Chi, H. J. *et al.*: *Korean J. Pharmacog.* **1981**, 12, 19.
[2] Cao, R. L. *et al.*: *Zhonghua Pifuke Zazhi* **1957**, 4, 286.
[3] Zheng, M. S. *et al.*: *J. Trad. Chin. Med.* **1988**, 8, 203.
[4] Fukushima, M. *et al.*: *Shoyakugaku Zasshi* **1989**, 43, 142.

[J.X. Guo]

301.   *Abutilon theophrastii* **Medic.**   (Malvaceae)
              [=*A. avicennae* Gaertn.]

Qing-ma (C), Ichibi (J), Eo-jeo-gwi (K)

Seed (CP)
  Local Drug Name: Qing-ma-zi (C), Dung-kwai-gee (H), Kei-ma (J), Gyeong-sil (K).
  Processing: Eliminate foreign matter (C, K).
  Method of Administration: Oral (decoction: C, H, K).
  Folk Medicinal Uses:
                1) Dysentery with bloody purulent stools (C, K).
                2) Urinary infection (C, H, J).
                3) Carbuncles and boils (C).
                4) Nebula (C).
                5) Constipation (J).

Scientific Research:
Chemistry
   1) Aliphatic acid: linoleic acid [1].
   2) Fatty oils [2].
   3) Globulin C [2].

Literature:
[1] Carmody, D. R. *et al.*: *Oil & Soap* **1945**, 22, 263.
[2] *"Quanguo Zhongcaoyao Huibian"* **1975**, Vol. 1, 197, 514.

[J.X. Guo]

302.   *Althaea rosea* **Cavanil** (Malvaceae)

Shu-kui (C), Tachi-aoi (J), Jeop-si-ggot (K)

Flower
Local Drug Name: Shu-kui-hua (C), Shoku-ki-ka (J), Chok-gyu-hwa (K).
Processing: Dry in shade (C, J, K).
Method of Administration: Oral (decoction: C, J, K); Topical (paste or decoction: C).
Folk Medicinal Uses:
       1) Dyschesia and difficult urination (C).
       2) Globus hystericus (C).
       3) Tetrodontoxism (C).
       4) External use for carbuncle (C).
       5) Edema (J).
       6) Rubella (J).
       7) Measles (J).
       8) Gonorrhoea (K).
       9) Menostasis, leukorrhea (K).
     10) Monoxenia (K).
     11) Scrofula (K).

Root
Local Drug Name: Chok-gyu-geun (K).
Processing: Dry under the sun (K).
Method of Administration: Oral (decoction, K).
Folk Medicinal Uses:
       1) Acute gastritis (K).
       2) Leukorrhea (K).

Scientific Research:
Chemistry
   1) Flavonoids: rutin, chrysin, kaempferol, robinetin, acacetin, phloretin [1].
   2) Fatty acids: palmitic acid, myristic acid, stearic acid, oleic acid, linoleic acid [2–3].
   3) Mucilages: althaea-mucilage R [4].
   4) Sterols: cholesterol, ergosterol, campesterol, sitosterol, stigmasterol [6, 8].

5) Anthocyans: cyanidin-3-glucoside, delphinidin-3-glucoside, malvidin-3,5-diglucoside [7].
6) Polysaccharides [9].

Pharmacology
1) Antiulcer effect (polysaccharides) [5, 9].

Literature:

[1] Srivastava, S. K.: *Indian Drugs* **1984**, 21, 468.
[2] Karawya, M. S.: *Egypt. J. Pharm. Sci.* **1979**, 20, 291.
[3] Gopalakrishnan, N.: *Phytochemistry* **1982**, 21, 2205.
[4] Tomoda, M.: *Chem. Pharm. Bull.* **1983**, 31, 2677.
[5] Manicheva, O. A.: *Rastit. Resur.* **1984**, 20, 256.
[6] Chouhan, U. K.: *J. Sci. Res.(Bhopal, India)* **1984**, 6, 49.
[7] Dokl. *Akad. Nauk Az. SSR* **1984**, 40, 76.
[8] Chauhan, U. K.: *Proc. Natl. Acad. Sci. India, Sect. B* **1984**, 54, 236.
[9] Barnaulov, O. D.: *Rastit. Resur.* **1985**, 21, 329-340.

[C.K. Sung]

303.   *Aquilaria sinensis* **(Lour.) Gilg**   (Thymelaeaceae)

Bai-mu-xiang (C), Toe-chum-heung (H), Baek-mok-hyang (K)

Related plant: *A. agallocha* Roxb.

Wood containing resin (CP)
Local Drug Name: Chen-xiang (C), Toe-chum-heung (H), Jin-ko (J), Chim-hyang (K).
Processing: Remove the white rotten-wood, split to small pieces, break to pieces or pulverize to fine powder before use (C).
Method of Administration: Oral (decoction: C, H, J, K; powder: H).
Folk Medicinal Uses:
1) Distension and pain in the chest and abdomen (C, H, J, K).
2) Vomiting or hiccup due to cold in the stomach (C, H, J, K).
3) Asthma in deficiency syndrome of the kidney (C, H).
4) Belching (H).
5) After birth (J).

Scientific Research:
Chemistry
1) Essential Oils: agarol [1], benzylacetone, *p*-methoxybenzy-lacetone [2], α-agarofuran, β-agarofuran, dihydroagarofuran [3], nor-ketoagarofuran, 4-hydroxydihdroagaro-furan, 3,4-dihydroxydihydroagarofuran [4], agarospirol [5], baimuxinic acid, baimuxinal [6], baimuxinol, dehydrobaimuxinol [7], sinenofuranal, sinenofuranol, dihydro-karanone [8], isobaimuxinol, anisic acid [9], baimuxifuranic acid [10].
2) Chromones: 2-(2-phenylethyl)chromone, 6-methoxy-2-(2-phenylethyl)chromone, 6,7-dimethoxy-2-(2-phenylethyl) chromone, 6-methoxy-2-[2-(3'-methoxyphenyl)-ethyl] chromone, 6-hydroxy-2-(2-phenylethyl)chromone, 6-hydroxy-2-[2-(2-(4'-

methoxyphenyl)ethyl chromone [11], 5,8-dihydroxy-2-[2-(4'-methoxyphenyl)-ethyl]chromone, 6,7-dimethoxy-2-[2-(4'-methoxyphenyl)ethyl]chromone [12].

Pharmacology
   1) Analgesic effect [13].

Literature:

[1] Jain, T. C. *et al.*: *Tetrahedron Letters* **1959**, 13.
[2] Kariyone, T. *et al.*: *"Shoyakugaku"* **1963**, 8.
[3] Maheshwan, M. L. *et al.*: *Tetrahedron* **1963**, 19, 1079.
[4] Maheshwan, M. L. *et al.*: *Tetrahedron* **1963**, 19, 1519.
[5] Varma, K. R. *et al.*: *Tetrahedron* **1965**, 21, 115.
[6] Yang, J. S. *et al.*: *Yaoxue Xuebao* **1983**, 18, 191.
[7] Yang, J. S. *et al.*: *Yaoxue Xuebao* **1986**, 21, 516.
[8] Xu, J. F. *et al.*: *Zhiwu Xuebao* **1988**, 30, 635.
[9] Yang, J. S. *et al.*: *Yaoxue Xuebao* **1989**, 24, 264.
[10] Yang, J. S. *et al.*: *Chin. Chem. Lett.* **1992**, 3, 983.
[11] Yang, J. S. *et al.*: *Yaoxue Xuebao* **1989**, 24, 678.
[12] Yang, J. S. *et al.*: *Yaoxue Xuebao* **1990**, 25, 186.
[13] Yoneda, K.: *Shoyakugaku Zasshi* **1986**, 40, 259.

[J.X. Guo]

304.   *Daphne genkwa* Sieb. et Zucc.   (Thymelaeaceae)

Yuan-hua (C), Yuan-far (H), Fuji-modoki (J), Pat-ggot-na-mu (K)

Flower (CP)
   Local Drug Name: Yuan-hua (C), Yuan-far (H), Gen-ka (J), Weon-hwa (K).
   Processing: 1) Eliminate foreign matter (C, K).
                      2) Stir-fry with vinegar until vinegar (C).
   Method of Administration: Oral (decoction or powder: C, H, J, K).
   Folk Medicinal Uses:
                      1) Anasarca, hydrothorax and ascites with dyspnea (C, J, K).
                      2) Constipation (C, J, K).
                      3) Oliguria (C, J, K).
                      4) External use for scabies, tinea and frostbite (C, K).
                      5) Edema (H).
   Contraindications: Contraindicated in pregnancy. Incompatible with licorice (C).

Scientific Research:
   Chemistry
      1) Flavonoids: apigenin [1], genkwanin [2], yuenkanin, 3-hydroxygenkwanin [3],
         luteolin, luteolin-7-methyl ether [4].
      2) Diterpenes: genkwadaphnin [5], yuanhuacine, yuanhuadine, yuanhuafine [6],
         yuanhuatine [7], yuanhuapine [8].

3) Volatile oils: α-furanaldehyde, phenylformaldehyde, dodecaldehyde, pentadecane, trimethylpyrazine, 2,5-dimethyl-3-(3-methylbutyl)-pyrazine, decanoic acid, dodecanoic acid, tridecanoic acid [9].

4) Others: sitosterol, benzoic acid [1].

Pharmacology

1) Diuretic effect [10].

2) Antimycotic effect [11].

3) Antitussive effect [12].

4) Abortifacient effect [13].

5) Sedative effect [14].

6) Antileukemic effect [5].

7) Xanthine oxidase inhibitory effect [4].

Literature:

[1] Nakao, M. *et al.*: *Yakugaku Zasshi* **1932**, 52, 341.
[2] Nakao, M. *et al.*: *Yakugaku Zasshi* **1932**, 52, 903.
[3] Li, S. F. *et al.*: *Zhongcaoyao* **1983**, 14(9), 8.
[4] Tadataka, K. *et al.*: *Chem. Pharm. Bull.* **1983**, 31, 3984.
[5] Kasai, R. *et al.*: *Phytochemistry* **1981**, 20, 2592.
[6] Wang, C. R. *et al.*: *Huaxue Xuebao* **1982**, 40, 835.
[7] Hu, B. H. *et al.*: *Yaoxue Tongbao* **1984**, 19(6), 50.
[8] Ouyang, S. H. *et al.*: *Huaxue Xuebao* **1986**, 44, 843.
[9] Liu, J. *et al.*: *Zhongguo Zhongyao Zazhi* **1993**, 18, 25.
[10] Ma, T. X. *et al.*: *Henan Yixueyuan Xuebao* **1960**, (7), 30.
[11] Cao, R. L. *et al.*: *Zhonghua Pifuke Zazhi* **1957**, 4, 286.
[12] Research Group: *Zhongcaoyao Tongxun* **1973**, (5), 7.
[13] Wang, Z. H.: *Zhonghua Fuchanke Zazhi* **1979**, 14(2), 125.
[14] Wei, C. W. *et al.*: *Zhongcaoyao* **1981**, 12(3), 27.

[J.X. Guo]

305. *Citrullus lanatus* **(Thunb.) Matsum. et Nakai**   (Cucurbitaceae)
[=*C. vulgaris* Schrad.]

Xi-gua (C), Sight-gwar (H), Suika (J), Su-bak (K)

Fruit

Local Drug Name: Xi-gua (C), Sight-gwar (H), Sui-ka (J), Seo-gwa (K).

Processing: Fresh.

Method of Administration: Oral (fresh: J, K).

Folk Medicinal Uses:

1) Nephritis (J, K).

2) Edema (J, K).

3) Febrile disease (H).

Fruit juice

Local Drug Name: Sui-ka-to (J).

Processing: Boil down into glutinous candy (J).

Method of Administration: Oral (J).
Folk Medicinal Uses:
        1) Nephritis (J).
        2) Edema (J).

Pericarp
  Local Drug Name: Xi-gua-pi (C), Sight-gwar-pay (H), Sui-ka-hi (J), Seo-gwa-pi (K).
  Processing: Dry under the sun (C, J, K).
  Method of Administration: Oral (decoction: C, J, K), (fresh: H).
  Folk Medicinal Uses:
        1) Nephritis (C, J, K).
        2) Edema (C, H, J, K).

Scientific Research:
  Chemistry
    1) Amino acid: citrulline [1].
    2) Triterpenoids: bryonolic acid (cell culture) [2–3].
  Pharmacology
    1) Antiallergic (bryonolic acid) [2–3].

Literature:
[1] Wada, M.: *Proc. Imp. Acad. (Jap.),* **1930**, 6, 15.
[2] Tabata, M. *et al.*: *J. Nat. Prod.*, **1993**, 56, 165.
[3] Cho, H. J. *et al.*: *Phytochemistry* **1993**, 33, 1407.

                [T. Kimura]

306.   *Momordica charantia* L.   (Cucurbitaceae)

       Ku-gua (C), Foo-gwar (H), Tsuru-reishi (J), Yeo-ju (K)

Fruit
  Local Drug Name: Ku-gua (C), Foo-gwar (H), Ku-ka (J), Go-gwa (K).
  Processing: Remove foreign matter, dry under the sun or use when fresh.
  Method of Administration: Oral (decoction: C, H, J, K); Topical (paste: H).
  Folk Medicinal Uses:
        1) Fever of heatstroke (C, H).
        2) Pharyngitis (H).
        3) Ringworm infection (H).
        4) Pyodermas (H).
        5) Miliaria (H).
        6) Toothache (C).
        7) Enteritis (C).
        8) Dysentery (C).
        9) Hematochezia (C).
       10) Sudamen (C).
       11) Furuncle (C).
       12) Diarrhea (J).

13) Congestion (J).

14) Eye disease (K).

Root

Local Drug Name: Ku-gua-gen (C), Foo-gwar-gun (H).

Processing: Remove foreign matter, dry under the sun.

Method of Administration: Oral (decoction: C, H).

Folk Medicinal Uses:

1) Diarrhea (C, H).

2) Amoebic dysentery (C, H).

Scientific Research

Chemistry

1) Glycoprotein: α-momorcharin, β-momorcharin [1–2].

Pharmacology

1) Fertility regulating effect [8].

2) Antilipolytic effect [4, 14, 20].

3) Insulin-like effect [3, 17].

4) Hemolytic effect [18].

5) Immunosuppressive effect [21].

6) Ribosome-inactivating effect [6].

Literature

[1] Yeung, H. W. *et al.*: *Int. J. Pept. Protein Res.* **1986**, 28, 518.

[2] Yeung, H. W. *et al.*: *Planta Med.* **1987**, 53, 164.

[3] Ng, T. B. *et al.*: *J. Ethnopharmacol.* **1986**, 15, 107.

[4] Ng, T. B. *et al.*: *Gen. Pharmac.* **1987**, 18, 275.

[5] Ng, T. B. *et al.*: *J. Ethnopharmacol.* **1987**, 21, 55.

[6] Yeung, H. W. *et al.*: *Int. J. Pept. Protein Res.* **1988**, 31, 265.

[7] Ng, T. B. *et al.*: *J. Ethnopharmacol.* **1987**, 21, 21.

[8] Law, L. K. *et al.*: *J. Reprod. Fert.* **1983**, 69, 597.

[9] Tam, P. P. L. *et al.*: *J. Reprod. Fert.* **1984**, 71, 567.

[10] Chan, W. Y. *et al.*: *Contraception* **1984**, 29, 91.

[11] Chan, W. Y. *et al.*: *Contraception* **1985**, 31, 83.

[12] Yeung, H. W. *et al.*: *Advances in Chinese Medicinal Materials Research* [Chang, H. M. *et al.* (eds.)] World Scientific Publ. Co., Singapore, **1985**, 311.

[13] Tam, P.P.L. *et al.*: *Advances in Chinese Medicinal Materials Research* [Chang, H. M. *et al.* (eds.)] World Scientific Publ. Co., Singapore, **1985**, 335.

[14] Wong, C. M. *et al.*: *J. Ethnopharmacol.* **1985**, 13, 313.

[15] Chan, W. Y. *et al.*: *Contraception* **1986**, 34, 537..

[16] Kubota, S. *et al.*: *Biochimica et Biophysica Acta* **1986**, 871, 101.

[17] Ng, T. B. *et al.*: *Int. J. Peptide Protein Res.* **1986**, 28, 163.

[18] Ng, T. B. *et al.*: *J. Ethnopharmacol.* **1986**, 18, 55.

[19] Ng, T. B. *et al.*: *J. Ethnopharmacol.* **1986**, 18, 45.

[20] Ng, T. B. *et al.*: *Can. J. Biochem. Cell. Biol.* **1986**, 64, 766.

[21] Leung, S. O. *et al.*: *Immunopharm.* **1987**, 13, 159.

[P.P.H. But]

307. *Momordica cochinchinensis* (Lour.) Spr. (Cucurbitaceae)

Mu-bie (C), Muk-bit-gee (H), Nanban-karasu-uri (J), Mok-byeol (K)

Seed (CP)
Local Drug Name: Mu-bie-zi (C), Muk-bit-gee (H), Moku-betsu-shi (J), Mok-byeol-ja (K).
Processing: Eliminate fruit pulp, clean, dry under the sun.
Method of Administration: Oral (decoction or powder: C, H, J, K).
Folk Medicinal Uses:

     1) Sores and inflammatory swelling (C, H).
     2) Boils, pyodermas (H).
     3) Mastitis (C, H).
     4) Scrofula, furuncle (C, H, K).
     5) Ringworm infections (H).
     6) Freckles (H).
     7) Sebacious cysts (H).
     8) Hemorrhoids (C, H).
     9) Hemangiomas (H).
    10) Acute fistula (C).
    11) Neurodermatitis (C).
    12) Scald (C).
    13) Hypertension (J).
    14) Edema (J).
    15) Rheumatalgia (J, K).
    16) Suppuration (J).
Side effects: Poisonous.

Scientific Research
Chemistry
    1) Triterpenoid: momordic acid [1].
    2) oleanolic acid, amino acid [1–2].
    3) Diterpenes: columin [3].
    4) Saponin: momordins I, III, II (hemsloside Ma_1) [4], momordica saponins I–II [5].
    5) Glycoprotein: momorcochin [8], cochinchinin [10].
    6) Cu, Fe, Mn, Zn [11].
Pharmacology
    1) Hypoglycemic effect [6].
    2) Hemolytic effect [7].
    3) Abortifacient effect [8].
    4) Ribosome-inactivating effect [9–10].
    5) Inhibitory effect on protein-synthesis [10].

Literature
[1] Murakami, M. *et al.*: *Tetrahedron Lett.* **1966**, (42), 5137.
[2] Duong Tan, P. *et al.*: *Wiss. Z. Univ. Rostock, Math.-Naturwiss. Reihe* **1969**, 18(1/2) (Pt. 1), 151.
[3] Waterman, P. G. *et al.*: *Planta Med.* **1985**, (2), 181.
[4] Iwamoto, M. *et al.*: *Chem. Pharm. Bull.* **1985**, 33, 1.
[5] Iwamoto, M. *et al.*: *Chem. Pharm. Bull.* **1985**, 33, 464.
[6] Reza-Ul-Jalil, *et al.*: *J. Bangladesh Acad. Sci.* **1986**, 10(1), 25.

[7] Ng, T. B. *et al.*: *J. Ethnopharmacol.* **1986**, 18, 55.

[8] Yeung, H. W. *et al.*: *Int. J. Pept. Protein Res.* **1987**, 30, 135.

[9] Wang, R. H. *et al.*: *Junshi Yixue Kexueyuan Yuankan* **1993**, 17, 246.

[10] Zheng, S. *et al.*: *Shengwu Huaxue Yu Shengwu Wuli Xuebao* **1992**, 24, 311.

[11] Itokawa, H. *et al.*: *Shoyakugaku Zasshi* **1980**, 34, 155.

[P.P.H. But]

308. *Trichosanthes cucumeroides* Maxim. (Cucurbitaceae)

Wang-gua (C), Wong-gwar (H), Karasu-uri (J)

Seed

Local Drug Name: O-ga-nin (J).

Processing: Dry under the sun (J).

Method of Administration: Oral (decoction; J).

Folk Medicinal Uses:

        1) Cough (J).

        2) Sputum (J).

Root

Local Drug Name: Wang-gua-gen (C), Wong-gwar-gun (H), O-ga-kon (J).

Processing: Dry under the sun (J). Cut into section and dry (C).

Method of Administration: Oral (decoction: C, H, J); Topical (paste: C, fresh: H).

Folk Medicinal Uses:

        1) Constipation (J).

        2) Jaundice (J).

        3) Menstrual disorder (J).

        4) Snake-bite (C, H).

        5) Acute tonsillitis, pharyngitis (C).

        6) Carbuncle (C).

        7) Traumatic injury (C).

        8) Dysuria (C).

        9) Stomachache (C, H).

        10) Sore throat (H).

        11) Oligomenorrhea (H).

        12) Wound pain (H).

        13) Boils and pyodermas (H).

Starch

Local Drug Name: Ten-ka-fun (J), Cheon-hwa-bun (K).

Processing: Precipitation of ground and diluted fresh root (J).

Method of Administration: Topical (powder: J, K).

Folk Medicinal Uses:

        1) Perspiration (J, K).

        2) Miliaria, prickly heat (J, K).

        3) Diabetes (K).

Scientific Research:
Chemistry
  1) Flavonoids: Kaempferitrin [1–2].
  2) Fatty acid: Trichosanic acid [3].

Literature:

[1] Nakaoki, T. *et al.*: *Yakugaku Zasshi* **1956**, 76, 347.
[2] Nakaoki, T. *et al.*: *Yakugaku Zasshi* **1957**, 77, 108.
[3] Crombie, L. *et al.*: *J. Chem. Soc.* **1957**, 1632.

[T. Kimura]

309.   *Lythrum salicaria* **L.** (Lythraceae)

Qian-gu-cai (C), Ezo-misohagi (J), Teol-bu-cheo-ggot (K)

Related plant: *Lythrum anceps* (Koehne) Makino: Misohagi (J), Bu-cheo-ggot (K).

Whole herb
  Local Drug Name: Qian-gu-cai (C), Sen-kutsu-Sai (J), Cheon-gul-chae (K).
  Processing: Dry under the sun (C, J, K). Use in fresh (C).
  Method of Administration: Oral (decoction: C, J, K). Topical (paste: C).
  Folk Medicinal Uses:
          1) Diarrhea, dysentery (C, J, K).
          2 Melena (J).
          3) Metrorrhagia (J).
          4) Cystitis (J).
          5) Hematochezia (C).
          6) Traumatic injury (C).
  Contraindication: Pregnancy (C).

Scientific research
Chemistry
  1) Glycoside: salicarin [1].
  2) Sterol: β-sitosterol [1].

Literature

[1] Zhou, T.Y. et al.: In: Wu, Z. Y. (Eds.) *Xinhua Bencao Gangyao,* Shanghai Science and
    Technology Press, Shanghai, **1990**, 3, 188.

[T. Kimura]

310.   *Trapa bicornis* **Osbeck,** *T. bispinosa* **Roxb.** (Trapaceae)
        T. bispinosa **Roxb. var.** *iinumai* **Nakino**

Ling (C), Ling (H), Hishi (J), Ma-reum (K)

Related plant: *T. maximowiczii* Korsch.: Xi-guo-ye-ling (C).

Fruit
 Local Drug Name: Ling (C), Ling (H), Ryo-jitsu (J), Neung (K).
 Processing: Dry under the sun (C, J, K). Use in fresh (C).
 Method of Administration: Oral (decoction; C, H, J, K), (cooked fruit; H).
 Folk Medicinal Uses:
 　　　　　　1) Gastric ulcer and cancer (C, J, K).
 　　　　　　2) Mammary cancer (C, J).
 　　　　　　3) Uterine cancer (C, J).
 　　　　　　4) Dysentery (C, H).
 　　　　　　5) Common cold (K).

Scientific Research:
 Chemistry
 　1) Tannins: trapanin A, trapanin B, cornusiins A, B, C and D, gemin D, casuarinin,
 　　casuarictin, tellimagrandin I, pedunculagin [1].

Literature:
 [1] Hatano, T. *et al.*: *Chem. Pharm. Bull.*, **1990**, 38, 2707. (*T. japonica* = *T. bispinosa* var.
 　iinumai)

　　　　　　　　　　　　　　　　　　　　　　　　　　　　　[T. Kimura]

311.　　　*Cynomorium songaricum* **Rupr.**　(Cynomoriaceae)

　　　　　Suo-yang (C), Sor-yeung (H), Sa-yo (J), Soae-yang (K)

Herb (CP)
 Local Drug Name: Suo-yang (C), Sor-yeung (H), Sa-yo (J), Soae-yang (K).
 Processing: Wash, soften thoroughly, cut into thin slices, and dry (C, K).
 Method of Administration: Oral (decoction: C, H, J, K).
 Folk Medicinal Uses:
 　　　　　　1) Aching and weakness of the loins and knees (C, H, J, K).
 　　　　　　2) Impotence, spermatorrhea (C, H, J, K).
 　　　　　　3) Constipation (C, H, J, K).

Scientific Research:
 Chemistry
 　1) Flavonoids: anthocyanin [1], naringenin [2].
 　2) Triterpenes: ursolic acid [3], acetyl ursolic acid, ursa-12-ene-28-oic acid, 3β-propane-
 　　dioic acid monoester [4].
 　3) Steroids: β-sitosterol, daucosterol [3], β-sitosterol palnitate [4].
 　4) Amino acids: glycine, alanine, valine, serine, cystine, arginine, lysine, glutamic acid,
 　　asparagine, phenylalanine, tyrasine, proline, histidine, isoleucine [3].
 　5) Volatile oils: ethyl acetate, acetic acid, 1,1-diethoxy-ethane, pyridine, *n*-hexanal, 2-
 　　furaldehyde, 2-furancarbinol, 2-heptanone, *n*-heptanal, 2,3,5-trimethyl-pyrazine, 2-

ethyl-hexarol, tetramethyl-pyrazine, *n*-nonanal, ethyl octanoate, methyl *n*-nonanoate, ethyl nonanoate, tetradecanoic acid, methyl hexadecanoate, dibutyl phthalate, ethyl hexadecanoate, palmitic acid, 9-octadecenoic acid [5], palmitic acid [5, 7].

6) Carbohydrate: sucrose [4].

7) Condensed tannins [6].

8) Aliphatic compounds: oleic acid, linoleic acid, dodecane, tridecane, tetradecane, pentadecane, tricosane, pentadecadiene, hexadecane, heneicosane, pentacosane, heptocosane, nonacosane [7].

9) Inorganic elements: K, P, Ca, Mg [8], Cu, Zn, Fe, Al, Co, Mn, Mo, Rb, V, SO_4^{2-}, PO_4^{3-}, F^-, Cl^-, NO_3^- [9].

Pharmacology

1) Catharsis effect [10].

2) Immunoregulatory effect [11–12].

3) Dual effect on the serum cortisol cotent [13].

4) Increasing effect on hypoxia tolerance [14].

5) Antiplatelet effect [14].

6) Anti-senility effect [15].

7) Inhibitory effect on reverse transcriptase and DNA polymerase [16].

Literature:
[1] Kouppert, K.: *Chem. Zentr.* **1941**, 1 1711.
[2] Shibata, H.: *Guovai Yixue, Zhongyi Zhongyao Fence* **1989**, 11(6), 36.
[3] Zhang, S. J. *et al.*: *Zhongguo Yaoxue Zazhi* **1991**, 26, 649.
[4] Ma, C. M. *et al.*: *Yaoxue Xuebao* **1993**, 28, 152.
[5] Zhang, S. J. *et al.*: *Zhongguo Zhongyao Zazhi* **1990**, 15(2), 39.
[6] Zhang, B. S. *et al.*: *Zhongyaocai* **1991**, 14(9), 36.
[7] Huneck, S.: *Phamazie* **1990**, 45, 297.
[8] Daniel, S.: *Bull. Soc, Bot. Fr.* **1966**, 113, 439.
[9] Zhang, B. S. *et al.*: *Zhongyaocai* **1990**, 13(10), 36.
[10] Zhang, B. S. *et al.*: *Xibei Yaoxue Zazhi* **1989**, 4(1), 6.
[11] Shi, G. G. *et al.*: *Zhongguo Yiyao Xuebao* **1989**, 4(3), 27.
[12] Zhen, Y. X. *et al.*: *Gansu Zhongyi Xueyuan Xuebao* **1991**, 8(4), 28.
[13] Li, M. Y. *et al.*: *Gansu Zhongyi Xueyuan Xuebao* **1991**, 8(1), 50.
[14] Yu, P. F. *et al.*: *Zhongguo Zhongyao Zazhi* **1994**, 19, 244.
[15] Zhang, B. S. *et al.*: *Zhongyaocai* **1993**, 16(10), 32.
[16] Ono, K.: *Chem. Pharm. Bull.* **1989**, 37, 1810.

[J.X. Guo]

312. *Aucuba japonica* **Thunb.** (Cornaceae)

Aoki (J), Sik-na-mu (K)

Leaf

Local Drug Name: Ao-ki (J), Cheon-gak-pan (K).

Processing: Fresh (J).

Method of Administration: Topical (fresh leaf or ground leaf: J); Oral (pill: J).
Folk Medicinal Uses:
        1) Scald, burns (J, K).
        2) Frostbite (J, K).
        3) Abscess (J).
        4) Beriberi (J).
        5) Edema (J).
        6) Gastrointestinal disorder (J, K).
        7) Mushroom poisoning (K).

Scientific Research:
Chemistry
  1) Iridoids: Aucubin [1], eucommiol, eucommioside II [2].
  2) E-phytol, phytone, bis-(2-ethylhexyl)-phthalate, friedelin [5].
Pharmacology
  1) Antidote for fatal mushroom poisoning caused by *Amanita phalloides* [3].
  2) Antiinflammatory effect (E-phytol, phytone, bis-(2-ethylhexyl)-phthalate, friedelin)
    [4–5].

Literature:
[1] Fujise, S. *et al.*: Chem. & Ind. 1959, 954; **1960**, 289; Kashi., **1960**, 81, 677; 1716; 1720; 1723; **1961**, 82, 221; 222; 367; 370; 750; 1110; Uda, T. *et al.*: Kashi., **1960**, 81, 1865; Wendt, M. W. *et al.*: *Helv. Chim. Acta*, **1960**, 43, 1440; Grimshaw, J. *et al.*: *Chem. & Ind.* **1960**, 656; Birch, A. J. *et al.*: *J. Chem. Soc.* **1961**, 5194; Haegle, W. *et al.*: *Tetrahed. Lett.* **1961**, 110; Ohara, H.: *Kashi.*, **1961**, 82, 58; 60; 62; 65.
[2] Bernini, R. *et al.*: *Phytochemistry* **1984**, 23, 1431.
[3] Chang, I. M. *et al.*: *Yakhak Hoechi* **1984**, 28, 35.
[4] Shimizu, M. *et al.*: *Shoyakugaku Zasshi* **1993**, 47, 1.
[5] Shimizu, M. *et al.*: *Biol. Pharm. Bull*, **1994**, 17, 665.

[T. Kimura]

313.   *Aralia elata* **(Miq.) Seem.**   (Araliaceae)
           [=*A. mandshurica* Rupr. et Maxim.]

Liao-dong-cong-mu (C), Taranoki (J), Du-reup-na-mu (K)

Root bark, stem bark
Local Drug Name: Long-ya-cong-mu (C), So-kon-pi (J), Chong-mok-pi (K).
Processing: Dry under the sun (C, J, K).
Method of Administration: Oral (decoction; C, J, K).
Folk Medicinal Uses:
        1) Articular rheumatism (J).
        2) Nephritis (J).
        3) Diabetes (C, J).
        4) Hepatitis (C, J).
        5) General weakness (J, K).
        6) Anxiety neurosis (J).

7) Gastroduodenal ulcer (C).
8) Acute and chronic gastritis (C, K).
9) Rheumatic arthritis (C).
10) Edema (C).
11) Gastric cancer (K).
12) Jaundice (K).

Scientific Research:
Chemistry
1) Saponins: araloside A, B, C [1], elatoside A, B, E [2–3], tarasaponin I, II, III [4] and
   four other triterpenoid saponins [6].
2) Triterpenoid: hederagenin [5].
Pharmacology
1) Inhibition of ethanol absorptin in rat (elatoside A, B) [2].

Literature:
[1] Kochetkov, N. K. *et al.*: *J. Gen. Chem. (U. S. S. R.)* **1960**, 30, 658; *Zhur. Obshchei Khim.*
    1961, 31, 655; *Tetrahedron Lett.* **1962**, 713; Khorlin, A. Y. *et al.*: *Izv. Akad. Nauk. S.*
    S. S. R. Ser.Khim., **1964**, 1338; Sokolov: *Lekartsv. Sregstvaiz Rast.,* **1962**, 270.
[2] Yoshikawa, M., *et al.*: *Chem. Pharm. Bull.* **1993**, 41, 2069.
[3] Yoshikawa, M., *et al.*: *Chem. Pharm. Bull.* **1994**, 42, 1354.
[4] Sakai, S., *et al.*: *Phytochem.* **1994**, 35, 1319; Nakajima, Y. *et al.*: *Phytochemistry* **1994**,
    36, 119.
[5] Shibata, S. *et al.*: *Shoyakugaku Zasshi* **1964**, 17, 50.
[6] Saito, S. *et al.*: *Chem. Pharm. Bull.,* **1990**, 38, 411.

[T. Kimura]

314.   *Centella asiatica* **(L.) Urb.**   (Umbelliferae)

Ji-xue-cao (C), Bunk-die-woon (H), Tsubo-kusa (J), Byeong-pul (K)

Herb (CP)
Local Drug Name: Ji-xue-cao (C), Bunk-die-woon (H), Seki-setsu-so (J), Jeok-seol-cho (K).
Processing: Eliminate foreign matter, wash clean, cut into sections, and dry in the sun (C, K).
Method of Administration: Oral (decoction: C, H, J, K); Topical (fresh leaf juice: H, J, K).
Folk Medicinal Uses:
1) Jaundice caused by damp-heat (C).
2) Heat stroke with diarrhea (C).
3) Urolithiasis and hematuria (C, H, K).
4) Carbuncles and boils, traumatic injuries (C, J, K).
5) Infectious hepatitis (H).
6) Measles (H).
7) Common cold (H).
8) Tonsillitis (H).
9) Bronchitis (H).
10) Urinary tract infection (H).

11) Hematemesis (H).
12) Food poisoning (H).
13) Hemorrhage (K).

Scientific Research:
Chemistry
  1) Triterpenoid saponins: thankuniside [1], madacassoide [2], isothankuniside [3], asiaticoside, brahmoside, brahminoside [4], hydroxy-asiaticoside [13].
  2) Triterpenes: madagascaric acid [2], asiatic acid, brahmic acid, isobrahmic acid, betulinic acid [5–6], methyl thankunate, methyl isothankunate [7–8], madecassic acid [9].
  3) Sugars: centellose, mesoinositol [6], polysaccharide [13].
  4) Volatile oils [8].
  5) Fatty oils [8].
  6) Flavonoids: kaempferol, quercetin [4], 3-glucosylquercetin, 3-glucosylkaempferol, 7-glucosylk-aempferol [10].
  7) Alkaloid: hydrocotyline [11].
  8) Steroid: sitosterol.
  9) Others: vellarin pectine, vitamin C, carotene.
Pharmacology
  1) Effect on wound healing [9].
  2) Bacteriostatic effect [12].
  3) Antiulcer effect [13].

Literature:
[1] Dutta, T. *et al.*: *J. Sci. Ind. Res (India)* **1962**, 21B, 239.
[2] Pinhas, H. *et al.*: *Bull. Chim. Fr.* **1967**, 1888.
[3] Dutta, T. *et al.*: *Indian J. Chem.* **1968**, 6(9), 543.
[4] Rao, P. S. *et al.*: *Curr. Sci.* **1969**, 38(4), 77.
[5] Singh, B. *et al.*: *Phytochemistry* **1968**, 7, 1385.
[6] Singh, B. *et al.*: *Phytochemistry* **1969**, 8, 917.
[7] Dutta, T. *et al.*: *Indian J. Chem.* **1967**, 5, 586.
[8] List, P. H. *et al.*: *Hagers Handbuch der Pharmazeutischen Praxis* Bd 3 (Springer-verlag) **1972**, 792.
[9] Tsurumi, K. *et al.*: *Oyo Yakuri* **1973**, 7, 833.
[10] Prum, N. *et al.*: *Pharmazie* **1983**, 38, 427.
[11] Basu, N. K. *et al.*: *Quart. J. Pharm. Pharmacol.* **1947**, 20, 135.
[12] Ninghua County Hospital: *Yiyao Weishen* (Fujian Weishenju) **1971**, (1), 49.
[13] Gu, Q.M. *et al.*: *Progress in Drug Development from Medicinal Plants.* Proceedings of UNESCO Regional Symposium on Drug Development from Medicinal Plants. Oct. 25-27, 1996, Hangzhou, China, **1996**, 268.

[J.X. Guo]

315.   *Changium smyrnioides* **Wolff** (Umbelliferae)

Ming-dang-shen (C), Ming-dong-sum (H), Min-to-jin (J)

Root (CP)

Local Drug Name: Ming-dang-shen (C), Ming-dong-sum (H), Min-to-jin (J).
Processing: Wash clean, soften thoroughly, cut into thick slices, and dry (C).
Method of Administration: Oral (decoction: C, H, J).
Folk Medicinal Uses:

1) Cough caused by heat in the lung (C, H, J).
2) Vomiting, regurgitation, anorexia and dryness of the mouth (C, H, J).
3) Bloodshot eyes and vertigo (C).
4) Boils and sores (C).

Scientific Research:

Chemistry

1) Organic acids [1].
2) Sugars [1].
3) Volatile oils [1–3].

Literature:

[1] *"Zhongguo Jinji Zhiwuzhi"* **1961**, 1835.
[2] Jing, R. L. *et al.*: *Nanjing Yaoxueyuan Xuebao* **1964**, (10), 35.
[3] Nanjing College of Pharmacy: *Yaoxue Xuebao* **1966**, 8, 100.

[J.X. Guo]

316. *Coriandrum sativum* **L.** (Umbelliferae)

Yuan-sui (C), Yuan-shui (H), Koendoro (J), Go-su (K)

Fruit

Local Drug Name: Yuan-sui (C), Yuan-shui-gee (H), Ko-zui-shi (J), Ho-yu-ja (K).
Processing: Dry under the sun (C, J).
Method of Administration: Oral (decoction: C, J, K).
Folk Medicinal Uses:

1) Gastrointestinal disorder (C, J, K).
2) Meteorism (J, K).
3) Small pox (K).
4) Indigestion (H).
5) Anorexia (H).
6) Stomachache (H).

Whole herb

Local Drug name: Yuan-sui (C), Yuan-shui (H).
Processing: Dry under the sun (C, H).
Method of Administration: Oral (decoction: C, H); Topical (decoction: C).
Folk Medicinal Uses:

1) Measles without adequate eruption (C, H).
2) Common cold or influenza without sweat (C, H).

Scientific Research:
Chemistry
1) Monoterpenes: *d*-linalool, *p*-cymene, α-pinene, β-pinene, limonene, geraniol, geranyl
   acetate, borneol, nerolidol, thymol dipentene, α-terpinene, β-terpinene [1–2].
2) Aromatic compounds: coriandrin [3–4], coriandron A, coriandron B [5], anethole [6].
3) Flavonoids: [7].
4) Alyphatic compounds: *trans*-2-tridecene-1-ol, tridecen-2-al-1, decanal [1–2, 8–9],
   6-octadecenoic acid [10].
5) Triterpenoids: coriandrinol [11].
6) Sugar: D-mannitol [7].

Pharmacology
1) Antiviral (coriandrin) [2].

Literature:

[1] Schratz, E. *et al.*: *Planta Med.* **1966**, 14, 310.
[2] Makarova, G. M. etal.: *Farmatsevt. Zh. (Kiev)* **1959**, 14, 43.
[3] Kraus, G. A. *et al.*: *Chem.* **1994**, 59, 4735.
[4] Ceska, O. *et al.*: *Phytochemistry* **1988**, 27, 2083.
[5] Baba, K. *et al.*: *Phytochemistry* **1991**, 30, 4143.
[6] Rasmussen, S. *et al.*: *Medd. Nor. Farm. Selsk.* **1972**, 34, 33.
[7] Faroog, M. O. *et al.*: *Arch. d. Pharm.* **1961**, 294, 138.
[8] Reisch, J. *et al.*: *Naturwiss.* **1965**, 52, 642.
[9] Reisch, J. *et al.*: *Planta Med.* **1966**, 14, 326.
[10] Lee, L. T. *et al.*: *Hua Hsueh* **1973**, 52.
[11] Vaghani, D. D. *et al.*: *Curr. Sci.* **1958**, 27, 388.

[T. Kimura]

317.   *Hydrocotyl sibthorpioides* Lam.   (Umbelliferae)
                H. wilfordi Maxim.

Tian-hu-shui (C), Tin-woo-shui (H), Chidomegusa (J), Pi-mak-i-pul (K)

Whole plant
Local Drug Name: Tian-hu-shui (C), Tin-woo-shui (H), Ten-ko-zui (J), Cheon-ho-yu (K).
Processing: Eliminate foreign matters and dry, or use fresh.
Method of Administration: Oral (decoction: C, H, J, K); Topical (juice: C, H, J, K).
Folk Medicinal Uses:
1) Hepatitis (C, H, J).
2) Liver cirrhosis and ascites (C, H).
3) Gall stone (C, H).
4) Urethritis (C, H).
5) Influenza (C, H).
6) Pertussis (C, H).
7) Stomatitis (C, H).
8) Pharyngitis (C, H).
9) Tonsillitis (C, H).

10) Paronychia (H).
11) Eczema (H).
12) Herpes zoster (H).
13) Epistaxis (H, K).
14) Urinary tract stone (C, H).
15) Hemorrhage (K).
16) Traumatic injury (J).
17) Erysipelas (C).

Scientific Research
Chemistry
1) Flavonoids: quercetin, quercetin 3-galactoside (hyperin), quercetin 3-O-β-D-(6"-caffeoyl-galactoside), isorhamnetin [1–2],

Literature
[1] Nakaoki, T. *et al.*: *Yakugaku Zasshi* **1960**, 80, 1473.
[2] Shigematsu, N. *et al.*: *Phytochemistry* **1982**, 21, 2156.

[P.P.H. But]

318.   *Ligusticum chuanxiong* **Hort.** (Umbelliferae)
[=*L. wallichii* Franch.]

Chuan-xiong (C), Chuan-gung (H)

Related Plant: *Cnidium officinale* Makino: Yang-chuan-xiong (C), Senky (J), Cheon-gung (K).

Rhizome (CP)
Local Drug Name: Chuan-xiong (C), Chuan-gung (H), Sen-ky (J), Cheon-gung (K).
Processing: Steam for a short time then dry under the sun.
Method of Administration: Oral (decoction; C, H, J, K).
Folk Medicinal Uses:

        1) Anemia (H, J, K).
        2) Menstrual disorder, amenorrhea, dysmenorrhea (C, H, J, K).
        3) Pain (H, J, K).
        4) Abdominal pain with mass formation (C, J).
        5) Pricking pain in the chest and costal regions (C).
        6) Swelling and pain due to traumatic injury (C).
        7) Rheumatic arthralgia (C).
        8) General weakness (H, J, K).
        9) Feeling of cold (H, J, K).

Scientific Research:
Chemistry
1) Phthalides: Cnidilide, neocnidilide, ligustilide, senkyunolide E, O, N and P [1–2], 4-hydroxy-3-butyl phthalide [3].
2) Ferulic acid, chrysophanic acid, sedanonic acid [3].

3) Alkaloid: tetramethylpyrazine (ligustrazine), perlolyrine (1(5-hydroxymethyl-2-furyl)-9H-pyridine-(3,4,6)indole) [4–5].

Pharmacology
　1) Hypotensive effect [4, 14–15].
　2) Cardiotonic effect [4, 6].
　3) Vasodilatory effect [6]
　4) Inhibitory effect on platelet aggregation [6, 9].
　5) Improve microcirculation [7–8].
　6) Anti-atherosclerosis effect [10–11].
　7) Inhibitory effect on vascular smooth muscle cell proliferation [12].
　8) Immunopotentiation effect [13].
　9) Calcium antagonist effect [15].

Literature:
[1] Naito, T. *et al.*: *Heterocycles* **1991**, 32, 2433.
[2] Naito, T. *et al.*: *Phytochemistry* **1992**, 31, 639.
[3] Beijing Institute of Pharmaceutical Industries: *Yueh Hsueh Hsueh Pao* **1979**, 14, 670.
[4] Beijing Institute of Pharmaceutical Industries: *Yueh Hsueh Tung Pao* **1980**, 15, 471.
[5] Beijing Institute of Pharmaceutical Industries: *Zhonghua Yixue Zazhi* **1977**, 57, 420.
[6] Beijing Institute of Pharmaceutical Industries: *Zhonghua Yixue Zazhi* **1977**, 57, 464.
[7] Shi, Y.M. *et al.*: *Zhonghua Yixue Zazhi* **1980**, 60, 623.
[8] Xue, Q.F. *et al*: *Zhonghua Yixue Zazhi* **1986**, 66, 334.
[9] Yu, H.P. *et al*: *Zhongxiyi Jiehe Zazhi* **1991**, 11, 291.
[10] Shi, L. *et al.*: *Zhongyao Yaoli Yu Linchang* **1989**, 5(5), 18.
[11] Shi, L. *et al.*: *Zhongyao Yaoli Yu Linchang* **1988**, 4(2), 14.
[12] Yu, X.J. *et al.*: *Hunan Yike Daxue Xuebao* **1992**, 17, 350.
[13] Hu, L.P. *et al.*: *Shanghai Zhongyiyao Zazhi* 1993, (4), 46.
[14] Qian, X.H. *et al.*: *Zhongxiyi Jiehe Zazhi* **1991**, 11, 533.
[15] Pang, P.K.T. *et al.*: *Planta Med.* **1996**, 62, 431.

[T. Kimura]

319.　　　*Pyrola japonica* **Klenze ex Alefeld**　(Pyrolaceae)

Ri-ben-lu-ti-cao (C), Ichiyakuso (J), No-ru-bal (K)

Herb
Local Drug Name: Ichi-yaku-so (J), Nok-su-cho (K).
Processing: Dry under the sun (J, K).
Method of Administration: Oral (decoction: J, K).
Folk Medicinal Uses:
　　　　　1) Rheumatism (C, J).
　　　　　2) Beriberi (J).
　　　　　3) Arthritis (C, J).
　　　　　4) Cystitis (J).
　　　　　5) Bruise (J).
　　　　　6) Snake bite (J).

7) Traumatic injury (J).

8) Edema (K).

Scientific Research:

Chemistry

1) Benzene derivatives.: 4-hydroxy-1-β-D-glucopyranosyloxy-5-methyl-2-(*trans,cis*-8-hydroxy-3,7-dimethyl-2,6-octadienyl) benzene [1].

2) Saponin: pirolatin [2–4].

Literature:

[1] Inouye, H. *et al.*: *Chem. Ber.* **1968**, 101, 4057.

[2] Inouye, H. *et al.*: *Chem. Pharm. Bull.* **1964**, 12, 255.

[3] Inouye, H. *et al.*: *Chem. Pharm. Bull.* **1964**, 12, 533.

[4] Inouye, H. *et al.*: *Chem. Pharm. Bull.* **1964**, 12, 888.

[C.K. Sung]

320.   *Diospyros kaki* **Thunb.**   (Ebenaceae)

Shi (C), Chi (H), Kaki (J), Gam-na-mu (K)

Fruit calyx (CP)

Local Drug Name: Shi-di (C), Chi-dight (H), Shi-tei (J), Si-che (K).

Processing: Dry under the sun (C, J).

Method of Administration: Oral (decoction; C, H, J, K).

Folk Medicinal Uses:

1) Hiccup (C, H, J, K).

2) Belching (H, J, K).

3) Nausea (K).

Leaf

Local Drug Name: Shi-ye (C), Shi-yo (J), Si-yeop (K).

Processing: Cut into pieces, then dry under the sun (C, J, K).

Method of Administration: Oral (tea or decoction; J, K; powder: C).

Folk Medicinal Uses:

1) Cough (J, K).

2) Bleeding of peptic ulcer (J).

3) Metrorrhagia (J).

4) Hypertension (C, J, K).

5) Arteriosclerosis (J).

6) Hemoptysis (J).

Fruit

Local Drug Name: Shi-zi (C), Chi (H), Si-byeong (K).

Processing: Peal the outer layer and dry (K).

Method of Administration: Oral (fresh or dried; H, K).

Folk Medicinal Uses:

1) Lung abscess (H).

2) Cough (C, H, K).

3) Alcoholism (K).
4) Acute gastritis (K).
5) Dysentery (K).
6) Hemoptysis (K).
7) Hematemesis (K).
8) Hypertension (C).

Scientific Research:
Chemistry
1) Steroids: β-sitosterol (wood) [1] .
2) Triterpenoids: betulinic acid, oleanolic acid, ursolic acid [2–3].
3) Naphthoquinones: diospyrol, mamegakinone, isodiospyrin, bisdiospyrin [4–5], plumbagin, diospyrin, neodiospyrin, 7-methyljuglone [6].
4) Flavonoid: lipeol [6], astragalin [7].
Pharmacology
1) Inhibitory effect on β-hexosaminidase release from rat basophilic leukemia cells [8].

Literature:
[1] Row, L. R. *et al.*: *Current Sci. (India)* **1964**, 33, 367.
[2] Iseda, S. *et al.*: *Yakugaku Zasshi* **1955**, 75, 230.
[3] Matsuura, S. *et al.*: *Yakugaku Zasshi* **1971**, 91, 905
[4] Yoshihira, K. *et al.*: *Tetrahedron Lett.* **1967**, 4857.
[5] Yoshihira, K. *et al.*: *Tetrahedron Lett.* **1970**, 7.
[6] Yoshihira, K. *et al.*: *Chem. Pharm. Bull.* **1971**, 19, 851.
[7] Nakaoiki, T. *et al.*: *Yakugaku Zasshi* **1960**, 80, 1298.
[8] Kataoka, M. *et al.*: *Natural Medicines* **1996**, 50, 344.

[T. Kimura]

321. *Buddleja officinalis* **Maxim.** (Loganiaceae)

Mi-meng-hua (C), Mut-mung-far (H), Wata-fujiutsugi (J), Mil-mong-hwa (K)
Flower (CP)
Local Drug Name: Mi-men-hua (C), Mut-mung-far (H), Mitsu-mo-ka (J), Mil-mong-hwa (K).
Processing: Eliminate foreign matter, and dry (C, K).
Method of Administration: Oral (decoction: C, H, J, K).
Folk Medicinal Uses:
1) Inflammation of the eye with lacrimation and photophobia (C, H, J, K).
2) Blurred vision in deficiency syndrome of the liver (C, H, K).
3) Nebula (C, H).

Scientific Research:
Chemistry
1) Flavonoids: linarin (buddleoside, acaciin) [1].
2) Triterpenes: mimengosides A, B [2].
3) Luteolin, luteolin-7-*O*-β-D-glucopyranoside, salidroside, verbacoside, isoaceteoside, echinacoside, apigenin, apigenin-7-*O*-β-D-glucopyranoside, acacetin, acacetin-7-*O*-

α-L-rhamnopyranosyl-(6-1)-β-D-glucopyranoside [4], 6'-N-pyridine-verbacoside, [5].

Pharmacology
1) Antiinflammatory effect [3].
2) Effect on smooth muscle [3].
3) Effect on central nervous system [3].
4) Uretic effect [3].
5) Anti-hepatotoxic effect [4].
6) Inhibitory effect on aldose reductase [4].
7) Antibacterial effect [5].
8) Anticancer effect [5].

Literature:
[1] Xu, L. X. *et al.*: *Yaowu Fenxi Zazhi* **1987**, 7, 106.
[2] Ding, N. *et al.*: *Chem. Pharm. Bull.* **1992**, 40, 780.
[3] *"Zhongyao Zhi"* **1994**, Vol. 5, 311.
[4] Matsuda, H. *et al.*: *Biol. Pharm. Bull.* **1995**, 18, 463.
[5] Zhao, Y.Y. *et al.*: *Progress in Drug Development from Medicinal Plants*. Proceedings of UNESCO Regional Symposium on Drug Development from Medicinal Plants. Oct. 25-27, 1996, Hangzhou, China, **1996**, 284.

[J.X. Guo]

322.   *Apocynum venetum* **L.**   (Apocynaceae)

Luo-bu-ma (C), Lor-boe-mar (H), Gal-jeong-hyang-pul (K)

Leaf (CP), **Whole plant**
Local Drug Name: Luo-bu-ma-ye (C), Lor-boe-mar (H), Ra-hu-ma (J), Na-po-ma (K).
Processing: Eliminate foreign matter, and dry (C, K).
Method of Administration: Oral (decoction: C, H, K).
Folk Medicinal Uses:
        1) Dizziness, palpitation and insomnia due to hyperactivity of the 'liver' (C, H, K).
        2) Edema with oliguria (C, K).
        3) Hypertension (C, H, J, K).
        4) Neurasthenia (C).
        5) Nephritic edema (C, J, K).

Scientific Research:
Chemistry
1) Amino acids: glutamic acid, alanine, valine [1].
2) Anthraquinone [1].
3) Tannins: catechin [1], gallotannin [2].
4) Flavonoids: rutin [1], isoquercetin [3], hyperoside (hyperin) [4], trifolin, astragalin [5].
5) Steroid: b-sitosterol [4].
6) Organic acids: succinic acid, chlorogenic acid [4].

7) Sugars: sucrose, D-*l*-bornesitol [4], meso-inositol [6].

8) Triterpenes: β-amyrin [4], lupeol [7], lupenyl palimtate [8].

9) Aliphatic compounds: myristoyl palmitate, hexadecyl palmitate [6].

10) Alcohols: triacontanol [6].

11) Alkanes: nonacosane, hentriacontane [6].

12) Inorganic constituent: KCl [6].

13) Long-chain fatty acid [7].

14) Coumarins: isofraxidin, scopoletin [7].

Pharmacology

1) Antihypertensive effect [1].

2) Sedative effect [7].

3) Effect on function of trachea (quercetin) [9].

4) Immunostimulant and inhibitory effect on the mutagenic of cyclophosphamide [10].

Literature:

[1] Northwestern Institute of Botany (China): *Zhongcaoyao Tongxun* **1972**, (4), 12.

[2] Jiang, D. F. *et al.*: *Zhongyao Tongbao* **1988**, 13, 548.

[3] Zhang, Z. J. *et al.*: *Zhongcaoyao Tongxun* **1974**, (1), 21.

[4] Nishibe, S. *et al.*: *Yakugaku Zasshi* **1978**, 98, 1395.

[5] Nishibe, S. *et al.*: *Shoyakugaku Zasshi* **1993**, 47, 27.

[6] Wang, M. S. *et al.*: *Nanjing Yaoxueyuan Xuebao* **1985**, 16(4), 35.

[7] Chen, M. H. *et al.*: *Zhongguo Zhongyao Zazhi* **1991**, 16, 609.

[8] Jiang, P. F. *et al.*: *Zhongyao Tongbao* **1985**, 10, 222.

[9] Dept. of Pharmacotherapeutics, Hebei New Medical College: *Xinyiyaoxue Zazhi* **1973**, 11, 24.

[10] Hang, B. Q. *et al.*: *Zhongguo Yaoke Daxue Xuebao* **1987**, 18, 144.

[J.X. Guo]

323. *Cynanchum atratum* **Bge.** (Asclepiadaceae)

Bai-wei (C), Bark-mei (H), Funabara-so (J), Baek-mi-ggot (K)

Related plant: *C. versicolor* Bge.: Man-sheng-bai-wei (C).

Root (CP)

Local Drug Name: Bai-wei (C), Bark-mei (H), Byaku-bi (J), Baek-mi (K).

Processing: Eliminate foreign matter, wash clean, soften thoroughly, cut into sections, and dry (C, K).

Method of Administration: Oral (decoction: C, H, J, K).

Folk Medicinal Uses:

1) Febrile diseases with invasion of the pathogenic factors into the blood (C, H, J, K).

2) Fever due to deficiency of yin or deficiency of blood after delivery (C, H).

3) Acute urinary infection, dysuria with hematuria (C, K).

4) Carbuncles and other subcutaneous pyogenic infections (C, H, K).

5) Rheumatism (H).

6) Edema (J).

Scientific Research:

Chemistry

    1) Volatile oils [1].

    2) Steroid glycosides and steroid: glaucogenin A, glaucoside C, glaucoside H, cynatratio-side F [2], cynatratioside A, B, C, D, E [3], atratosides A, B, C, D [4].

    3) Others: cynanchol (a mixture) [5].

Pharmacology

    1) Antifebrile effect [6].

    2) Antiinflammatory effect [6].

Literature:

[1] *"Zhongcaoyao Youxiaochengfen De Yanjiu"*, **1972**, Vol. 1, 417.

[2] Zhang, Z. X. *et al.*: *Chem. Pharm. Bull.* **1985**, 33(10), 4188.

[3] Zhang, Z. X. *et al.*: *Chem. Pharm. Bull.* **1985**, 33(4), 1507.

[4] Zhang, Z. X. *et al.*: *Phytochemistry* **1988**, 27(9), 2935.

[5] *"Quanguo Zhongcaoyao Huibian"* **1975**, Vol. 1, 303.

[6] Xue, B.Y. *et al.*: *Zhongguo Zhongyao Zazhi* **1995**, 20, 751.

[J.X. Guo]

324. *Cynanchum glaucescens* (Decne.) Hand-Mazz. (Asclepiadaceae)

Yuan-hua-ye-bei-qian (C), Weon-hwa-yeop-baek-jeon (K)

Related plant: *C. stauntonii* (Decne.) Schltr. ex Levl.: Niu-ye-bei-qian (C), Yu-yeop-baek-jeon (K).

Rhizome (CP)

    Local Drug Name: Bai-qian (C, K), Bark-chin (H), Byaku-zen (J).

    Processing: 1) Eliminate foreign matter, wash clean, soften thoroughly, cut into sections, and dry (C, K).

              2) Stir-fry with honey until not sticky to fingers (C).

    Method of Administration: Oral (decoction: C, H, J, K).

    Folk Medicinal Uses:

              1) Cough with copious expectoration and dyspnea (C, H, J, K).

Scientific Research:

Chemistry

    1) Glycogenins: glaucogenin-A, glaucogenin-B [1].

    2) Glycosides: glaucogenin-C mono D-thevetoside [1], glaucoside-A, B, C, D, E [2], glaucoside-F, G [3], glaucoside-H, I, J [4].

    3) Disaccharide: glaucobiose [5].

Pharmacology

    1) Expectorant effect [6].

    2) Antitussive effect [6].

    3) Antiasthmatic effect [6].

    4) Antiinflammatory effect [6].

Literature:

[1] Nakagawa, T. *et al.: Tetrahedron Lett.* **1982**, 23, 757.

[2] Nakagawa, T. *et al.: Tennen Yuki Kagobutsu Toronkai Koen Yoshisha,* 24th, **1981**, 79.

[3] Nakagawa, T. *et al.: Chem. Pharm. Bull.* **1983**, 31, 879.

[4] Nakagawa, T. *et al.: Chem. Pharm. Bull.* **1983**, 31, 2244.

[5] Nakagawa, T. *et al.: Tetrahedron Lett.* **1982**, 23, 5431.

[6] Liang, A.H. *et al.: Zhongguo Zhongyao Zazhi* **1995**, 20, 178.

[J.X. Guo]

325. *Cynanchum paniculatum* (Bunge) Kitag. (Asclepiadaceae)
[=*Pycnostelma paniculatum* (Bunge) K. Schum.]

Xu-chang-qing (C), Liu-diu-juk (H), Suzu-saiko (J), San-hae-bak (K)

Root (CP)

Local Drug Name: Xu-chang-qing (C), Liu-diu-juk (H), Jo-cho-kei (J), Seo-jang-gyeong (K).

Processing: Eliminate foreign matter, wash clean rapidly, cut into sections, and dry in the shade (C, K).

Method of Administration: Oral (decoction: C, J, K); Topical (decoction: J).

Folk Medicinal Uses:

        1) Rheumatic arthralgia (C, H, J, K).

        2) Epigastric pain and distension (C, H, J, K).

        3) Toothache (C, J, K).

        4) Lumbago (C, K).

        5) Traumatic injury (C, H, K).

        6) Urticaria (C, K).

        7) Eczema (C, K).

        8) Snake bite (H).

        9) Herpes zoster (H).

        10) Ascites (H).

        11) Cirrhosis (H).

        12) Dysmenorrhea (H).

        13) Gastric ulcer (H).

Scientific Research:

Chemistry

    1) Phenols: paeonol [1], iso-paeonol [2].

    2) Glycosides: cyanpanosides A-C [3], neocynapanoside A [4].

    3) Aliphatic compounds: crythritol, triacontane, stearic acid decyl ester, hexadecene [2].

    4) Steroid: sitosterol [2].

Pharmacology

    1) Antiseptic effect (paeonol) [5].

    2) Blood-lipiod lowering effect [6].

    3) Analgesic effect (iso-paeonol) [7].

    4) Gastrointestinal motility inhibitory effect (iso-paeonol, paeonol) [7].

Literature:

[1] Lin, Y. X. *et al.*: *Yaoxue Xuebao* **1963**, 10, 576.

[2] Lou, F. C. *et al.*: *Zhonggou Yaoke Daxue Xuebao* **1989**, 20, 167.

[3] Sugama, K. *et al.*: *Chem. Pharm. Bull.* **1986**, 34, 4500.

[4] Sugama, K. *et al.*: *Phytochemistry* **1988**, 27, 3984.

[5] *Igaku Chuo Zasshi* **1963**, 184, 125.

[6] Basic Theory Group: *Xin Yiyaoxue Zhazhi* **1977**, 4, 31.

[7] Sun, F. Z. *et al.*: *Zhongguo Zhongyao Zazhi* **1993**, 18(6), 362.

[J.X. Guo]

326. *Cynanchum stauntoni* Schltr. ex Levl. (Asclepiadaceae)

Liu-ye-bai-qian (C), Bark-chin (H), Byakuzen (J), Baek-jeon (K)

Rhizome (CP)

Local Drug Name: Bai-qian (C), Bark-chin (H), Byaku-zen (J), Baek-jeon (K).

Processing: Eliminate foreign matter, wash clean, soften thoroughly, cut into sections, and dry (C), stir-fry with honey (C), dry under the sun (K).

Method of Administration: Oral (decoction: C, H, J, K).

Folk Medicinal Uses:

> 1) Cough (C, H, J, K).
> 2) Sputum (C, H, J, K).
> 3) Asthma (J, K).

Scientific Research:

Chemistry

> 1) Triterpenoid: hancockinol [1].
> 2) Fatty acid, β-sitosterol [1].

Pharmacology

> 1) Antitussive effect [2].
> 2) Expectorant effect [2].
> 3) Antiinflammatory effect [2].

Literature:

[1] Qiu, S.X., *et al.*: *Zhongguo Zhongyao Zazhi* **1994**, 19, 488.

[2] Liang, A.H., *et al.*: *Zhongguo Zhongyao Zazhi* **1996**, 21, 173.

[3] Liu, D.X., *et al.*: *Zhongguo Zhongyao Zazhi* **1990**, 15, 617.

[4] Yin, X.J., *et al.*: *Mutat. Res.* **1991**, 260, 73.

[C.K. Sung]

327. *Rubia cordifolia* L., *R. akane* Nakai (Rubiaceae)

Qian-cao (C), Chin-cho (H), Akane (J), Ggok-du-seo-ni (K)

Root (CP)

Local Drug Name: Qian-cao (C), Chin-cho (H), Sei-so (J), Cheon-cho-geun (K).
Processing: Wash clean, cut into slices, and dry under the sun (C, J, K).
Method of Administration: Oral (decoction: C, J, K); Topical (powder or decoction: C).
Folk Medicinal Uses:

        1) Dysmenorrhea (C, H, J, K).
        2) Epistaxis (C, H).
        3) Uterine bleeding (C, H).
        4) Amenorrhea with blood stasis (C, H).
        5) Arthralgia, traumatic swelling and pain (C, H).
        6) Hemoptysis, hematemesis (C, H, J).
        7) Analgesic (K).
        8) Hepatitis (C, H).
        9) Dermatitis (H).

Scientific Research:

Chemistry
   1) Cyclic hexapeptides: RA-I, II, III, IV, V, VII [1–4, 7].
   2) Lignans [8].
   3) Anthraquinones: 2-ethoxycarbonyl-1-hydroxyanthraquinone [9].
   4) Polysaccharide [10].
Pharmacology
   1) Antineoplastic effect (cyclic hexapeptides) [5–6].

Literature:

[1] Itokawa, H. *et al.*: *Chem. Pharm. Bull.* **1986**, 34, 3762.
[2] Itokawa, H. *et al.*: *Chem. Pharm. Bull.* **1983**, 31, 1424.
[3] Itokawa, H. *et al.*: *Proceedings of the 13th International Congress on Chemotherpy* edited by Spitzy, K. G. and Karrer, K. Egermann, Vienna, **1983**, 284/100-284/113
[4] Itokawa, H. *et al.*: *Planta Med.* **1984**, 50, 313.
[5] Itokawa, H. *et al.*: *Chem. Pharm. Bull.* **1984**, 32, 284.
[6] Itokawa, H. *et al.*: *Proceedings of the 13th International Congress on Chemotherpy* edited by Spitzy, K. G. and Karrer, K. Egermann, Vienna, **1983**, 284/114-284/116
[7] Itokawa, H. *et al.*: *Tennen Yuki Kagobutsu Toronkai Koen Yoshishu* **1990**, 32, 72.
[8] Park, M. K. *et al.*: *Arch. Pharmacal Res.* **1990**, 13, 289.
[9] Okuyama, E. *et al.*: *Phytochemistry* **1990**, 29, 3973.
[10] Huang, R.Q. *et al.*: *Yaoxue Tongbao.* **1995**, 30(suppl.), 3.

        [C.K. Sung]

328.   *Arnebia euchroma* **(Royle) Johnst.** (Boraginaceae)
[=*Macrotomia euchroma* Pauls.]

Xing-jiang-zi-cao (C), Gee-cho (H)

Related plants: *Lithospermum erythrorhizon* Sieb. et Zucc.: Zi-cao (C), Ji-chi (K);
    A. guttata Bunge: Nei-meng-zi-cao (C).

Root (CP)

Local Drug Name: Zi-cao (C), Gee-cho (H), Nan-shi-kon (J).

Processing: Eliminate foreign matter, and cut into thick slices or sections (C).

Method of Administration: Oral (decoction: C, H); Topical (water or vegetable oil extract: C; ointment: J).

Folk Medicinal Uses:

   1) Purpura dark in colour due to presence of exuberant toxic heat in blood (C, H).

   2) Measles with inadequate eruption (C, H, J).

   3) Sores (C, H, J).

   4) Eczema (C, H, J).

   5) Scalds and burns (C, H, J).

   6) Hemorrhoid (J).

   7) Congelation (J).

Scientific Research:

Chemistry

   1) Naphthoquinones: shikonin, teracrylshikonin, β-hydroxyisovaleryshikonin, acetylshi-konin [1], dehydro-alkannin [2], isobutylshikonin, isovalerylshikonin, α-methyl-*n*-butylshikonin, β,β-dimethylacrylshikonin, deoxyshikonin [3–5], β,β-dimethyl-acryl-alkannin, β-hydroxyisovalerylalkannin, 1-methoxyacetylshikonin, β-acetoxy-isovalerylalkannin [6], L-alkannin [7].

   2) Benzoquinones: arnebinone, arnebinol, shikonofurans B and C, *dl-O*-methyllasiodi-plodin [8], arnebifuranone [9].

   3) Triterpenoids: tormentic acid, 2α-hydroxyursolic acid [10].

   4) Alkaloids: O^9-angeloyretronecine, O^7-angeloyretronecine [11].

Pharmacology

   1) Inhibitory effect on prostaglandin biosynthesis [8].

   2) Inhibitory effect on capillary permeability, edema and granuloma [12].

   3) Antiinflammatory effect [12].

   4) Fertility lowering effect [13–14].

   5) Antibacterial and antiviral effect [15–17].

   6) Antipyretic effect [18].

Literature:

   [1] Morimato, J. *et al.*: *Tetrahedron Letters* **1966**, 31, 3677.

   [2] Kyogoku, K. *et al.*: *Shoyakugaku Zasshi* **1973**, 27, 24.

   [3] Bandynkova, V. A. *et al.*: *Tr. Vses. S'ezda Farm.* **1970**, 1st, 253.

   [4] Konoshima, M. *et al.*: *Shoyakugaku Zasshi* **1974**, 28(1), 75.

   [5] Morimato, J. *et al.*: *Tetrahedron Letters* **1965**, 52, 47.

   [6] Fu, S. L. *et al.*: *Zhongcaoyao* **1986**, 17, 434.

   [7] Li, Z. L. *et al.*: *Yaowu Fengxi Zazhi* **1986**, 6(1), 41.

   [8] Yao, X. S. *et al.*: *Tennen Yuki Kagobustu Toronkai Koen Yoshishu* **1983**, 26, 134.

   [9] Yao, X. S. *et al.*: *Tetrahedron Letters* **1984**, 25(48), 5541.

   [10] Yang, M. H. *et al.*: *Planta Med.* **1992**, 58(2), 227.

   [11] Roeder, E. *et al.*: *Planta Med.* **1993**, 59, 192.

   [12] Lin, Z. B. *et al.*: *Beijing Yixueyuan Xuebao* **1980**, 12(2), 101.

   [13] Xie, L. X. *et al.*: *Shangyi Xuebao* **1959**, 6, 601.

   [14] Cheng, S. Q.: *Sichuang Yixueyuan Xuebao* **1959**, 3, 13.

   [15] Zhang, M. Z.: *Zhonghua Pifuke Zazhi* **1953**, 1, 21.

[16] Zhang, M. *et al.*: *Zhongcaoyao* **1989**, 20, 449.
[17] Tanaka, Y.: *Yakugaku Zasshi* **1972**, 92, 52.
[18] Xie, L. X. *et al.*: *Shanxi Yixue Zazhi* **1959**, 3, 13.

[J.X. Guo]

329.   *Elsholtzia ciliata* **(Thunb.) Hylander**   (Labiatae)

Tu-xiang-ru (C), Toe-heung-yu (H), Naginata-koju (J), Hyang-yu (K)

Herb
Local Drug Name: Tu-xiang-ru (C), Toe-heung-yu (H), Ko-ju (J), Hyang-yu (K).
Processing: Dry under the sun (C, H, K), or use in fresh (C).
Method of Administration: Oral (decoction: C, H, J, K).
Folk Medicinal Uses:
　　　　　　　　　　1) Common cold in summer (C, H).
　　　　　　　　　　2) Fever without perspiration (C, H).
　　　　　　　　　　3) Heat stroke (C, H).
　　　　　　　　　　4) Acute enterogastritis (C, H).
　　　　　　　　　　5) Choking sensation in chest (C).
　　　　　　　　　　6) Ozostomia (C).
　　　　　　　　　　7) Difficult urination (C).
　　　　　　　　　　8) Bad breath (H).
　　　　　　　　　　9) Paralysis (H).
　　　　　　　　　　10) Oliguria (H).
　　　　　　　　　　11) Pyodermas (H, external use).
　　　　　　　　　　12) Anasarca (J).
　　　　　　　　　　13) Neuralgia (J).
　　　　　　　　　　14) Rheumatism (J).
　　　　　　　　　　15) Lumbago (J).
　　　　　　　　　　16) Abdominal pain (J, K).
　　　　　　　　　　17) Vomiting (J, K).
　　　　　　　　　　18) Perspiration (K).
　　　　　　　　　　19) Diarrhea (K).

Scientific Research:
　Chemistry
　　1) Flavonoids: 5-hydroxy-6-methylflavanone-7-O-α-D-galactopyranoside, 5-hydroxy-6,7-imethoxyflavone, 5-hydroxy-7,8-dimethoxyflavone, 5-hydroxy-7,4'-dimethoxy-flavanonol, 5,7-dimethoxy-4'-methoxyflavone [1], 5,7-dihydroxy-4'-methoxyflavone, 5-hydroxy-7,4'-methoxyflavone, acacetin-7-O-β-glucoside [2].
　　2) Hydrocarbons: 6-methyl-tritriacontane, 13-cyclohexyl-hexoacosane [2].
　　3) Sterols: β-sitosterol, β-sitosterol-β-D-glucoside [2].
　　4) Fatty acids: palmitic acid, linoleic acid, linolenic acid [2].
　　5) Triterpenes: ursolic acid [2].

Literature:
[1] Zheng, S. *et al.*: *Gaodeng Xuexiao Huaxue Xuebao* **1989**, 10, 866.
[2] Zheng, S. *et al.*: *Zhiwu Xuebao* **1990**, 32, 215.

[C.K. Sung]

330. *Elsholtzia splendens* Nakai ex F. Maekawa (Labiatae)

Hai-zhou-xiang-ru (C), Heung-yu (H), Nishiki-ko-ju (J), Ggot-hyang-yu (K)

Herb (CP)
Local Drug Name: Xiang-ru (C), Heung-yu (H), Ko-ju (J), Hyang-yu (K).
Processing: Remove remaining roots and foreign matter, cut into sections (C, K).
Method of Administration: Oral (decoction: C, H, J, K).
Folk Medicinal Uses:
　　　　1) Attack of summer heat and damp manifested by chills and fever (C, H, J, K).
　　　　2) Headache (C, H, J, K).
　　　　3) Abdominal pain (C, H, J, K).
　　　　4) Vomiting (C, H, J, K).
　　　　5) Diarrhea (C, H, J, K).
　　　　6) Oliguria and no sweating (C, J).
　　　　7) Edema (H).

Scientific Research:
Chemistry
　1) Volatile oils: carvaerol, thymol, *p*-cymene, γ-terpinene, α-caryophyllene, α-hellandrene [1], elsholtzia ketone [2].
Pharmacology
　1) Antiviral effect [3].

Literature:
[1] Li, W. Z. *et al.*: *Yaoxue Xuebao* **1983**, 18(5), 363.
[2] Zhu, G. P. *et al.*: *Yaoxue Xuebao* **1992**, 27(4), 287.
[3] Institute of Chinese Materia Medica: *Xin Yiyaoxue Zazhi* **1973**, (12), 38.

[J.X. Guo]

331. *Lycopus cavaleriei* Leveille (Labiatae)
[=*L. coreanus* Levl., *L. ramosissimus* (Makino) Makino]

Swip-ssa-ri (K)

Related Plant: *Lycopus lucidus* Turcz.: Shirone (J).

Herb
Local Drug Name: Taku-ran (J), Taek-ran (K).
Processing: Dry under the sun (K).
Method of Administration: Oral (decoction: J, K).
Folk Medicinal Uses:
1) Female disease (J, K).
2) Menstrual disorder (J).
3) Disease after child birth (K).
Contraindications: Pregnancy.

Scientific Research:
Chemistry
1) Saponins.
2) Flavonoids.
Pharmacology
1) Cardiotonic effect.

Literature:
[1] Lee, H.K. *et al.*: *Kisul Yon'guso Pogo* **1963**, 2, 76.

[C.K. Sung]

332.   ***Ocimum basilicum* L.**   (Labiatae)

Luo-le (C), Law-luck (H), Kamiboki (J)

Related plant: *Ocimum basilicum* L. var. *pilosum* (Willd.) Benth.: Luo-le (C).

Whole herb
Local Drug Name: Luo-le (C), Law-luck (H), Ra-roku (J).
Processing: Dry under the sun (J, C).
Method of Administration: Oral (decoction; C, H, J); Topical (paste of fresh herb or
decoction: C).
Folk Medicinal Uses:
1) Dyspepsia (C, H, J).
2) Diarrhea (C, J, H).
3) Menstrual disorder (H, J).
4) Nephropathy (J).
5) Common cold caused by wind and cold (C, H).
6) Headache (C, H).
7) Stomach and abdominal distention (C).
8) Stomachache (C, H).
9) Traumatic injury (C, H).
10) Rheumatic arthritis (C, H).
11) Enteritis (H).
12) Snake bite (C).
13) Eczema (C).
14) Dermatitis (C).

Fruit
  Local Drug Name: Luo-le-zi (C), Ra-roku-shi (J).
  Processing: Dry under the sun (J).
  Method of Administration: Oral (Decoction: H, J).
  Folk Medicinal Uses:
                        1) Cataract (J).
                        2) Sore eye (H).
                        3) Corneal opacity (H).

Scientific Research:
  Chemistry
     1) Monoterpenes: *trans*-α-ocimene, *trans*-β-ocimene, *cis*-α-ocimene, *cis*-β-ocimene, α-myrcene, β-myrcene [1].
     2) Sugars: planteose [2].

Literature:
[1] Ohloff, G. *et al.*: *Ann* **1964**, 83, 675
[2] French, D. *et al.*: *Biochem. Biophys.* **1959**, 85, 471.

[T. Kimura]

333.   *Phlomis umbrosa* **Turcz.**   (Labiatae)

                        Zao-su (C), Sok-dan (K)

Root
  Local Drug Name: Zao-su (C), Sok-dan (K).
  Processing: Dry under the sun (K).
  Method of Administration: Oral (decoction: K).
  Folk Medicinal Uses:
                        1) Hemorrhage (K).
                        2) Tineapedis (K).
                        3) Common cold (C).
                        4) Bronchitis (C).

Scientific Research:
  Chemistry
     1) Organic acids: succinic acid [1].
     2) Miscellaneous: bentonicine [1].

Literature:
  [1] Zhu, D. *et al.*: *Zhongcaoyao* **1984**, 15, 380.

[C.K. Sung]

334. *Rabdosia japonica* Hara (Labiatae)
[=*Isodon japonicus* Hara, *Prectranthus japonicus* Koidz.]

Hikiokoshi (J), Bang-a-pul (K)

Related Plant: *Isodon glaucocalyx* (Maxim.) Kudo (*Prectranthus glaucocalyx* Maxim.):
Xiang-cha-cai (C).

Whole herb
Local Drug Name: En-mei-s (J), Yeon-myeong-cho (K).
Processing: Dry under the sun.
Method of Administration: Oral (decoction: J, K).
Folk Medicinal Uses:
        1) Dyspepsia (J, K).
        2) Anorexia (J, K).
        3) Abdominal pain (J, K).

Scientific Research:
Chemistry
   1) Diterpenes: Enmein, enmein-3-acetate[1-2], isodocarpin, nodosin, isodotricin, oridonin, ponicidin, epinodosinol, sodoponin, isodoacetal, nodosinin, odocinin [3], isodonal [4].
Pharmacology
   1) Antibacterial (enmein, oridonin).
   2) Antitumor (enmein, oridonin).
Literature:
[1] Fujita, E. *et al.*: *Chem. Comm.* **1967**, 252;
[2] Fujita, E. *et al.*: *Yakugaku Zasshi* **1967**, 87, 1076.
[3] Fujita, E. *et al.*: *Tetrahedron Lett.* **1966**, 3153.
[4] Kubota, T. *et al.*: *Tetrahedron Lett.* **1967**, 3781.

[T. Kimura]

335. *Capsicum annuum* L. (Solanaceae)
[=*C. frutescens* L.]

La-jiao (C), Lart-jiu (H), Togarashi (J), Go-chu (K)

Fruit (JP)
Local Drug Name: La-jiao (C), Lart-jiu (H), Togarashi (J), Go-chu (K).
Processing: Dry under the sun (C, J, K).
Method of Administration: Oral (tincture: C, H, J, K; powder: H, J, K); Topical (tincture: J; ointment: C).
Folk Medicinal Uses:
        1) Myalgia (C, H, J, K).
        2) Frostbite (C, H, J, K).

3) Areatic alopecia (J, K).

4) Dyspepsia (C, H, J, K).

5) Stomach ache due to cold syndrome of stomach (C).

6) Disorder of the stomach-qi (C).

7) Neuralgia (K).

8) Sputum (K).

9) Common cold (K).

10) Dysentery (H, K).

11) Lumbago (K).

Contraindications: Gastroduodenal ulcer, acute gastritis, pulmonary tuberculosis, hemorrhoid (C).

Scientific Research:

Chemistry

1) Acid amides: capsaicin-I, capsaicin-II (dihydrocapsaicin) [1], capsi-amide [2], capsianside [3].

2) Carotenoids: α-carotene, β-carotene, β-carotene monoepoxide, xanthophyll, violaxanthin, foliaxanthin, α-cryptoxanthin, β-cryptoxanthin, antheraxanthin, foliachrome [10], capsanthin [4, 12], capsorubin [11–13], nigroxanthin, cucurbitaxanthin B [5], cryptocapsin [13].

3) Steroid glycosides: capsicosides A, B, C, D [9].

Pharmacology

1) Tendency of stomac movement inhibition (ethanol extract) [6].

2) Local and general hypesthesia (capsaicin) [7].

3) Apnea, bradycardia, hypotonia (capsaicin) [7].

4) Sensory deprivation (capsaicin) [8].

Literature:

[1] Kosuge, S. *et al.*: *Nogeishi* **1958**, 32, 578; 32, 720; **1960**, 34, 811; **1961**, 35, 596; 35, 923; *Agric. Biol. Chem.* **1970**, 34, 248; Bennet, D. T. *et al.*: *J. Chem. Soc.* (C) **1968**, 442; Crombie, L. *et al.*: *J. Chem. Soc.* **1955**, 1025.

[2] Takahashi, M. *et al.*: *Yakugaku Zasshi* **1977**, 97, 758.

[3] Yahara, S. *et al.*: *Tetrahedron Lett.* **1988**, 29, 1943.

[4] Biacs, P. A. *et al.*: *J. Agric. Food Chem.* **1989**, 37, 350.

[5] Deli, J. *et al.*: *Chimia* **1994**, 48, 102; *Helv. Chim. Acta* **1993**, 76, 952.

[6] Sone, Y.: *Tohoku J. Exptl. Med.* **1936**, 29, 321.

[7] Molnar, J.: *Arzneim.-Forsch.* **1965**, 15, 718.

[8] Jansco, N. *et al.*: *Naunyn-Schmiedebergs Arch. exp. Pathol. Phrmakol* **1959**, 236, 142; Yaksh, T.L. *et al.*: *Science* **1979**, 206, 481.

[9] Yahara, S. *et al.*: *Phytochemistry* **1994**, 37, 831.

[10] Cholnosky, L. *et al.*: *Acta Chim. Acad. Sci. Hung.* **1958**, 16, 227.

[11] Zechmeister, L. *et al.*: *Ann.* **1934**, 509, 269; **1935**, 516, 30; **1940**, 543, 248; Karrer, P. *et al.*: *Helv. Chim. Acta* **1935**, 18, 1303; **1951**, 34, 2159; Grangaud, R. *et al.*: *Soc. Biol. Filiales*, **1952**, 146, 1577; Cholnosky, L. *et al.*: *Ann.* **1957**, 606, 194.

[12] Entschel, R. *et al.*: *Helv. Chim. Acta* **1960**, 43, 89.

[13] Barber, M. S. *et al.*: *Proc. Chem. Soc.* **1960**, 19.

[T. Kimura]

336.   *Hyoscyamus niger* **L.**   (Solanaceae)

Lang-dang (C), Hiyosu (J), Sa-ri-pul (K)

Seed (CP)
Local Drug Name: Tian-xian-zi (C), Ten-sen-shi (J), Cheon-seon-ja (K).
Processing: Dry in the sun (C).
Method of Administration: Oral or topical (decoction: C, K).
Folk Medicinal Uses:
　　　　　1) Gastric spasm and pain (C).
　　　　　2) Rheumatalgia (C, K).
　　　　　3) Asthma and cough (C).
　　　　　4) Traumatic injury (C).
　　　　　5) Schizophrenia (C).
Contraindication: Heart diseases, tachycardia, glaucoma, pregnancy.
Side effects: Neurological poisoning.

Scientific Research
Chemistry
　　1) Alkaloid: atropine, hyoscine, hyoscine N-oxide, hyoscyamine, skimmianine, atropine,
　　　　apohyoscine, apoatropine, α-belladonine, β-belladonine [1–3].
Pharmacology
　　1) Analgesic effect.

Literature
　[1] Phillipson, J. D. *et al.*: *J. Pharm. Pharmacol.* **1973**, 25(suppl.), 116P.
　[2] Phillipson, J. D. *et al.*: *Phytochemistry* **1975**, 14, 999.
　[3] Sharova, E. G. *et al.*: *Khim. Prir. Soedin.* **1977**, (1), 126.

[P.P.H. But]

337. *Physalis alkekengi* **L. var.** *franchetii* **(Mast.) Makino**   (Solanaceae)

Suan-jiang (C), Suan-cheung (H), Hozuki (J), Ggwa-ri (K)

Root, Rhizome
Local Drug Name: Suan-jiang-gen (C), Suan-cheung (H), San-sh o-kon (J), San-jang-geun
　　　　　　　(K).
Processing: Dry under the sun.
Method of Administration: Oral (decoction: J, K).
Folk Medicinal Uses:
　　　　　1) Fever (J, K).
　　　　　2) Cough (J, K).
　　　　　3) Diarrhea (J).
　　　　　4) Edema (J).

Whole herb
Local Drug Name: Suan-jiang (C), San-sho (J), San-jang (K).
Processing: Dry under the sun.
Method of Administration: Oral (decoction: J, K).
Folk Medicinal Uses:

       1) Fever (J, K).
       2) Cough (J, K).
       3) Diarrhea (J).
       4) Edema (J, K).
       5) Sore finger (K).
       6) Sore throat (K).
       7) Laryngitis (K).
       8) Carbuncle (K).

Persistent Calyx or **Persistent Calyx with Fruit** (CP)
Local Drug name: Jin-deng-long (C), Gwae-geum-deung (K).
Processing: Dry (C, K).
Method of Administration: Oral (decoction: C, K); Topical (paste: C).
Folk Medicinal Uses:

       1) Sore throat and hoarsenese of voice (C, K).
       2) Cough with yellow sticky sputum (C).
       3) Dysuria (C).
       4) Eczema (C).
       5) Edema (K).
       6) Jaundice (K).

Scientific Research:
Chemistry
  1) Steroids: physalin A [1], physalin B [2], 4-desmethylsterols [3], physalin N, physalin
     O, physalin P [4–5].
Pharmacology
  1) Cell differentiation inducer (physalin A) [1].

Literature:
[1] Sunayama, R. *et al.*: *Phytochemistry* **1993**, 34, 529.
[2] Kawai, M. *et al.*: *Bull. Chem. Soc. Japan* **1994**, 67, 222.
[3] Itoh, T. *et al.*: *Steroids* **1977**, 30, 425.
[4] Kawai, M. *et al.*: *Bull. Chem. Soc. Japan* **1993**, 66, 1299.
[5] Kawai, M. *et al.*: *Phytochemistry* **1993**, 31, 4229.

                          [T. Kimura]

338.   *Veronicastrum sibiricum* **(L.) Pennell** (Scrophulariaceae)

Cao-ling-xian (C), Naeng-cho (K)

Related plant: *Veronicastrum sibiricum* (L.) Pennell var. *japonicum* (Nakai) Hara: Kugaiso
      (J).

Herb:
Local Drug Name: Cao-ling-xian (C), Zan-ryu-ken (J), Cham-ryong-geom (K).
Processing: Dry under the sun (C, J, K) or use in fresh (C).
Method of Administration: Oral (decoction: C, J, K); Topical (paste of fresh herb: C).
Folk Medicinal Uses:

> 1) Common cold (C, K).
> 2) Rheumatalgia (C, J).
> 3) Myoneuralgia (C).
> 4) Cystitis (C).
> 5) Traumatic bleeding (C).
> 6) Arthritis (J).
> 7) Gout (J).

Scientific Research:
Chemistry
  1) Phenyl propanoids: isoferulic acid [1–2], 3,4-dimethoxycinnamic acid [2].
  2) Triterpenoids: 3-O-acetyloleanolic acid [2].
  3) Steroids: β-sitosterol, daucosterol [2–3], campesterol, campesteryl 3-O-D-glucoside, stigmasterol [3].
  4) Iridoids: minecoside, 6-O-veratryl catalpol ester, calalpol, aucubin, 6-deoxy-8-isoferuloyl harpagide [3–4].
  5) Sugars: D-mannitol [2–3].
Pharmacology
  1) Antiinflammatory effect [1].
  2) Analgesic effect [1].

Literature:
[1] Zhou, B *et al.*: *Zhongguo Zhongyao Zazhi* **1992**, 17(2), 102.
[2] Zhou, B *et al.*: *Zhongguo Zhongyao Zazhi* **1992**, 17(1), 35.
[3] Lee, S. Y. *et al.*: *Saengyak Hakhoechi* **1987**, 18(3), 168.
[4] Lee, S. Y. *et al.*: *Saengyak Hakhoechi* **1988**, 19(1), 34.

[C.K. Sung]

339.   *Campsis grandiflora* **(Thunb.) Loisel.**   (Bignoniaceae)
           C. chinensis **Voss.** [=*C. radicans* (L.) Seem.]

Ling-xiao-hua (C), Ling-siu-far (H), Nozenkazura (J), Neung-so-hwa (K)

Flower (CP)
Local Drug Name: Ling-xiao-hua (C), Ling-siu-far (H), Ryo-sho-ka (J), Neung-so-hwa (K).
Processing: Dry under the sun.
Method of Administration: Oral (decoction: C, H, J, K).
Folk Medicinal Uses:

> 1) Irregular menses, amenorrhea (C, H, J, K).
> 2) Urticaria (C, H, J).
> 3) Leukorrhea (C, H, K).
> 4) Hypogastric pain (C, H).

     5) Traumatic injury (C, J).
     6) Bruise (J).
Contraindications: Debility, pregnancy.

Root
 Local Drug Name: Zhi-wei-gen (C), Ling-siu-far-gun (H), Ja-wi-geun (K).
 Processing: Dry under the sun.
 Method of Administration: Oral or topical (decoction: C, K).
 Folk Medicinal Uses:
     1) Rheumatalgia (C, H, K).
     2) Acute gastroenteritis (C, H).
     3) Traumatic injury (C, H).

Scientific Research
 Chemistry
  1) Glycosides: campneosides I-II, acteoside [1].
  2) Iridoid glucoside: tecomoside, cachinesides I-V [2–3], campenoside, 5-
   hydroxycampeno-side [6], campsiside, 5-hydroxycampsiside [7].
  3) Flavanone disaccharides: naringenin 7-O-α-L-rhamnosyl(1→4)rhamnoside, dihydro-
   kaempferol 3-O-α-L-rhamnoside 5-O-β-D-glucoside [4].
  4) β-sitosterol, apigenin [5].
  5) Alkaloid: boschniakine [7].
 Pharmacology
  1) Apigenin showed analgesic, antiinflammatory, and bronchial dilatory effects [5].

Literature
 [1] Imakura, Y. *et al.*: *Phytochemistry* **1985**, 24, 139.
 [2] Imakura, Y. *et al.*: *Phytochemistry* **1984**, 23, 2263.
 [3] Imakura, Y. *et al.*: *Heterocycles* **1986**, 24, 2593.
 [4] Ahmad, M. *et al.*: *J. Chem. Res., Synop.* **1991**, (5), 109.
 [5] Chen, J. B. *et al.*: *Zhongcaoyao* **1981**, 12, 372.
 [6] Kobayashi, S. *et al.*: *Heterocycle* **1981**, 16, 1475.
 [7] Imakura, Y. *et al.*: *Chem. Pharm. Bull.* **1985**, 33, 2220.

                    [P.P.H. But]

340. *Androgrnphis paniculata* **(Burm.f.) Nees** (Acanthaceae)

       Chuan-xin-lian (C), Chuan-sum-lin (H), Sen-shin-ren (J)

Herb (CP)
 Local Drug Name: Chuan-xin-lian (C), Chuan-sum-lin (H), Sen-shin-ren (J).
 Processing: Eliminate foreign matter, wash clean, cut into sections, and dry (C).
 Method of Administration: Oral (decoction, powder: C, H); Topical (powder: C).
 Folk Medicinal Uses:
     1) Influenza with fever, sore throat, ulcers in the mouth or on the tongue
      (C, H).
     2) Acute or chronic cough (C).

3) Colitis, dysentery (C, H).

4) Urinary infection with difficult painful urination (C).

5) Carbuncles, sores, venomous snake bite (C, H).

6) Pulmonary tuberculosis (H).

Scientific Research:

Chemistry

1) Flavonoids: andrographidines A-F [1], apigenin-4',7-di-*O*-methyl ether, 5-hydroxy-2',3',7,8-tetramethoxy-flavone [2], apigenin-4,7-dimethylether, mono-*O*-methyl-wightin, panicolin A [3], 2',5-dihydroxy-7,8-dimethoxyflavone, 5-hydroxy-2',7,8'-trimethoxyflavone, 5-hydroxy-7,8-dimethoxyflavone [4], 5-hydroxy-2',3,7,8-tetra-methoxyflavone, 5-hydroxy-7,8-dimethoxy-flavanone [5], oroxylin, wogonin [6].

2) Diterpenes: andrographinin, andropanoside, 14-deoxy-12-methoxyandrographolide [7], andrographiside, deoxyandrographiside, 3,4-dideoxyandrographolide [8], androgra-pholide [9], 11,12-didehydro-14-deoxyandrographolide, 14-deoxy-19-β-D-gluco-side-andrographolide [10], 14-deoxy-11-oxy-andrographolide [11], 14-deoxy-andro-grapholide [12], deoxy-andrographolide, deoxyandrographolide 19-β-D-glucopy-ranoside [13], neo-andrographolide [14], andrographoside, 14-deoxy-andrographo-side [15], ninandrographolide [16].

3) Sesquiterpenes: γ-bisabolene [17], 2-*cis*-6-*trans*-farnesol, 2-*trans*-6-*trans*-farnesol [18], paniculide A, paniculide B, paniculide [19].

4) Monoterpenes: carvacrol [20], procumbide [21].

5) Phenylpropanoids: eugenol [20], caffeic acid, chlorogenic acid, di-*O*-caffeoyl-quinic acid [22],.

6) Alkanes: hentriacontane, tritriacontane [20].

7) Steroid: α-1-sitosterol [3].

8) Organic acid: myristic acid [20].

Pharmacology

1) Anaphylactic response [23].

2) Antiischemic effect (flavonoids) [24].

3) Cyclic AMP stimulation (flavonoids) [24].

4) Cyclic GMP inhibition (flavonoids) [24].

5) Platelet aggregation inhibition (flavonoids) [24].

6) Prostaglandin synthesis stimulation (flavonoids) [24].

7) Thromboxane B-2 synthesis inhibition (flavonoids) [24].

8) Cytotoxic effect [25].

9) Reverse transcriptase inhibition [25].

10) Antiviral effect [25–26].

11) Antitumor effect [27].

12) Cell differentiation induction [28].

13) Antiascariasis effect [29].

14) Antitoxic effect [30].

15) Cardiac depressant effect [30].

16) Hypotensive effect [30].

17) Smooth muscle stimulant effect [30].

18) Antibacterial effect [31].

19) Alkaline phosphatase stimulation [32].

20) Glutamate-oxaloacetate-transaminase stimulation [32].

21) Glutamate-pyruvate-transaminase stimulation [32].

22) Plasma bilirubin increase [32].

23) Nematocidal effect [33].

24) Abortifacient effect [34].

25) Antimutagenic effect [35].

26) Antidiarrheal effect [36].

27) Hypertriglyceridemia effect [37].

28) Antihepatotoxic effect [37–38, 48].

29) Antimalarial effect [39].

30) Antipyretic effect [40].

31) Antibiotic inducing effect [41].

32) Delayed type cutaneous hypersensitivity stimulation [41].

33) Macrophage migration stimulation [41].

34) Mitogenic effect [41].

35) Phagoccytosis rate increased [41].

36) Antiandrogetic effect [42].

37) Antigonadotropin effect [42].

38) Antispermatogetic effect [42].

39) Antifilarial effect [43].

40) Antiinflammatory effect [44].

41) Smooth muscle relaxant effect [45].

42) Toxicity assessment [45].

43) Vasodilator effect [45].

44) Barbiturate sleeping time decreased [46].

45) Choleretic effect [46].

46) Blood system effects [47].

47) Sialidase inhibition [47].

Literature:

[1] Kuroyanagi, M. *et al.*: *Chem. Pharm. Bull.* **1987**, 35, 4429.

[2] Govindachari, T. R. *et al.*: *Indian J. Chem.* **1969**, 7, 306.

[3] Ali, M. E. *et al.*: *Pak. J. Sci. Ind. Res.* **1972**, 15, 33.

[4] Jalal, M. A. *et al.*: *Phytochemistry* **1979**, 18, 149.

[5] Gupta, K. K. *et al.*: *Phytochemistry* **1983**, 22, 314.

[6] Zhu, P. *et al.*: *Zhongcaoyao* **1984**, 15, 375.

[7] Fujita, T. *et al.*: *Chem. Pharm. Bull.* **1984**, 32, 2117.

[8] Hu, C. Q. *et al.*: *Zhongcaoyao* **1981**, 12, 531.

[9] Tuu, N. V. *et al.*: *Tap Chi Puoc Hoc* **1984**, 2, 7.

[10] Chaichantipyuth, C. *et al.*: *Asian J. Pharm. Suppl.* **1986**, 6(8), 59.

[11] Balmain, A. *et al.*: *J. Chem. Soc. Perkin. Trans. I* **1973**, 1247.

[12] Medforth, C. J. *et al.*: *J. Chem. Soc. Perkin. Trans. I* **1990**, 6, 1011.

[13] Chen, W. M. *et al.*: *Phanta Med.* **1982**, 45, 245.

[14] Chan, W. R. *et al.*: *Tetrahedron Lett.* **1968**, 4803.

[15] Hu, C. Q. *et al.*: *Yaoxue Xuebao* **1982**, 17, 435.

[16] Meng, Z. M. *et al.*: *Nanjing Yaoxueguan Xuebao* **1982**, 1, 15.

[17] Overton, K. H. *et al.*: *Chem. Commun.* **1976**, 105.

[18] Overton, K. H. *et al.*: *Biochem. J.* **1974**, 144, 585.

[19] Allison, A. J. *et al.*: *Chem. Commun.* **1968**, 1493.

[20] Ojha, T. N. *et al.*: *Acta Cienc Indica [Ser] Chem.* **1983**, 9(1/4), 239.

[21] Abeysekera, A. M. *et al.*: *Fitoterapia* **1990**, 61(5), 473.

[22] Satyanarayana, O. *et al.*: *Leather Sci.* **1978**, 25.

[23] Guo, Z. X.: *J. Clinical Dermatology* **1987**, 16(4), 218.

[24] Zhao, H. Y. *et al.*: *Chung-hua I Hsueh Tsa Chi* **1991**, 104(9), 70.

[25] Yao, X. T. *et al.*: *Virology* **1992**, 187(1), 56.

[26] Chang, R. S. *et al.*: *Antiviral Res.* **1988**, 9, 163.

[27] Itokawa, H. *et al.*: *Shoyakugaku Zasshi* **1990**, 44, 58.

[28] Taki, T. *et al.*: *J. Pharmacobio. Dyn.* **1984**, 10(3), 60.

[29] Kaleysa Raj, R.: *Indian J. Physiol. Pharmacol.* **1975**, 19, 47.

[30] Nazimudeen, S. K. *et al.*: *Indian J. Pharm. Sci.* **1978**, 40, 132.

[31] Nakanishi, K. *et al.*: *Chem. Pharm. Bull.* **1965**, 13, 882.

[32] Sharma, A. *et al.*: *Fitoterapia* **1991**, 62, 131.

[33] Ali, M. A. *et al.*: *Shoyakugaku Zasshi* **1991**, 45, 206.

[34] Chen, Z. Z. *et al.*: *Zhongcaoyao* **1982**, 13(5), 32.

[35] Liu, D. X. *et al.*: *Chung-kuo Chung Yao Tsa Chi* **1990**, 15, 617.

[36] Gupta, S. *et al.*: *Int. J. Crude Drug Res.* **1990**, 28, 273.

[37] Handa, S. S. *et al.*: *Indian J. Med. Res.* **1990**, 92(4), 276.

[38] Bhaumik, A. *et al.*: *J. Res. Indian Med.* **1993**, 12(1), 33.

[39] Misra, P. *et al.*: *Int. J. Pharmacog.* **1991**, 29(1)19.

[40] Vedavathy, S. *et al.*: *J. Ethnopharmacol.* **1991**, 33, 193.

[41] Puri, A. *et al.*: *J. Nat. Prod.* **1993**, 56, 995.

[42] Akbarsha, M. A. *et al.*: *Indian J. Exp. Biol.* **1990**, 28, 421.

[43] Dutta, A. *et al.*: *J. Helminthol.* **1982**, 56, 81.

[44] Thamlikitkul, V. *et al.*: *J. Med. ASSN Thailand* **1991**, 74, 437.

[45] Feng, P. C. *et al.*: *J. Pharm. Pharmacol.* **1962**, 14, 556.

[46] Chaudhuri, S.K. *et al.*: *Indian J. Exp. Biol.* **1978**, 16, 830

[47] Zhao, H. A. *et al.*: *Muench Med. Wochenschr* **1990**, 132, 132.

[48] Chander, R. *et al.*: *Int. J. Pharmacognosy* **1995**, 33, 135.

[J.X. Guo]

341.   *Cistanche deserticola* **Y.C.Ma**   (Orobanchaceae)

Rou-cong-rong (C), Yuk-sung-yung (H), Jong-yong (K)

Related plant: *C. salsa* (C. A. Mey.) G. Beck.

Herb (CP)

Local Drug Name: Rou-cong-rong (C), Yuk-sung-yung (H), Niku-ju-yo (J), Yuk-jong-yong (K).

Processing: Eliminate foreign matter, wash clean, soften thoroughly, cut into thick slices, and dry, or stew or steam with wine (C).

Method of Administration: Oral (decoction: C, H, J, K).

Folk Medicinal Uses:

        1) Impotence, infertility (C, H, K).

        2) General weakness with aching of the loins and knees (C, H, J, K).

        3) Constipation (C, K).

        4) Lumbago (H).

        5) Leukorrhea (H).

Scientific Research:

Chemistry

   1) Terpines: 8-hydroxygeraniol-1-β-D-glucoside, 8-epiloganic acid [1], cistanin, cistachlorin [2].

   2) Organic acid: succinic acid [2].

   3) Sugar: D-mannitol [2–3].

   4) Amino acids [3].

   5) Steroids: β-sitosterol, β-sitosterd-β-D-glucoside [2], daucosterol [4].

   6) Alcohol: triacontanol [4].

   7) Alkaloid: betaine [4].

   8) Other: acteoside [4].

Pharmacology

   1) Antihypertensive effect [5].

   2) Salivant effect [5].

   3) Respiratory paralysis.

Literature:

[1] Kobayashi, H. *et al.*: *Yakugaku Zasshi* **1983**, 103, 508.

[2] Hiromi, K. *et al.*: *Chem. Pharm. Bull.* **1984**, 32, 1729.

[3] Luo, S. F.: *Zhongyao Tongbao* **1986**, 11, 681.

[4] Chen, M. H. *et al.*: *Zhongguo Zhongyao Zazhi* **1993**, 18, 424.

[5] Liu, S. S.: *"Zhongyao Yanjiu Wenxian Zhaiyao"* **1963**, 258.

                [J.X. Guo]

342.   *Lonicera japonica* **Thunb.** (Caprifoliaceae)

Ren-dong (C), Gum-ngun-far (H), Suikazura (J), In-dong (K)

Stem, Branch (CP)

  Local Drug Name: Ren-dong-teng (C), Yun-dung-teng (H), Nin-do (J), In-dong (K).

  Processing: Dry under the sun (C, J).

  Method of Administration: Oral (decoction: C, H, J, K).

  Folk Medicinal Uses:

          1) Suppuration (J, K).

          2) Infectious diseases as a blood cleanser (J, K).

          3) Arthritis (H, J).

          4) Epidemic febrile diseases (C).

          5) Acute dysentery (C).

          6) Carbuncles (C).

          7) Sores (C).

          8) Acute arthritis with redness swelling and pain of joint (C).

Flower (CP)

  Local Drug Name: Jin-yin-hua (C), Gum-ngun-far (H), Kin-gin-ka (J), Geum-eun-hwa (K).

  Processing: Dry under the sun, or dry after fumigating with sulfur (C).

  Method of Administration: Oral (decoction: C, H, J, K).

Folk Medicinal Uses:

1) Suppuration (J, K).
2) Infectious diseases as a blood cleanser (J, K).
3) Arthritis (J).
4) Carbuncles, boils (C).
5) Erysipelas (C).
6) Acute or bacillary dysentery (C, H).
7) Upper respiratory tract infection (C, H).
8) Influenza (H).
9) Epidermic febrile diseases (C).
10) Acute conjunctivitis (H).
11) Lobar pneumonia (H).
12) Lung empyema (H).
13) Acute mastitis (H).
14) Pyodermas (H).
15) Acute appendicitis (H).
16) Enteritis (H).
17) Cervical erosion (H).

Scientific Research:

Chemistry
1) Saponin:. loniceroside A [1], 3-O-α-L-rhamnosyl(1→2)-α-L-arabinopyranosyl
      hederagenin 28-O-β-D-xylopyranosyl(1→6)-β-D-glucopyranosyl ester, etc. [5].
2) Flavonoids: lonicerin [2], luteorin [3].
3) Tannins.
Pharmacology
1) Antibacterial [4].
2) Hepatoprotective effect [5].

Literature:

[1] Son, K. H., *et al.*: *Phytochemistry* **1994**, 35, 1005.
[2] Nakaoki, T. *et al.*: *Yakugaku Zasshi* **1961**, 81, 558.
[3] Nakaoki, T. *et al.*: *Yakugaku Zasshi* **1960**, 80, 1743.
[4] Sun, Y.B. *et al.*: *Zhongguo Zhongyao Zazhi* **1996**, 21, 242.
[5] Lou, H. *et al.*: *Progress in Drug Development from Medicinal Plants*. Proceedings of
      UNESCO Regional Symposium on Drug Development from Medicinal Plants. Oct.
      25-27, 1996, Hangzhou, China, **1996**, 344.

[T. Kimura]

343.   *Sambucus racemosa* **L. subsp.** *sieboldiana* **(Miq.) Hara**
     [=*S. sieboldiana* (Miq.) Blume ex Graebn.]   (Caprifoliaceae)

Jie-gu-mu (C), Niwatoko (J), Ddak-chong-na-mu (K)

Related Plant: *Sambucus williamsii* Hance: Jie-gu-mu (C); *S. buergeriana* Bl.:

Stem

Local Drug Name: Jie-gu-mu (C), Sek-kotsu-boku (J), Jeop-gol-mok (K).
Processing: Dry under the sun.
Method of Administration: Oral (decoction: J, K).
Folk Medicinal Uses:
  1) Bruise (J, K).
  2) Fracture (J, K).
  3) Nephritis (J, K).
  4) Edema (J, K).
  5) Articular rheumatism (J, K).
  6) Gastrectasis (K).

Leaf

Local Drug Name: Sek-kotsu-boku-yo (J), Jeop-gol-mok-yeop (K).
Processing: Dry under the sun.
Method of Administration: Oral (decoction: J, K).
Folk Medicinal Uses:
  1) Bruise (J, K).
  2) Fracture (J, K).
  3) Nephritis (J, K).
  4) Edema (J, K).
  5) Articular rheumatism (J, K).

Flower

Local Drug Name: Sek-kotsu-boku-ka (J), Jeop-gol-mok-hwa (K).
Processing: Dry under the sun.
Method of Administration: Oral (decoction: J, K).
Folk Medicinal Uses:
  1) Nephritis (J, K).
  2) Edema (J, K).
  3) Articular rheumatism (J, K).

Whole herb

Local Drug Name: Jie-gu-mu (C).
Processing: Dry under the sun (C).
Method of Administration: Oral (decoction: C); Topical (paste: C).
Folk Medicinal Uses:
  1) Fracture (C).
  2) Traumatic injury and bleeding (C).
  3) Rheumatic arthritis (C).
  4) Gout (C).
  5) Acute and chronic nephritis (C).
  6) Osteoarthritis deformans (C).

Scientific Research:

Chemistry
  1) Triterpenoids: α-Amyrin, betulin, oleanolic acid, ursolic acid [1].
  2) Steroids: β-sitosterol [1–2].
  3) Flavonoids: Kaempferol, quercetin, panacenoside [3].
  4) Tannins.

Literature:
[1] Inoue, T, *et al.*: *Hoshi Yakkadaigaku Kiyo*, **1962**, 11, 17.
[2] Yagi, A. *et al.*: *Shoyakugaku Zasshi* **1970**, 24, 44.
[3] Yagi, A. *et al.*: *Yakugaku Zasshi* **1970**, 90, 1053.

[T. Kimura]

344.   *Patrinia scabiosaefolia* **Fisch.**   (Valerianaceae)

Huang-hua-long-ya (C), Ominaeshi (J), Ma-ta-ri (K)

Related Plant: *Patrinia villosa* Juss.: Bai-hua-bai-jiang (C), Otokoeshi (J).

Root
Local Drug Name: Bai-jiang-cao (C), Hai-sho-kon (J), Pae-jang (K).
Processing: Dry under the sun (C, J).
Method of Administration: Oral (decoction: C, J, K); Topical (paste: C).
Folk Medicinal Uses:

         1) Appendictis (C, J, K).
         2) Diarrhea (J, K).
         3) Leukorrhea (J, K).
         4) After birth (C, J, K).
         5) Eye diseases (C, J).
         6) Dysentery (C).
         7) Hepatitis (C).
         8) Enteritis (C).
         9) Sputum (K).
      10) Neuralgia (K).

Scientific Research:
Chemistry
    1) Saponin: patrinoside C, C1, D, D1 [1], scabioside A-G, sibirosides A, B, C [2],
      patrinia-glycosides A-I, B-I, B-II [5], sulfapatrinosides I, II [6], 3-O-α-L-arabino-
      pyranosyl hederagenin 28-O-β-D-glucopyranosyl-(1→6)-β-D-glucopyranoside, 3-
      O-β-D-glucopyranosyl-(1→3)-α-L-rhamnopyranosyl-(1→3)-α-L-arabinopyranosyl
      oleanolic acid, and its 28-O-β-D-glucopyranosyl-(1→6)-β-D-glucopyranoside [3].
    2) Triterpenoids: oleanolic acid, hederagenin [1].
    3) Iridoids: patrinoside [4].
    4) Essential oil: patrinene, isopatrinene.
Pharmacology
    1) Cat attractive [7].

Literature:
[1] Sidorovich, T. N.: *Apotech Delod.* **1966**, 15, 38.
[2] Bukharov, V. G. *et al.*: *Fiz. Khim. Akad. Nauk. SSR.* **1971**, 123.
[3] Choi, J. S. *et al.*: *Planta Med.* **1987**, 53, 62.
[4] Taguchi, H. *et al.*: *Chem. Pharm. Bull.* **1974**, 22, 1935; **1979**, 27, 1275.
[5] Nakanishi, T. *et al.*: *Chem. Pharm. Bull.* **1993**, 41, 183.

[6] Inada, A. *et al.*: *Chem. Pharm. Bull.* **1989**, 36, 4269.
[7] Motomura, I.: *Shokubutsu Kenkyu Zasshi* **1968**, 43, 124.

[T. Kimura]

345. *Dipsacus asperoides* C.Y. Cheng et T.M. Ai (Dipsacaceae)

Chuan-xu-duan (C), Juk-duan (H), Cheon-sok-dan (K)

Root (CP)
Local Drug Name: Xu-duan (C), Juk-duan (H), Sok-dan (K).
Processing: Wash clean, soften thoroughly, cut into thin slices, and dry (C).
Method of Administration: Oral (decoction: C, H, J, K).
Folk Medicinal Uses:

      1) Aching and weakness of the loins and knees (C, H, J, K).
      2) Rheumatic arthralgia (C, H, J, K).
      3) Abnormal uterine bleeding or excessive menstrual flow (C, J).
      4) Traumatic injury (C, H, J, K).

Scientific Research:
Chemistry
    1) Triterpenes: akebia saponin D, akebia saponin D-4'-*O*-acetate [1], 3-*O*-(4-*O*-acetyl)-
        α-L-arabinopyranosyl-hederagenin-28-*O*-β-D-glucopyranosyl(1→6)-β-D-glucopy-
        ranoside, 3-*O*-α-L-arabinopyranosyl-oleanolic acid-28-*O*-β-D-glucopyranosyl-
        (1→6)-β-D-glucopyranoside [2], 3-*O*-[β-*O*-xylopyranosyl(1→4)-β-D-glucopy-
        ranosyl-(1→4)][α-L-rhamnopyranosyl(1→3)]-β-D-glucopyranosyl(1→3)-α-L-
        rhamno-pyranosyl(1→2)-α-arabinopyranosyl-hederagenin, 3-*O*-[β-D-xylopyrano-
        syl(1→4)-β-D-glucopyranosyl(1→4)][α-L-rhamnopyranosyl (1→3)]-β-D-gluco-
        pyranosyl (1→3)-α-L-rhamnopyranosyl (1→2)-α-L-arabinopyranosyl-hedera-
        genin-28-*O*-β-D-glucopyranosyl (1→6)-β-D-glucopyranosyl-ester [3], 3-*O*-[β-D-
        glucopyranosyl (1→4)][α-L-rhamnopyranosyl(1→3)]-β-D-gluco-pyranosyl
        (1→3)-α-L-rhamnopy-ranosyl(1→2)-α-arabinopyranosyl-hederagenin, 3-*O*-[β-D-
        glucopyranosyl(1→4)] [α-L-rhamnopyranosyl (1→3)]-β-D-glucopyranosyl
        (1→3)-α-L-rhamnopyranosyl (1→2)-α-arabinopyranosyl-hederagenin-28-*O*-β-D-
        glucopyranosyl (1→6)-β-S-glucopyranosyl ester, 3-*O*-L-β-D-xylopyranosyl
        (1→4)-β-S-glucopyranosyl(1→4)] [α-L-rhamnopyranosyl(1→3)]-β-S-glucopy-
        ranosyl(1→3)-α-L-rhamnopyranosyl (1→2)-α-arabinopyranosyl-oleanolic acid-
        28-*O*-β-D-glucopyranosyl(1→6)-β-D-glucopyranosyl ester [4], hederagenin,
        hederagenin 3-*O*-α-L-arabinoside, 3-*O*-α-L-arabinopyranosyl-hederagenin 28-*O*-
        β-D-glucopyranosyl ester, hederagenin 28-*O*-β-D-glucopyranosyl (1→6)-β-D-
        glucopyranosyl ester (dipsacus saponin A) [5].
    2) Iridoid glycosides: sweroside, loganin, cantleyoside [1].
    3) Steroids: daucosterol, β-sitosterol [2].
    4) Sugar: sucrose [2].
Pharmacology
    1) Protective effect on vitamin E deficiency [6].

Literature:

[1] Kouno, I. *et al.*: *Phytochemistry* **1990**, 29, 338.

[2] Zhang, Y. W. *et al.*: *Yaoxue Xuebao* **1991**, 26, 676.

[3] Zhang, Y. W. *et al.*: *Yaoxue Xuebao* **1992**, 27, 912.

[4] Zhang, Y. W. *et al.*: *Yaoxue Xuebao* **1993**, 28, 358.

[5] Jurg, K. Y. *et al.*: *Arch. Pharmacol. Res.* **1993**, 16, 32.

[6] Ni, Z. Q. *et al.*: *Chin. J. Physiol.* **1941**, 16, 379.

[J.X. Guo]

346. *Codonopsis pilosula* (Franch.) Nannf. (Campanulaceae)

Dang-shen (C), Dong-sum (H), Hikage-no-tsuru-ninjin (J), Man-sam (K)

Related plants: *C. pilosula* Nannf. var. *modesta* (Nannf.) L.T. Shen: Su-hua-dang-shen (C); *C. tangshen* Oliv.: Chuan-dang-shen (C).

Root (CP)

Local Drug Name: Dang-shen (C), Dong-sum (H), To-jin (J), Man-sam (K).

Processing: Eliminate foreign matter, wash clean, soften thoroughly, cut into thick slices, and dry (C, K).

Method of Administration: Oral (decoction: C, H, J, K).

Folk Medicinal Uses:

1) Weakness of the spleen and the lung manifested by shortness of breath (C, H, J, K).

2) Cough (C, K).

3) Palpitation (C, K).

4) Anorexia (C, J, K).

5) Loose stools (C).

6) Diabetes caused by internal heat (C).

7) General weakness (J).

8) Puerperium (K).

Contraindication: Incompatible with herbs derived from *Veratrum* spp. (C).

Scientific Research:

Chemistry

1) Sugars and glycosides: gluose, sucorse, fructuse, inulin [1], heteropolysaccharide CP_1, CP_2, CP_3, CP_4 [2], *n*-hexyl-β-D-glucopyranoside, ethyl-α-D-fructofuranoside [3], syrigin [3–5], (*E*)-2-hexenyl-β-D-glucopyranosyl-(1→2)-β-D-glucopyranoside, (*E*)-2-hexenyl-α-L-arabinopyranosyl-(1→6)-β-D-glucopyranoside, hexyl-β-D-glucopy-ranosyl-(1→6)-β-D-glucopyranoside, hexyl-β-D-glucopyranosyl-(1→2)-β-D-glucopyranoside, (6R,7R)-*trans,-trans,-trans*-tetradeca-4,12-diene-8,10-diyne-1,6,7-triol-*O*-β-D-glucopyranoside, (*Z*)-3-hexenyl-β-D-glucopyranoside, (*E*)-2-hexenyl-β-D-glucopyranoside, tangshenoside I, II, III, IV [4–5], compound F [6].

2) Steroids: α-spinasterol, stigmasterol, Δ^7-stigmasterol [7], Δ^7-stigmasteryl-β-D-glucoside [8], α-spina-steryl-β -D-glucoside , stigmasteryl-β-D-glucoside, stigmasta-7,22-diene-3-one, stigmasta-5,22-diene-3-one, stimasta-7-ene-3-one [9].

3) Alkaloids and nitrogen compounds: nicotinic acid, 5-hydroxy-2-pyridinmethand [3], $C_{11}H_8N_2$ [7], *n*-butyl-allophanate [10], choline [11], codopiloic acid [12].

4) Triterpenoids: taraxerol [9–10], taraxeryl acetate, friedelin [10].

5) Essential oils: palmitate acid, etc [13].

6) Trace elements: K, Na, Ca, Mg, Fe, Cu, Co, Zn, Mn, Cr, Mo, Sn, Sr, Al [1].

7) Amino acids: Lys, Thr, Val, Met, Ile, Leu, Phe, Asp, Ser, Glu, Glg, Ala, Cgs, Tyr, His, Arg, Pro, Asp-NH$_2$, Glu-NH$_2$ [1, 11, 14].

8) Others: 2-furancarboxylate, atractylenolide II, III, syringaldehyde, diethylphthalate, vanillic acid [3], methyl palmitate [7], 5-(hydroxymethyl)-2-furaldehyde, 5-(methoxymethyl)-2-furaldehyde [15].

Pharmacology

1) Antihypertensive effect [16].

2) Inhibitory effect on heart [17–18].

3) Blood picture altering effect [17–18].

4) Thromoboplastic effect [18].

5) Blood sugar elevating effect [18].

6) Intensive effect on uterine contraction [18].

7) Immunoenhancement [19].

8) Antiinflammatory effect [19].

9) Regulatory effect on gastrointestinal kinesis [19–20].

10) Ulcer-preventive effect [21].

11) Antagonistic effect on oxygen deficit [22].

12) Accelerated respiration [23].

13) Inhibitory effect on mobility [24].

14) Inhibitory effect on central nervous system [25].

15) Memory improving effect [26].

16) Analgesic effect [27].

17) Radiation protective effect [28].

18) Senility preventive effect [29].

Literature:

[1] Cai, D. G. *et al.*: *Zhongcaoyao* **1982**, 13(10), 10.

[2] Zhang, S. C. *et al.*: *Zhongcaoyao* **1987**, 18(3), 2.

[3] Wan, Z. T. *et al.*: *Zhongguo Yaokedaxue Xuebao* **1988**, 19(1), 61.

[4] Mizutani, K. *et al.*: *Chem. Pharm. Bull.* **1988**, 36(7), 2689.

[5] Masa Michi Yu Da, *et al.*: *Phytochemistry* **1990**, 29(6), 1989.

[6] Tanaka, O.: *Gendai Toyo Igaku* **1990**, 11(4), 103.

[7] Chen, H. S. *et al.*: *Zhongcaoyao* **1985**, 16(7), 7.

[8] Wan, H. K. *et al.*: *Zhongcaoyao* **1985**, 16(11), 4.

[9] Wan, Y. Z. *et al.*: *Zhongcaoyao* **1986**, 17(15), 41.

[10] Wan, Y. Z. *et al.*: *Zhongcaoyao* **1982**, 13(1), 1.

[11] Sa, D. Z. *et al.*: *Beijing Zhongyixueyuan Xuebao* **1987**, 10(6), 36.

[12] Wan, H. K. *et al.*: *Zhongcaoyao* **1991**, 22(5), 195.

[13] Liao, J. *et al.*: *Zhongcaoyao* **1987**, 18(9), 2.

[14] Hang, G. R. *et al.*: *Zhongcaoyao* **1991**, 22(9), 422.

[15] Lee, I. R.: *Yakhak Hoe Chi* **1978**, 22(1), 1.

[16] Liu, S. S. *et al.*: *"Zhongyao Yanjiu Wenxian Zhaiyao"* **1963**, 533.

[17] Zhao, S. X. *et al.*: *Huadong Yaoxueyuan Xuebao* **1956**, (1), 37.

[18] Wan, S. M. *et al.*: *Shanxi Yiyao* **1973**, (9), 22.

[19] Liu, G. Z. *et al.*: *Zhongxiyijiehe Zazhi* **1983**, 3(2), 114.

[20] Wu, P., et at.: *Zhongyao Tongbao, Zhongyao Lilun Zongkan* **1986**, (6), 147.

[21] Li, H. *et al.*: *Zhongxiyijiehe Zazhi* **1987**, 7(3), 166.

[22] Wan, K. Z. *et al.*: *Zhongyao Tongbao* **1986**, 11(8), 53.

[23] Zhang, Z. W. *et al.*: *Haerbin Zhongyi* **1963**, (3), 43.

[24] Pan, S. Y. *et al.*: *Zhongcaoyao* **1987**, 18(7), 19.

[25] Sun, Y. *et al.*: *Jilin Zhongyiyao* **1989**, (5), 36.

[26] Zhang, L. *et al.*: *Zhongyao Yaoli Yu Linchuang* **1990**, 6(6), 9.

[27] Research Group: *Xin Yiyaoxue Zazhi* **1974**, (12), 39.

[28] Liu, G. Z. *et al.*: *Zhongguorenmingjiefangjun Junshiyixuekexueyuan Yuankan* **1981**, (3), 303.

[29] He, J. Y. *et al.*: *Beijing Zhongyixueyuan Xuebao* **1988**, 11(5), 38.

[J.X. Guo]

347. *Artemisia asiatica* **Nakai** (Compositae)
[=*A. vulgaris* auct. non L.]

Ngie (H), Ssuk (K)

Herb

Local Drug Name: Ngie (H), Ae-yeop (K).

Processing: Dry under the sun (K).

Method of Administration: Oral (decoction: H, K); Topical (moxibustion: H).

Folk Medicinal Uses:

      1) Hemorrhage (K).

      2) Diarrhea (K).

      3) Common cold (K).

      4) Fever (K).

      5) Dysentery (H, K).

      6) Swelling (K).

      7) Abdominal pain (H, K).

      8) Uterine bleeding (H).

      9) Dysmenorrhea, irregular menses (H).

      10) Arthralgia (H).

      11) Pruritus (H).

      12) Eczema (H).

Scientific Research:

Chemistry

    1) Essential oils: thujone, caryophyllene, farnesol [1–3], benzaldehyde, pinene [2], 2-pyrrolodione, cineole, 1-acetylpiperidine, camphor, myrcene [2–3].

    2) Coumarin [2–3].

Pharmacology

    1) Bacteriocidal effect [1].

    2) Antimutagenic effect (myrcene, cineole, camphor, caryophyllene, coumarin, farnesol) [3].

Literature:
[1] Kim, Y.-S. *et al.*: *Han'guk Yongyang Siklyong Hakhoechi* **1994**, 23, 994.
[2] Kim, Y.-S. *et al.*: *Han'guk Yongyang Siklyong Hakhoechi* **1994**, 23, 261.
[3] Kim, J. O. *et al.*: *Han'guk Yongyang Siklyong Hakhoechi* **1992**, 21, 308.

[C.K. Sung]

348.   *Artemisia capillaris* Thunberg   (Compositae)

Yin-chen-hao (C), Yun-chan-hoe (H), Kawara-yomogi (J), Sa-cheol-ssuk (K)

Related plant: *Artemisia scoparia* Waldst. et Kit.: Bin-hao (C)

Young Herb (CP)
Local Drug Name: Yin-chen (C), Yun-chan-hoe (H), Men-in-chin (J), In-jin-ho (K).
Processing: Dry under the sun (C, H, J, K).
Method of Administration: Oral (decoction: C, H, J, K); Topical (hot decoction: C, H).
Folk Medicinal Uses:

1) Jaundice (C, H, J, K).
2) Inflammation (J, K).
3) Infectious icteric hepatitis (C, H).
4) Sores with exudation and itching (C).
5) Pruritus (H).
6) Dysuria (H).
7) Hepatitis (J).
8) Swelling (K).

Contraindications: Deficiency jaundice.

Flower bud
Local Drug Name: Inchin-ko (J).
Processing: Dry under the sun (J).
Method of Administration: Oral (decoction: J).
Folk Medicinal Uses:

1) Jaundice (J).
2) Hepatitis (J).

Contraindications: Deficiency jaundice.

Scientific Research:
Chemistry

1) Polyacetylenes: capillarin, dehydrofalcarinone, dehydrofalcarinol[1], norcapillene [2], capillanol [3], methoxycapillene [4], neocapillene [5, 19], capillene, capillone, capillin [23].
2) Terpenes: α-pinene, β-pinene, *p*-cymene, Δ^3-carene, α-terpineol, bornyl acetate, methyleugenol [24], β-elemene, β-caryophylene [1].
3) Flavones: cirsilineol, cirsimaritin, genkwanin, rhamnocitrin [6], arcapillin, eupatolitin [7–8].
4) Chromenes: capillarisin [9, 20–22, 27, 31], 7-methylcapillarisin [29].

5) Coumarins: scoparone [1, 10–11, 22], 6,7-dimethoxyesculetin [27].

6) Phenylpropanoids: capillartemisin A, B [12, 27], capillarol [21].

7) Organic acids: chlorogenic acid, caffeic acid.

8) Fatty acids: stearic acid, palmitic acid, oleic acid, linoleic acid, arachidic acid.

9) Plant hormones: abscisic acid, gibberellin A_3 [23].

Pharmacology

1) Increase of bile excretion (essential oil, capillarisin, capillartemisin A and B, scoparone, 6,7-dimethylesculetin) [9, 13–14, 20, 27].

2) Hepatoprotective effect (methanol extract, eupatolitin, arcapillin, scoparone) [7, 15–17].

3) Antiinflammatory effect (scoparone) [10].

4) Analgesic effect (scoparone) [10].

5) Treatment of biliary ascariasis (decoction) [18].

6) Antifungal effect (capillin).

7) Diuretic effect (water and alcohol extract).

8) Hypotensive effect [32].

9) Antipyretic effect.

10) Antianginal effect (scoparone) [25].

11) Hypolipemic effect [26].

12) Blood platelet aggregation inhibitory effect [26].

13) Antitumor effect (capillarisin, Capi-N, Capi-N-lys) [28].

14) Aldose reductase inhibitory effect (capillarisin, 7-methylcapillarisin) [29].

15) Vascular-dilatory effect (scoparone) [30].

Literature:

[1] Harada, R. *et al.*: *Phytochemisty* **1982**, 21, 2009.

[2] Miyazawa, M. *et al.*: *Phytochemisty* **1976**, 15, 223.

[3] Miyazawa, M. *et al.*: *Phytochemisty* **1975**, 14, 1874.

[4] Miyazawa, M. *et al.*: *Phytochemisty* **1975**, 14, 1126.

[5] Miyazawa, M. et al: *Phytochemisty* **1976**, 15, 1987.

[6] Komiya, T. *et al.*: *Yakugaku Zasshi* **1976**, 96, 855.

[7] Kiso, Y. *et al.*: *Heterocycles* **1982**, 19, 1615.

[8] Namba, T. *et al.*: *Phytochemistry* **1983**, 22, 1057.

[9] Komiya, T. *et al.*: *Chem. Pharm. Bull.* **1975**, 23, 1387.

[10] Yamahara, J. *et al.*: *Yakugaku Zasshi* **1982**, 102, 285.

[11] Singh, G. *et al.*: *Chem. Ind.* **1954**, 1294.

[12] Kitagawa, I. *et al.*: *Chem. Pharm. Bull.* **1983**, 31, 352.

[13] Aburada, M. *et al.*: *Yakugaku Zasshi* **1976**, 96, 147.

[14] Komiya, T. *et al.*: *Yakugaku Zasshi* **1976**, 96, 841.

[15] Kimura, Y. *et al.*: *Chem. Pharm. Bull.* **1985**, 33, 2028.

[16] Kiso, Y. *et al.*: *Planta Med.* **1984**, 50, 81.

[17] Hikino, H.: *Chin. Pharm. Bull.* **1985**, 20, 415.

[18] Wang, S. M. *et al.*: *Zhejiang J. Trad. Chin. Med.* **1985**, 20, 64.

[19] Yano, K.: *Phytochemistry* **1975**, 14, 1783.

[20] Ohshio, H. *et al.*: *Japan. Kokai* **76 09,709**, 26 Jan. **1976**, Appl. 74 81,370, 15 Jul. **1974**; 5 pp.

[21] Ueda, J. *et al.*: *Agric. Biol. Chem.* **1986**, 50, 3083.

[22] Miyachi, H. *et al.*: *Yakugaku Zasshi* **1987**, 107, 435.

[23] Ueda, J. *et al.*: *Agric. Biol. Chem.* **1987**, 51, 595.

[24] Yano, K. *et al.*: *J. Agric. Food Chem.* **1987**, 35, 889.

[25] Yamahara, J. *et al.*: *Chem. Pharm. Bull.* **1989**, 37, 1297; **1989**, 37, 485.

[26] Liu, Y.: U. S. US **4,842,859**, 27 Jun. **1989**, Appl. 905,554, 08 Sep. **1986**, 6 pp

[27] Hoshino, T. *et al.*: *Jpn. Kokai Tokkyo Koho* JP **01,285,118**, 16 Nov. **1989**, Appl. 88/114,171, 11 May **1988**; 7 pp.

[28] Xu, Q. *et al.*: *Wakan Iyaku Gakkaishi* **1989**, 6, 1.

[29] Yamaguchi, T. *et al.*: *Jpn. Kokai Tokkyo Koho* JP **01,228,914**, 12 Sep. **1989**, Appl. 88/53,551, 09 Mar. **1988**; 5 pp.

[30] Yamahara, J. *et al.*: *J. Ethnopharmacol.* **1989**, 26, 129.

[31] Tashiro, Y. *et al.*: *Jpn. Kokai Tokkyo Koho* JP **02,142,781**, 31 May **1990**, Appl. 88/296,096, 25 Nov. **1988**; 3 pp.

[32] Sharma, M.L.: *Indian J. Pharmacol.* **1985**, 17, 219.

[C.K. Sung]

349.   *Atractylodes japonica* Koidz.   (Compositae)

Guan-cang-zhu (C), Okera (J), Sap-ju (K)

Related plant: *Atractylodes macrocephala* Koidz. (*A. ovata* DC.): Bai-zhu (C), Bark-suet (H), Obana-okera (J).

Rhizome
Local Drug Name: Wa-byaku-jutsu (J), Baek-chul (K).
Processing: Dry under the sun (J, K).
Method of Administration: Oral (decoction: J, K).
Folk Medicinal Uses:

1) Gastrointestinal disorder (J, K).
2) Gastric neurosis (J, K).
3) Edema (J, K).
4) Rheumatalgia, arthritis (J, K).
5) General weakness (J, K).
6) Diarrhea (K).
7) Neuralgia (K).
8) Mastitis (K).

Scientific Research:
Chemistry

1) Sesquiterpenoids: atractylon, 3β-hydroxyatractylon, 3β-acetoxyatractylon, 5α,10β-selina-4(14),7(11)-dien-8-one, atractylenolide I, II, III [1].
2) Aldehydes: acetaldehyde, 2-furaldehyde [2].
3) Polyacetylenes: diacetyl-atractylodiol [3], (4E,6E,12E)-tetradecatriene-8,10-diyne-1,3-diol diacetate, (6E,12E)-tetradecadiene-8,10-diyne-1,3-diol diacetate [4].
4) Sugars: atractan A, B, C [5].

Pharmacology

1) Weak diuretic effect (ethanol extract) [6].
2) Inhibition of stress ulcer (50% methanol extract) [7].
3) Inhibition of blood permeability induced by acetic acid (50% ethanol or methanol extract, eudesma-4(14),7(11)-dien-8-one, atractilenolide I) [8].

4) Inhibition of adjuvant arthritis (decoction) [9].

5) Prevention of carbon tetrachloride hepatitis (ethyl acetate extract, atractylon) [10].

6) Choleretic effect (ethyl acetate extract) [10].

7) Tendency of increasing bowel movement (benzene extract) [11].

8) Antitumor effect (decoction) [12].

9) Blood sugar lowering effect (atractan A, B, C) [13].

10) Reticulo-endothelial system stimulatroy effect (inulin) [14].

Literature:

[1] Hikino, H. *et al.*: *Chem. Pharm. Bull.* **1962**, 10, 640; Nishikawa, Y. *et al.*: *Shoyakugaku Zasshi* **1975**, 29, 139; Idem.: *Yakugaku Zasshi* **1976**, 96, 1089; **1977**, 97, 515.

[2] Takahashi, S. *et al.*: *Yakugaku Zasshi* **1959**, 79, 541.

[3] Yosioka, I. *et al.*: *Chem. Pharm. Bull.* **1974**, 22, 1943.

[4] Kano, Y. *et al.*: *Chem. Pharm. Bull.* **1989**, 37, 193.

[5] Konno, C. *et al.*: *Planta Med.* **1985**, 51, 102.

[6] Haginiwa, T. *et al.*: *Shoyakugaku Zasshi* **1963**, 17, 16; Tsurumi, S.: *Gifu Ikadaigaku Kiyo*, **1963**, 11, 129, 138.

[7] Kubo, M. *et al.*: *Yakugaku Zasshi* **1983**, 103, 442.

[8] Endo, K. *et al.*: *Chem. Pharm. Bull.*, **1979**, 27, 2954.

[9] Cho, S. G. *et al.*: *Shoyakugaku Zasshi* **1982**, 36, 78.

[10] Yamahara, J. *et al.*: *Shoyakugaku Zasshi* **1983**, 37, 17; Kiso, Y. *et al.*: *J. Nat. Prod.*, **1983**, 46, 651; Kiso, Y. *et al.*: *Planta Med.* **1985**, 51, 97.

[11] Yamahara, J. *et al.*: *Yakugaku Zasshi* **1977**, 97, 873.

[12] Hsue, C. *et al.*: *Wakan Iyakugaku Zasshi* **1986**, 3, 31.

[13] Konno, C. *et al.*: *Planta Med.* **1985**, 51, 102.

[14] Matsuda, H. *et al.*: *Yakugaku Zasshi* **1987**, 107, 429.

[T. Kimura]

350. *Carpesium abrotanoides* L. (Compositae)

Tian-ming-jing (C), Tin-ming-jing (H), Yabu-tabako (J), Dam-bae-pull (K)

Fruit (CP)

Local Drug Name: He-shi (C), Hok-sut (H), Kaku-shitsu (J), Hak-seul (K).

Processing: Eliminate foreign matter, and dry in the sun (C, K).

Method of Administration: Oral (decoction: C, H, J, K).

Folk Medicinal Uses:

1) Ascariasis, oxyuriasis, taeniasis (C, H, J, K).

2) Abdominal pain or infantile malnutrition due to intestinal parasitosis (C, K).

3) Pyoderma (H).

4) Trichiusis (H).

Leaf

Local Drug Name: Ten-mya-sei (J).

Processing: Air-dry (J).

Method of Administration: Topical (ointment: J).
Folk Medicinal Uses:
        1) Burns (J).
        2) Bruise (J).

Scientific Research:
Chemistry
    1) Sesquiterpene lactones: carabrone, carpesia-lactone [1], granilin [2], carpesiolin [3], carabrol, ivaxillin, 11(13)-dehydroivaxillin [14], isoivaxillin, 11(13)-dihydrotele-kin, telekin [5].
    2) Organic acids: capronic acid [6], valeric acid, oleic acid, d-linolenic acid.
    3) Steroid: stigmasterol [6].
    4) Others: cerotin, triacontane, hentriacontane [6].
Pharmacology
    1) Antiscolic effect [7–8].
    2) Effect on nervous system [9].
    3) Antifungal effect [3].
    4) Antibacterial effect [3].

Literature:
[1] Kariyone, T. *et al.*: *Yakugaku Zasshi* **1949**, 69, 317.
[2] Marayama, M. *et al.*: *Phytochemistry* **1975**, 14, 2247.
[3] Marayama, M. *et al.*: *Phytochemistry* **1977**, 16, 782.
[4] Marayama, M. *et al.*: *Phytochemistry* **1983**, 22, 2773.
[5] Dong, Y. F. *et al.*: *Zhiwu Xuebao* **1988**, 30, 71.
[6] Naito, S.: *Yakugaku Zasshi* **1955**, 75, 39, 325, 355.
[7] Zhu, Y.: *Zhongyao De Yaoli Yu Yingyong* **1954**, 12.
[8] Kaku, T.: *Yakugaku Zasshi* **1943**, 63, 252.
[9] *"Quanguo Zhonggcaoyao Huibian"* **1975**, 1, 911.

[J.X. Guo]

351.   *Carthamus tinctorius* L.   (Compositae)

Hong-hua (C), Hung-far (H), Beni-bana (J), It-ggot (K)

Flower (CP, JP)
Local Drug Name: Hong-hua (C), Hung-far (H), Ko-ka (J), Hong-hwa (K).
Processing: Dry under the sun or in shade (C, J).
Method of Administration: Oral (decoction: C, H, J, K).
Folk Medicinal Uses:
        1) Arteriosclerosis (J).
        2) Menstrual disorder, amenorrhea, dysmenorrhea (C, H, J, K).
        3) Feeling of cold (J).
        4) Climacterium (J).
        5) Retention of lochia (C).
        6) Formation of mass in the abdomen (C).

7) Traumatic injury or sores with swelling and pain (C, H).
8) Lochia (H).
9) Measles (K).
10) Throat fever (K).
11) Contusion (K).
12) Boil of breast (K).
Contraindication: Use with caution in pregnancy (C, H, J).

Scientific Research:
Chemistry
  1) Phenolic compounds: carthamin, saflor yellow [1], kinobeon A [3], safflomin C [11].
  2) Alkanes: 6R,8S- and/or 6S,8R-erythro-hentriacontane-6,8-diol [4].
  3) Glucoside: luteolin 7-glucoside [13].
  4) Glycoside: tinctormine [14].
  5) Serotonin derivatives: 4,4"-bis(*N-p*-coumaroyl)serotonin, 4-[*N*-(*p*-coumaroyl)-
      serotonin-4"-yl]-*N*-feruloylserotonin, 4,4"-bis(*N*-feruloyl)serotonin [15].
  6) C-glycosyl quinochalcone: carthamoside [17].
Pharmacology
  1) Blood flow increasing (water or ethanol extracts) [2].
  2) Preventing expansion of myocardiac infarction (95% ethanol extract) [5].
  3) Vasodilatory effect against angiotonic activities of adrenaline and noradrenaline (75%
      ethanol extract) [6]
  4) Inhibitiory effect on platelet aggregation (adenosine in the water extract) [7].
  5) Analgesic, sedative and Antiinflammatory effects (50% methanol or water extract) [8].
  6) Inhibition of blood permeability (water extract) [9].
  7) Antitumor effect against Ehrlich's ascites (water or methanol extract) [10].
  8) Antitumor promotion effect (extract and stigmasterol) [12].
  9) Calcium-antagonist effect [14].
  10) Antioxidant effect [15].

Literature:
[1] Obsra, H., *et al.*: *Chem. Lett.* **1978**, 643; **1979**, 201; *Bull. Chem. Soc. Japan* **1980**, 53, 289; Takahashi, Y., *et al.*: *Tetrahedron Lett.* **1984**, 25, 2471.
[2] Todoki, K. *et al.*: *Kanagawa Shigaku* **1983**, 18, 64.
[3] Wakayama, S. *et al.*: *Z. Naturforsch., Sect. C* **1994**, 49, 1.
[4] Akihisa, T. *et al.*: *Phytochemistry* **1994**, 36, 105, 153.
[5] Wang, B.-Z. *et al.*: *Yaoxue Xuebao*, **1979**, 14, 474.
[6] Li, S.-Y. *et al.*: *Zhonghua Yixue Zazhi* **1979**, 59, 550.
[7] Kutsuna, H. *et al.*: *Yakugaku Zasshi* **1988**, 108, 1101.
[8] Kasahara, Y. *et al.*: *Shoyakugaku Zasshi* **1989**, 43, 331.
[9] Kiyoshige, T. *et al.*: *Kiso to Rinsho* **1983**, 17, 3175.
[10] Kosuge, T. *et al.*: *Yakugaku Zasshi* **1985**, 105, 791.
[11] Onodera, J. *et al.*: *Chem. Lett.* **1989**, 1571.
[12] Kasahara, Y. *et al.*: *Phytotherapy Res.* **1994**, 8, 327.
[13] Shigematsu, N. *et al.*: *Phytochemistry* **1982**, 21, 2156.
[14] Meselhy, M.R. *et al.*: *Chem. Pharm. Bull.* **1992**, 40, 3355.
[15] Zhang, H.L. *et al.*: *Chem. Pharm. Bull.* **1996**, 44, 874.
[16] Hattori, M. *et al.*: *Phytochemistry* **1992**, 31, 4001.

[17] Che, Q.M. *et al.*: *Progress in Drug Development from Medicinal Plants.* Proceedings of UNESCO Regional Symposium on Drug Development from Medicinal Plants. Oct. 25-27, 1996, Hangzhou, China, **1996**, 372.

[18] Huang, X.L.: *Shoyakugaku Zasshi* **1992**, 46, 210.

[T. Kimura]

352.   *Centipeda minima* **(L.) A. Braun et Aschers.**   (Compositae)

E-bu-shi-cao (C), Ngor-but-sik-cho (H), Tokin-sô (J), Jung-dae-ga-ri-pul (K)

Herb (CP)
Local Drug Name: E-bu-shi-cao (C), Ngor-but-sik-cho (H), A-bul-sik-cho (K).
Processing: Eliminate soil, and dry in the sun (C, K).
Method of Administration: Oral (decoction: C, H, K); Topical (decoction: C, H).
Folk Medicinal Uses:
1) Headache, cough, expectoration and nasal obstruction in common cold (C, H, K).
2) Sinusitis with nasal discharge (C, H, K).
3) Rhinitis (H).
4) Bronchitis (H).
5) Pertussis (H).
6) Ascariasis (H).
7) Amebiasis (H).
8) Malaria (H).
9) Traumatic injury (H).
10) Arthritis (H).
11) Stomachache (H).
12) Diarrhea (H).
13) Vomiting (H).
14) Eye disorder (K).

Scientific Research:
Chemistry
1) Volatile oils: palmitic acid, α-pinene, β-pinene.
2) Organic acids [1–2].
3) Tannins [1–2].
4) Resins [1–2].
5) Steroids: taraxasterol, taraxasteryl palmitate, taraxasteryl acetate, campsterol, stigmasterol, β-sitosterol, arnidiol [1–2].
6) Akohols: hexacosanol [3].
7) Triterpenoid sapoins and sapogenins: taraxerol [1], lupeol, lupeyl acetate [3], 1α,3β,19α,23-tetrahydroxyurs-12-en-28-oic acid-28-*O*-β-d-xylopyranoside, 1β,2α,3β,19α,23-pentahydroxyurs-12-en-28-oic-acid-28-*O*-β-d-xylopyranoside, 3α,21α,22α,28-tetrahydroxyolean-12-en-28-*O*-d-xylopyranoside, 3α,16α,21α,22α,28-pentahydroxyolean-12-en-28-*O*-β-d-xylopyranoside [4], 2α,3β,23,19α-tetra-hydroxyurs-12-en-28-oic acid-28-*O*-β-D-xylopyranoside,

3α,21β,22α,28-tetrahy-droxyolean-12-en-28-*O*-β-D-xylopyranoside,
3β,16α,21β,22α,28-pentahydroxy-olean-12-en-28-*O*-β-D-xylopyranoside [5],
3α,21β,22α,28-tetrahydroxyolean-12-ene, 3α,16α,21β,22α,28-pentahydroxy-
olean-12-en-28-*O*-β-D-xylopyranoside [6].

8) Phenols and phenolic derivatives: 3,3',5,5'-tetramethoxystilbene, 2-isopropyl-5-
methylhydroquinone-4-*O*-β-D-xylopyranoside [5], 3,5,4'-trimethoxy-*trans*-stilbene
[6], 10-isobutyryloxy-8,9-epoxythymol isobutyrate, 9,10-diisobutyryloxy-8-hydro-
xythymol [7].

9) Ester: tetratiacontanyl nonadecanoate [5].

10) Ketone: 6-hydroxy-hexacos-*trans*-8-en-3-one [6].

11) Sesquiterpene lactones: arnicolide C, helenalin, florilenalin isobutyrate, florilenalin
isovalerate, florilenalin argelate [7], 6-*O*-senesioylplenolin [8], isobutyroylplenolin
[9], 6-*O*-angeloylplenolin [10].

12) Amide: aurantiamide acetate [8].

13) Flavonoids: quercetin 3,3'-dimethylether, quercetin 3-methylether, apigenin [8].

14) Other: brevifolin [7].

Pharmacology

1) Antiallergic effect [8–9].

2) Inhibitory effect on PAF binding to platelets [10].

3) Bacteriostatic effect [11].

4) Antitussive, expectorant and antiasthmatic effect [11].

Literature:

[1] Murakami, T.: *Yakugaku Zasshi* **1970**, 90, 846.
[2] Wei, J. X.: *Zhongcaoyao Tongxun* **1976**, 1, 44.
[3] Sen, A. B. *et al.*: *J. Indian Chem. Soc.* **1970**, 47, 96.
[4] Gupta, D. *et al.*: *Phytochemistry* **1989**, 28, 1197.
[5] Gupta, D. *et al.*: *Phytochemistry* **1990**, 29, 1945.
[6] Gupta, D. *et al.*: *Indian J. Chem., Sect. B* **1990**, 29B, 34.
[7] Bohlmaun, F. *et al.*: *Kexue Tongbao* **1984**, 29, 900.
[8] Wu, J. B. *et al.*: *Chem. Pharm. Bull.* **1985**, 33, 4091.
[9] Wu, J. B. *et al.*: *Chem. Pharm. Bull.* **1991**, 39, 3272.
[10] Iwakami, S. *et al.*: *Chem. Pharm. Bull.* **1992**, 40, 1196.
[11] *"Yixue Kexue Jisu Jinyan Zhongjie Jiaoliu Huiyi Ziliao Huibian"* **1959**, 48.

[J.X. Guo]

353.　　　*Chrysanthemum indicum* L.　(Compositae)

Ye-ju (C), Yair-guk-far (H), Aburagiku (J), Gam-guk (K)

Flower (CP)

Local Drug Name: Ye-ju-hua (C), Yair-guk-far (H), Ya-giku-ka (J), Gam-guk (K).

Processing: Dry under the sun (C, K) or dry after steaming (C), extract with sesame oil (J).

Method of Administration: oral (decoction: H, K); Topical (decoction or ointment: C, H, J).

Folk Medicinal Uses:

　　　　1) Hypertension (H, K).

　　　　2) Abdominal pain (K).

3) Lumbago (K).

4) Acute gastritis (K).

5) Boils (C).

6) Carbuncles (C).

7) Inflammation of the eye (C).

8) Headache and dizziness (C).

9) Traumatic injury (J).

10) Common cold (H).

11) Prevention of epidemic encephalitis (H).

12) Pyodermas (H).

13) Mastitis (H).

14) Hepatitis (H).

15) Dysentery (H).

16) Furunculosis (H).

17) Snake bites (H).

18) Traumatic injury (H).

Side Effects: Nausea, vomiting.

Scientific Research:

Chemistry

1) Sesquiterpene lactones: angeloylcumambrin B, arteglasin A, angeloylajadin [1], handelin [2–3], chrysetunone, tunefulin [4], cumambrin A [5].

2) Essential oils: camphor [6], chrysanthenone, β-caryophyllene oxide, limonene, α-pinene [7], β-pinene, camphene, myrcene, 3-carene, α-phellandrene, α-terpinene, γ-cymene, β-ocimene, terpinolene, borneol [8].

3) Flavones: acaciin [9], luteolin 7-O-β-D-glucopyranoside [10], acacetin 7-O-β-D-galactopyranoside [11]

4) Terpenes: indicumenone [12], α-amyrin, β-amyrin, α-amyrin acetate, β-amyrin acetate, friedelin [7].

5) Lignans: sesamin [7].

6) Sterols: β-sitosterol [7].

Pharmacology

1) Anaphylactic effect (arteglasin A) [13–15].

2) Inhibitior effect on platelet aggregation [16].

3) Antimicrobial effect.

4) Hypotensive effect.

Literature:

[1] Mladenova, K. et al.: Planta Med. **1985**, 51, 284.

[2] Chien, M. K. et al.: Acta Pharm. Sin. **1963**, 10, 129.

[3] Chen, Z. N. et al.: Acta Pharm. Sin. **1987**, 22, 67.

[4] Mladenova, K. et al.: Planta Med. **1988**, 54, 553.

[5] Yu, D. Q. et al.: Acta Pharm. Sin. **1987**, 22, 837.

[6] Tsumaki, T. et al.: Repts. Res. Sci. Dept. Kyushu Univ. **1947**, 1, 10.

[7] De Pascual, T. J. et al.: Riv. Ital. EPPOS **1980**, 62, 236.

[8] Stoianova-Ivanova, B. et al.: Planta Med. **1983**, 49, 236

[9] Xu, L. X. et al.: Acta Pharm. Sin. **1987**, 22, 318.

[10] He, Y. Q. et al.: J. Beijing Med. Coll. **1982**, 14, 259.

[11] Chatterjee, A. et al.: Phytochemistry **1981**, 20, 1760.

[12] Mladenova, K. et al.: Planta Med. **1987**, 53, 118.

[13] Hausen, B. M. *et al.*: *Arch. Dermatol. Res.* **1976**, 255, 111.
[14] Hausen, B. M. *et al.*: *Z. Immunitaetsforsch.* **1977**, [Suppl] 2, 133.
[15] Hausen, B. M. *et al.*: *Naturwissenschaften* **1975**, 62, 585.
[16] Schulz, K. H. *et al.*: *Arch. Dermatol. Forsch.* **1975**, 251, 235.
[17] Yang, J. L. *et al.*: *Acta Acad. Med. Sin.* **1982**, 4, 306.

[C.K. Sung]

354.   *Cichorium glandulosum* Boiss. et Hout   (Compositae)

Mao-ju-ju (C)

Related plants: *C. intybus* L.: Ju-ju (C), Kiku-nigana (J), Chi-ko-ri (K).

Herb (CP)
 Local Drug Name: Ju-ju (C).
 Processing: Eliminate foreign matter, cut into sections (C).
 Method of Administration: Oral (decoction: C, J).
 Folk Medicinal Uses:
              1) Jaundice caused by damp-heat (C, J).
              2) Epigastric pain with impairment of appetite (C).
              3) Edema with oliguria (C, J).
              4) Nephritis (J).

Scientific Research:
 Chemistry
    1) Sesquiterpenes: 8-deoxylactucin, lactucin, lactupicrin [1], cichoriolide A, cichorio-
       sides A, B, C [2], cichoralexin [3].
    2) Coumarins: cichorin, esculine, esculetin [4], cichoriin (6-hydroxy-7-*O*-glucosyloxy
       coumarin) [5].
    3) Flavonoids: apigenin, luteolin, 7-*O*-β-D-glucopyranoside, quercitrin, hyperin, apigenin
       7-*O*-L-arabinoside [6].
    4) Organic acids: caffeic acid, chlorogenic acid, neochlorogenic acid, dicaffeyltartaric
       acid, 3-feruloyl acid, 3-*p*-coumaroylquininic acid [7].
    5) Anthocyanins: cyanidin 3-*O*-β-(6-*O*-malonyl)-D-glucopyranoside [8].
    6) Carbohydrate: inulin [9].
    7) Polyphenolic compounds [10].
 Pharmacology
    1) Cholagogue effect (polyphenolic compounds) [10].

Literature:
[1] St. Pyrek, J.: *Phytochemistry* **1985**, 24, 186.
[2] Seto, M. *et al.*: *Chem. Pharm. Bull.* **1988**, 36, 2423.
[3] Monde, K. *et al.*: *Phytochemistry* **1990**, 29, 3449.
[4] Gorecki, P. *et al.*: *Herba Pol.* **1974**, 20, 339.
[5] Mrugasievicz, K. *et al.*: *Pul. PL* 122567 (cl. C07H17106), 16 Feb **1984**, Appl. 205837, 04
      Apr 1978; 2pp.
[6] Dem'yanenko, V. G. *et al.*: *Khim. Prir. Soedin* **1973**, 9, 119.

[7] Dem'yanenko, V. G. *et al.*: *Khim. Prir. Soedin* **1972**, 8, 796.

[8] Bridle, P. *et al.*: *Phytochemistry* **1984**, 23, 2968.

[9] Maly, E. *et al.*: *Czech. CS* 262, 630 (cl. A23L1/00), 14 Aug **1989**, Appl. 86/6,020, 15 Aug **1986**; 3pp.

[10] Dem'yanenko, V. G. *et al.*: U.S.S.R. 577,033 (cl. A61k35 /78), 25 Oct **1977**, Appl. 2,088,334, 30 Dec **1974**.

[J.X. Guo]

355.   *Cirsium setosum* **(Willd.) MB.**   (Compositae)
[=*Cephalanoplos setosum* (Bunge) Kitam, *Breea setosa* Kitam.]

Ci-er-cai (C), Ezo-no-kitsune-azami (J), Eong-geong-kwi-a-jae-bi (K)

Herb (CP)
Local Drug Name: Xiao-ji (C), Siu-gight (H), Sho-kei (J).
Processing: 1) Eliminate forengn matter, wash clean, soften briefly, cut into sections, and dry (C).
          2) Stir-fry the sections until turning blackish-brown (C).
Method of Administration: Oral (decoction: C, H); Topical (fresh herb: C).
Folk Medicinal Uses:
          1) Epistaxis, spitting of blood (C, H, J).
          2) Hematuria (C, H, J).
          3) Hematochezia (C, H, J).
          4) Abnormal uterine bleeding (C, H, J).
          5) Carbuncles, sores (C, H, J).
          6) Traumatic injury (C, H, J).

Scientific Research:
Chemistry
    1) Flavonoids: acacetin [1], linarin [2], acacetin-7-rhamnoglucoside, rutin [3].
    2) Organic acids: protocatechuic acid, caffeic acid, chlorogenic acid [3].
    3) Alkaloids, saponins [4].
Pharmacology
    1) Hemostatic effect [3].
    2) Elevating blood pressure [5].
    3) Antiinflammatory effect [6].
    4) Antibacterial effect [6].

Literature:
[1] Rendyuk, T.D. *et al.*: *Farmatsiya (Moscow)* **1978**, 27(2). 68.

[2] Rendyuk, T.D. *et al.*: *Acta Pharm. Jugosl.* **1977**, 27(3), 135.

[3] Li, Q.H.: *Zhongcaoyao* **1982**, 13(9), 9.

[4] Nanjing College of Pharmacy: *"Zhongcaoyao Xue"* **1980**, Vol. 3, 1166.

[5] Dept. of Pharmacology: *Shandong Yixueyuan Xuebao* **1959**, (7), 4.

[6] *"Zhongyao Zhi"* **1988**, Vol. 4, 11.

[J.X. Guo]

356. *Echinops latifolius* **Tausch.** (Compositae)

Shu-zhou-lou-lu (C), Lou-loe (H), Okuriru-higotai (J), Keun-jeol-gut-dae (K)

Related plant: *Rhaponticum uniflorum* (L.) DC.: Qi-zhou-lou-lu (C).

Root (CP)
Local Drug Name: Lou-lu (C), Lou-loe (H), Ro-ro (J), Nu-ro (K).
Processing: Eliminate foreign matter, cut into thick slices, and dry in the sun (C, K).
Method of Administration: Oral (decoction: C, H, J, K).
Folk Medicinal Uses:
        1) Mastitis with swelling and pain (C, H, J, K).
        2) Carbuncle (C, H, K).
        3) Scrofula and ulcers (C, H).
        4) Galactostasis (C, H, K).
        5) Arthritis with ankylosis (C, H, J).
Contraindication: Use with caution in pregnancy (C, J).

Scientific Research:
Chemistry
  1) Alkaloid: echinopsine [1].
  2) Thiophenes: 2,2',5'2"-terthienyl, cardopatine, 5-(buten-3-ynyl-1)-bithiophene, 2-(1,3-
     pentadiynyl)-5-(3,4-dihydroxy-butan-1-ynyl)-thiophene, 5-(3,4-dihydroxy-butan-
     1-ynyl)-2,2'-bithiophene [2].
  3) Steroids: β-sitosterol, daucosterol [2].
  4) Triterpene: taraxerol acetate [2].
  5) Aliphatic compounds: hentriacotane, tetracosanol, hexacosanol, heptacosanol,
     octacosanol, nonacosanol, triacontanol, dotriacontanol [2].
  6) Volatile oils [3].
Pharmacology
  1) Antifungal effect [4].

Literature:
[1] Hegnauer, R.: *Chemotaxonomie der Pflanzen* **1964**, 3, 516.
[2] Lu, H. C. *et al.*: *Zhongcaoyao* **1989**, 20, 482.
[3] Yu, D. W. *et al.*: *Zhonghua Yaoxue Zazhi* **1936**, 1, 201.
[4] Cao, R. L. *et al.*: *Zhonghua Pifuke Zazhi* **1957**, 4, 286.

[J.X. Guo]

357. *Elephantopus mollis* **H.B.K.** (Compositae)
(*E. tomentosa* auct. non L.)

Bai-hua-di-dan-cao (C), Bark-far-day-darm (H)

Root
Local Drug Name: Di-dan-cao (C), Bark-far-day-darm (H).

Processing: Dry under the sun.

Method of Administration: Oral (decoction: C, H).

Folk Medicinal Uses:

> 1) Febrile diseases (C, H).
> 2) Acute tonsillitis (C, H).
> 3) Laryngopharyngitis (C, H).
> 4) Hepatitis (C, H).
> 5) Pertussis (H).

Scientific Research

Chemistry

> 1) Lactone: molephantin, molephantinin, phantomolin, 2-epi-deoxyorthopapp-4*E*-enolide methacrylate, deoxyelephantopin, deoxyisoelephantopin, tomenphantopins A-B, dihydroelephantopin, phantomolin epoxide [1–5, 8–12], 2-hydroxy-2-deethoxyphantomolin [14].
> 2) Triterpenoids: β-amyrin acetate, lupeol acetate, epifriedelanol, lupeol [1, 14].
> 3) Steroid: stigmasterol [1].
> 4) 1-hydroxy-15-senecioyloxy-α-curcumene, polyynes [7].

Pharmacology

> 1) Antitumor effect [1, 4–5].
> 2) Antiinflammatory effect [6].
> 3) Hepatoprotective effect [13].

Literature

[1] Lee, K. H. *et al.*: *J. Pharm. Sc.* **1980**, 68, 1050.
[2] Banerjee, B. *et al.*: *Planta Med.* **1986**; 52, 29.
[3] Jakupovic K. *et al.*: *Phytochemistry* **1987**, 26, 1467.
[4] Hayashi, T. *et al.*: *Phytochemistry* **1987**, 26, 1065.
[5] Rustaiyan, A. *et al.*: *Lloydia* **1978**, 41, 649.
[6] Sung, C.Y. *et al.*: *Yaoxue Xuebao* **1963**, 10, 708.
[7] Bohlmann, F. et al.: *Chem. Ber.* **1976**, 109, 3956.
[8] McPhail, A.T. et al.: *Tetrahedron Lett.* **1974**, (32), 2739.
[9] Lee, K. H. et al.: *J. Chem. Soc., Chem. Commun.* **1973**, (14), 476.
[10] Lee, K. H. *et al.*: *J. Pharm. Sc.* **1975**, 64, 1077.
[11] Govindachari, T.R. *et al.*: *Indian J. Chem.* **1970**, 8, 762.
[12] Govindachari, T.R. *et al.*: *Indian J. Chem.* **1972**, 10, 272.
[13] Lin, C.C. *et al.*: *J. Ethnopharm.* **1995**, 45, 113.
[14] But, P. P. H. *et al.*: *Planta Med.* **1996**, 62, 474.

[P.P.H. But]

358. *Elephantopus scaber* **L.** (Compositae)

Di-dan-cao (C), Day-darm-cho (H)

Root, herb

Local Drug Name: Di-dan-cao (C), Day-darm-cho (H).

Processing: Eliminate foreign matter, wash clean, dry under the sun, or use in fresh.
Method of Administration: Oral (decoction: C, H); Topical (paste or fresh herb: C, H).
Folk Medicinal Uses:

1) Cmmon cold, influenza (C, H).
2) Acute tonsillitis (C, H).
3) Laryngopharyngitis (C, H).
4) Acute ictero-hepatitis (C, H).
5) Boils (C).
6) Eczema (C, H).
7) Conjunctivitis (H).
8) Epidemic encephalitis B (H).
9) Pertussis (H).
10) Cirrhosis (H).
11) Ascites (H).
12) Nephritis (H).
13) Furunculosis (H).
14) Toothache (C).
15) Centipede bite (C).

Scientific Research

Chemistry

1) Lactone: deoxyelephantopin, isodeoxyelephantopin [1, 18], elephantol methacrylate, elephantopin, [18], 11,13-dihydroxyelephantopin [2], scabertopin [21].
2) Amino acid [17].
3) Lupeol, stigmasterol, epifridelinol, triacontain-1-ol, dotriacontain-1-ol [2, 5, 9], 4,5-dicaffeoyl quinic acid, 3,5-dicaffeoyl quinic acid [6], deacylcyanopicrin, stigmasteryl-3-β-glucopyranoside, crepiside E, glucozaluzanin-C [3], luteolin-7-glucoside [19].

Pharmacology

1) Antitumor effect [4].
2) Aldose reductase inhibitory effect [6].
3) Antiinflammatory effect [7].
4) Antibacterial effect [8].
5) Hepatoprotectice effect [10–12].
6) Writhing, loss of muscle tone, ataxia, prostration [14].
7) Antipyretic effect [14].
8) Hypotensive effect [14].

Literature

[1] Kurokawa, T. K. et al.: Tetrahedron Lett. 1970, (33), 2863.
[2] De Silva, L. B. et al.: Phytochemistry 1982, 21, 1173.
[3] Hisham, A. K.et al.: Planta Med. 1992, 58, 474.
[4] Lee, K. H. et al.: J. Pharm. Sc. 1975, 64, 1572.
[5] Bohlmann, et al.: Phytochemistry 1980, 19, 2669.
[6] Ichikawa, K. et al.: Sankyo Kenkyusho Nempo 1991, 43, 99.
[7] Sung, C. Y. et al.: Yaoxue Xuebao 1963, 10, 708.
[8] Chen, C. P. et al.: J. Ethnopharm. 1989, 27, 285.
[9] Sim, K.Y. et al.: Phytochemistry 1969, 8, 933.
[10] Lin, C. C. et al.: Amer. J. Chin. Med. 1991, 19, 41.
[11] Ohta, S. et al.: Yakugaku Zasshi 1993, 113, 870.

[12] Laranja, S.M. *et al.*: *Rev. Assoc. Med. Bras. (Brazil)* **1992**, 38(1), 13.

[13] Hammer, M.L. *et al.*: *J. Ethnopharm.* **1993**, 40, 53.

[14] Poli, A. *et al.*: *J. Ethnopharm.* **1992** **37**, 71

[15] Laranja, S. M. *et al.*: *Mem. Inst. Oswaldo Cruz. (Brazil)* **1991**, 86(Suppl. 2), 237.

[16] Ruppelt, B. M. *et al.*: *Mem. Inst. Oswaldo Cruz. (Brazil)* **1991**, 86(Suppl. 2), 203.

[17] Narayana, B. M.: *Indian J. Exp. Biol.* **1980**, 18, 1346.

[18] Govindachari, T. R.: *Indian J. Chem.* **1972**, 10, 272.

[19] Ghanim, A.: *Indian J. Chem.* **1963**, 1, 320.

[20] Lin, C.C. *et al.*: *J. Chin. Med. (Taipei)* **1992**, 2, 33.

[21] But, P. P. H. *et al.*: *Phytochemistry* **1997**, 44, 113.

[P.P.H. But]

359.   *Eupatorium fortunei* **Turcz.**   (Compositae)

Pei-lan (C), Pui-larn (H), Fujibakama (J), Beol-deung-gol-na-mu (K)

Herb (CP)

Local Drug Name: Pei-lan (C), Pui-larn (H), Hai-ran (J), Pae-ran (K).

Processing: Eliminate foreign matter, wash clean, soften briefly, cut into sections, and dry in the sun (C, K).

Method of Administration: Oral (decoction: C, H, J, K).

Folk Medicinal Uses:

1) Accumulation of damp in the spleen and stomach marked by stuffiness in the epigastrium, nausea, sweet taste and sticky sensation in the mouth, foul breath and salivation (C, H).

2) Summer heat and damp marked by sensation of distension in the head and stuffiness in the chest (C, H, K).

3) Irregular menses (H).

4) Diabetes (J).

5) Anasarca (J).

6) Menstrual disorder (J).

7) Headache (K).

Scientific Research:

Chemistry

1) Volatile oils: *p*-cymene, neryl acetate, 5-methylthymol ether [1].

2) Steroids: taraxasteryl palmitate, taraxasteryl acetate, taraxasterol [2], stigmasterol, β-sitosterol [3].

3) Trierpenes: β-amyrin palmitate, β-amyrin acetate [3].

4) Organic acids: fumaric acid, succinic acid [2], palmitic acid [3].

5) Others: octacosanol [3], mannitol [2].

Pharmacology

1) Antiviral effect [4].

Literature:

[1] Liang, X. T. *et al.*: *Yaoxue Xuebao* **1959**, 7(4), 131.

[2] Yoshizaki, M. *et al.*: *Yakugaku Zasshi* **1974**, 94(3), 338.
[3] Lai, C. F. *et al.*: *Tai-wan Yao Hsueh Tsa Chih* **1978**, 30(2), 103.
[4] Wang, S. Y.: *Sc. Rec.,* **1958**, New Ser. 2(7), 233.

[J.X. Guo]

360.　　　　　　　　*Allium fistulosum* **L.**　(Liliaceae)

Cong (C), Chung (H), Negi (J), Pa (K)

Bulb
  Local Drug Name: Cong-bai (C), Chung-bark (H), So-haku (J), Chong-baek (K).
  Processing: Dry under the sun (C, H, J, K) or fresh (H).
  Method of Administration: Oral (decoction: H, J, K), topical (paste: C).
  Folk Medicinal Uses:
  　　　　　1) Common cold (C, H, J, K).
  　　　　　2) Headache (C, H, J, K).
  　　　　　3) Cough (J, K).
  　　　　　4) Oliguria (H, fresh, crush to apply around navel).
  　　　　　5) Ascariasis, intestinal obstruction (H, fresh, mash with sesame oil).
  　　　　　6) Eczema, hives, leg ulcer (H, boil in water to wash infected parts).
  　　　　　7) Nasal stuffness (H).
  　　　　　8) Metropathy (K).
  　　　　　9) Contusion, fracture (K).
  　　　　　10) Mastitis (K).
  　　　　　11) Acute gastritis (K).
  　　　　　12) Dysentery (K).

Root
  Local Drug Name: Chong-su (K).
  Processing: Dry under the sun (K).
  Method of Administration: Oral (decoction, K).
  Folk Medicinal Uses:
  　　　　　1) Common cold (K).
  　　　　　2) Fever (K).
  　　　　　3) Dysosmia (K).
  　　　　　4) Insomnia (K).

Scientific Research:
  Chemistry
  　　1) Cyclic sulfur compounds: *cis*-3,5-diethyl-1,2,4-trithiolane, *trans*-3,5-diethyl-1,2,4-
  　　　　trithiolane, *trans*- and *cis*-3-methyl-5-ethyl-1,2,4-trithiolane [1].
  　　2) Sulfur compounds: allicin, allyl sulfide.
  　　3) Fatty acids: palmitic acid [9], stearic acid, arachidic acid, oleic acid, linoleic acid [2–3].
  　　4) Vitamins: vitamins B_1, B_2, C [4–5], A.
  　　5) Sterols: cholesterol [6].
  　　6) Enzymes: alliin lyase [8].
  　　7) Miscellaneous: tridecan-2-one, 2,3-dihydro-2-octyl-5-methyl-3-furanone [7].

Pharmacology
  1) Antimicrobial effect (essential oils).

Literature:
[1] Kameoka, H. *et al.*: *Tennen Yuki Kagobutsu Toronkai Koen Yoshishu, 21st* **1978**, 199.
[2] Murata, N. *et al.*: *Plant Cell Physiol.* **1982**, 23, 1071.
[3] Nakatsu, S. *et al.*: *Kenkyu Hokoku - Miyazaki Daigaku Nogakubu* **1984**, 31, 21.
[4] Kitagawa, Y.: *Eiyo To Shokuryo* **1973**, 26, 551.
[5] Karba, I.P.: *Byul. VNII Rastenievodstva* **1978**, 78, 61.
[6] Itoh, H. *et al.*: *Phytochemistry* **1977**, 16, 140.
[7] Kameoka, H.: *Phytochemistry* **1984**, 23, 155.
[8] Fujita, M.: *Agric. Biol. Chem.* **1990**, 54, 1077
[9] Sanchez, M.A.: *An. Asoc. Quim. Argent.* **1988**, 76, 227.

[C.K. Sung]

361. *Allium macrostemon* **Bge.** (Liliaceae)

Xiao-gen-suan (C), Dol-dal-rae (K)

Related plants: *Allium chinense* G. Don (*A. bakeri* Regel): Rakkyo (J).

Bulb (CP)
  Local Drug Name: Xie-bai (C), Hie-bark (H), Gai-haku (J), Hae-baek (K).
  Processing: Wash clean, eliminate fibrous root, steam thoroughly or scald thoroughly in
              boiling water, and dry in the sun (C, K).
  Method of Administration: Oral (decoction: C, H, K).
  Folk Medicinal Uses:
                1) Angina pectoris (C, H, J).
                2) Cough and dyspnea caused by retained sputum (C, H, J).
                3) Tenesmus in dysentery (C, H, J).

Scientific Research:
  Chemistry
    1) Saponins: macrostemonoside A, D, E, F [1–3].
    2) Lipids: prostaglandin A-1, prostaglandin B-1 [4].
    3) Volatile oils: methyl allyl trisulfide, etc. [5].
  Pharmacology
    1) Antianginal effect [6].
    2) Cholecystokinin receptor binding effect [7].
    3) HMG-Co-A reductase inhibition [7].
    4) Cyclooxygenase inhibition (volatile oil) [8].
    5) Lipoxygenase stimulation (volatile oil) [8].
    6) Thromboxane B-2 synthesis inhibition (volatile oil) [8].
    7) Inhibitory effect on β-hexosaminidase release from rat basophilic leukemia cells [9].

Literature:
[1] Wu, Y. *et al.*: *Shenyang Yaoxueyuan Xuebao* **1992**, 91, 69.

[2] Peng, J. P. *et al.*: *Yaoxue Xuebao* **1992**, 27, 918.

[3] Peng, J. P. *et al.*: *Yaoxue Xuebao* **1993**, 28, 526.

[4] Sun, Q. L. *et al.*: *Zhongcaoyao* **1991**, 22(4), 150.

[5] Wu, Y. *et al.*: *Shengyang Yaoxueyuan Xuebao* **1993**, 10(1), 45.

[6] Chen, K.: *Amer. J. Chin. Med.* **1981**, 9, 193.

[7] Han, G. Q. *et al.*: *Int. J. Chinese Med.* **1991**, 16(1), 1.

[8] Gu, Y. Q. *et al.*: *Yaoxue Xuebao* **1988**, 23, 8.

[9] Kataoka, M. *et al.*: *Natural Medicines* **1996**, 50, 344.

[J.X. Guo]

362.　　　*Aloe vera* **L.,** *A. vera* **L. var.** *chinensis* **(Haw.) Berg.,**
　　　　　A. barbadensis **Miller,** *A. ferox* **Miller**　(Liliaceae)

Lu-hui (C), Lo-whui (H), Kidachi-aroe (J), Al-ro-e (K)

Leaf
  Local Drug Name: Lu-hui-ye (C), Loe-whui (H), No-hoe (K).
  Method of Administration: Oral (decoction: C, H, K); topical (powder: C).
  Folk Medicinal Uses:
　　　　　　1) Headache (H).
　　　　　　2) Dizziness (H).
　　　　　　3) Constipation (C, H, K).
　　　　　　4) Infantile convulsion (H).
　　　　　　5) Infantile malnutrition (H).
　　　　　　6) Pertussis (H).
  Contraindication: Pregnancy, weak in spleen and stomach.
Leaf exudate (CP, JP)
  Local Drug Name: Lu-hui (C), Loe-whui (H), Aroe (J), No-hoe (K).
  Processing: Use fresh or collect the sap, heat till thicken and cool for storage.
  Method of Administration: Oral (decoction: C, H, K).
  Folk Medicinal Uses:
　　　　　　1) Constipation (C, H, J, K).
　　　　　　2) Amenorrhea (C).
　　　　　　3) Infantile convulsion (C).
　　　　　　4) Hemorrhoid (C).
　　　　　　5) Rhinitis (C).
　　　　　　6) Scrofula (C).
　　　　　　7) Infantile malnutrition (C).
  Contraindication: Pregnancy, diarrhea, allergic reaction [7-9].

Leaf mucilage (JP)
  Local Drug Name: Lu-hui (C), Loe-whui (H), Aroe (J), No-hoe (K)
  Processing: Use fresh or collect the sap.
  Method of Administration: Oral (decoction: C, H, K); Topical (gel: C, H, J, K).
  Folk Medicinal Uses:
　　　　　　1) Pyodermas (H).
　　　　　　2) Burns (C, H, J, K).

3) Scalds (C, H, J, K).
4) Eczema (H).
6) Gastric ulcer (K).
7) Traumatic injury (K).

Flower
Local Drug Name: Lu-hui-hua (C), Loe-whui-Far (H).
Method of Administration: Oral (decoction: C, H).
Folk Medicinal Uses:
>> 1) Epistaxis (H).
>> 2) Hematuria (H).

Scientific Research:
Chemistry
   1) Anthrones: aloin (barbaloin), aloinoside A, aloinoside B, isobarbaloin.
   2) Anthraquinones: aloe-emodin [1], aloe-emodine diglucoside, aloe-emodin-8-
        monoglucoside.
   3) Resins: aloeresin A [2], aloenin.
   4) Polysaccharides: [3–4].
   5) Chromones: aloesin [5, 20], iso-aloesin [27].
   6) Lectin [16].
Pharmacology.
   1) Immunostimulatory effect [6].
   2) Prolonged survival in tumor-bearing mice but no anti-cancer effect [10].
   3) Neither antidiabetic effect nor antiulcer effect [11].
   4) Protective effect against UV-irradiation [12].
   5) Cathartic effect [13, 25-26].
   6) Antiinflammatory effect [14, 22-23].
   7) Wound healing effect [14, 18, 22-23].
   8) Hemagglutinating effect [16].
   9) Protective effect on skin against aging [17].
   10) Antitumor effect [19].
   12) Hypoglycemic effect [21].
   13) Antiviral effect [24].
   14) Potential risk for colorectal cancer [28].

Literature
[1] Tsukida, L. *et al.*: *Yakugaku Zasshi* **1954**, 74, 224.
[2] Gramatica, P. *et al.*: *Tetrahedron Lett.* **1982**, 2423.
[3] Wang, S. X. *et al.*: *Zhiwu Xuebao* **1989**, 31, 389.
[4] Gowa, C. *et al.*: *Carbohyd. Res.* **1979**, 72, 201.
[5] Yuan, A. X. *et al.*: *Zhongguo Zhongyao Zazhi* **1991**, 16, 292.
[6] Wang, S. X *et al.*: *Zhiwu Xuebao* **1989**, 31, 389.
[7] Morrow, D. M.: *Arch. Dermatol.* **1980**, 116, 1064.
[8] Hogan, D. J.: *Can. Med. Assoc. J.* **1988**, 138, 336.
[9] Sauchak, U. I.: *Vestn. Dermatol. Venerol.* **1977**, 12, 44.
[10] Jeong, H. Y. *et al.*: *Yakhak Hoeji* **1994**, 38, 311.
[11] Koo, M. W. L.: *Phytother. Res.* **1994**, 8, 461.
[12] Strickland, F. M. *et al.*: *J. Invest. Dermatol.* **1994**, 102, 197.
[13] Koch, A.: *Planta Med.* **1993**, 59(Suppl.), 689.

[14] Udupa, S. L.: *Fitoterapia* **1994**, 65, 141.

[15] Ahmad, S.: *Hamdard Med.* **1993**, 36(1), 108.

[16] Winters, W. D.: *Phytother. Res.* **1993**, 7(Suppl.), S23.

[17] Danhof, I. E.: *Phytother. Res.* **1993**, 7(Suppl.), S53.

[18] Heggers, J. P. *et al.*: *Phytother. Res.* **1993**, 7(Suppl.), S48.

[19] Soeda, M.: *Toho Igakkai Zasshi* **1969**, 16, 365.

[20] Haynes, L. J. *et al.*: *J. Chem. Soc., C.* **1970**, (18), 2581.

[21] Ajabnoor, M. A.: *J. Ethnopharmacol.* **1990**, 28, 215.

[22] Davis, R. H. *et al.*: *J. Am. Podiatr. Med. Assoc.* **1994**, 84, 77.

[23] Davis, R. H. *et al.*: *J. Am. Podiatr. Med. Assoc.* **1994**, 84, 614.

[24] Anonymous: *J. Am. Dent. Assoc.* **1994**, 125, 1308.

[25] Ishii, Y. *et al.*: *Biol. Pharm. Bull.* **1994**, 17, 495.

[26] Ishii, Y. *et al.*: *Biol. Pharm. Bull.* **1994**, 17, 651.

[27] Yuan, A. X.: *Zhongguo Zhongyao Zazhi* **1993**, 18, 609.

[28] Siegers, C. P. *et al.*: *Gut* **1993**, 34, 1099.

[P.P.H. But]

363. *Asparagus cochinchinensis* **(Lour.) Merrill** (Liliaceae)

Tian-dong (C), Tin-moon-dung (H), Kusasugikazura (J), Cheon-mun-dong(K)

Root (CP)

Local Drug Name: Tian-dong (C), Tin-moon-dung (H), Ten-mon-do (J), Cheon-mun-dong
(K).

Processing: Dry under the sun (K) or cut into thin slices and dry (C).

Method of Administration: Oral (decoction or juice: C, H, J, K).

Folk Medicinal Uses:
> 1) Cough (C, H, J, K).
> 2) Pulmonary tuberculosis (C, H, J, K).
> 3) Bronchitis (C, H, J, K).
> 4) Diphtheria (C, H).
> 5) Pertussis (C, H).
> 6) Rhinitis (C, H).
> 7) Diabetes mellitus (C, H, J, K).
> 8) Breast cancer (C, H).
> 9) Boils, pyodermas (H, topical).
> 10) Snake bites (H, topical).
> 11) Hematemesis (J, K).
> 12) Freckle on the face (K).
> 13) Constipation (C, H).
> 14) Diarrhea (J).

Contraindications: Diarrhea of debility and cold diseases.

Scientific Research:

Chemistry
> 1) Steroidal saponins: methylprotogracillin, pseudoprotodioscin, 20(22)-unsatd.
> furostanoside [1], 3-O-[α-L-rhamnopyranosyl-(1→4)-β-D-glucopyranosyl]-26-O-

(β-D-glucopyranosyl)-(25R)-furosta-5,20-diene-3β,26-diol, methylprotodioscin, pseudoprotodioscin [5], furostanol oligosides [7].

2) Steroidal sapogenins: sarsasapogenin [9].

3) Polysaccharides: asparagus polysaccharide A, B, C, D [2].

4) Amino acids [3-4]: citrulline, asparagine, serine, threonine, proline, glycine, alanine, valine, methionine, leucine, isoleucine, phenylalanine, tyrosine, aspartic acie, gluctamic acid, arginine, histidine, lysine, unidentified acidic amino acid [8].

5) Oligosaccharides: [10].

6) Trace elements [3]: Ge [6].

Pharmacology

1) Antiviral effect (spyrostane glycoside) [1].

2) Antitumor effect (polysaccharide) [2].

Literature:

[1] Aquino, R. *et al.*: *J. Chemother.* (Florence) **1991**, 3, 305.

[2] Du, X. *et al.*: *Shenyang Yaoxueyuan Xuebao*, **1990**, 7, 197.

[3] Wen, J. *et al.*: *Zhiwu Ziyuan Yu Huanjing* **1992**, 1(3), 55.

[4] Ni, J. *et al.*: *Zhongcaoyao* **1992**, 23, 182.

[5] Liang, Z. Z. *et al.*: *Planta Med.* **1988**, 54, 344.

[6] Chiang, H. C. *et al.*: *T'ai-wan Yao Hsueh Tsa Chih* **1986**, 38, 189.

[7] Konishi, T. *et al.*: *Chem. Pharm. Bull.* **1979**, 27, 3086.

[8] Tomoda, M. *et al.*: *Kyoritsu Yakka Daigaku Kenkyu Nempo* **1975**, 20, 9.

[9] Okanishi, T. *et al.*: *Chem. Pharm. Bull.* **1975**, 23, 575.

[10] Tomoda, M. *et al.*: *Chem. Pharm. Bull.* **1974**, 22, 2306.

[11] Ahmad, V.U. *et al.*: *Hamdard Medicus* **1996**, 39, 27.

[P.P.H. But & C.K.Sung]

364. *Convallaria keiskei* Miq. (Liliaceae)

Ling-lan (C), Suzuran (J), Eun-bang-ul-ggot (K)

Herb

Local Drug Name: Ling-lan (C), Suzu-ran (J), Yeong-ran (K).

Processing: Dry under the sun (C, K).

Method of Administration: Oral (decoction: C, J, K).

Folk Medicinal Uses:

1) Cardiac disorder (J, K).

2) Bed-wetting (K).

3) Congestive heart-failure (C).

4) Atrial fibrillation (C).

Side Effects: poisonous, drooling, nausea, vomiting, pulmonary and cardiac insufficiency.

Scientific Research:

Chemistry

1) Cardenolide glycosides: locundeside, convalloside, convallatoxoloside, neoconvallatoxoloside, neoconvalloside [1], rhodexin A [2], convallatoxin [6], periplogenin-3-O-α-L-rhamnopyranoside [7].

2) Nucleosides: thymidine [3].

3) Flavonoids: hyperoside, bioquercetin, keioside, biorobin (from leaf) [4].

4) Nucleoside: thymidine [5].

5) Steroidal saponins [8]: convallasaponin-A and -B [9].

Pharmacology

1) Cardiac stimulating activities (cardiac glycosides) [1, 6].

2) Active in acute and chronic liver and bile duct disease (flavonoids) [4].

Literature:

[1] Komissarenko, N. F. *et al.*: *Khim. Prir. Soedin.* **1986**, (2), 201.

[2] Komissarenko, N. F. *et al.*: *Khim. Prir. Soedin.* **1983**, (6), 790

[3] Yoshizawa, I. *et al.*: *Yakugaku Zasshi* **1978**, 98, 1129.

[4] Komissarenko, N. V. *et al.*: *Pastit. Resur.* **1992**, 28(1), 82.

[5] Yoshizawa, I. *et al.*: *Yakugaku Zasshi* **1978**, 98, 1129.

[6] Kazarinov, N. A. *et al.*: *Khim.-Farm. Zh.* **1969**, 3(6), 42.

[7] Komissarenko, N. F.: *Khim. Prir. Soedin.* **1968**, 4(4), 256.

[8] Yoshizawa, I. *et al.*: *Chem. Pharm. Bull.* **1967**, 15, 129.

[9] Kimura, M. *et al.*: *Chem. Pharm. Bull.* **1968**, 16, 25.

[C.K. Sung]

365.   *Hemerocallis fulva* L.   (Liliaceae)

Xuan-cho (C), Huan-cho (H), Hon-kanzo (J), Weon-chu-ri (K)

Related plant: *Hemerocallis fulva* L. var. *kwanso* Regel: Yabu-kanzo (J); *H. flava* L.:
Huang-hua-cai (C).

Root

Local Drug Name: Xuan-cao (C), Huan-cho-gun (H), Kanzo-kon (J), Hweon-cho-geun (K).

Processing: Dry under the sun (K).

Method of Administration: Oral (decoction: H, J, K).

Folk Medicinal Uses:

1) Jaundice (C, H, J, K).

2) Cystitis (C, H).

3) Oliguria (C, H).

4) Hematuria (C, H).

5) Epistaxis (H).

6) Melena (H).

7) Hemoptysis (H).

8) Hepatitis (H).

9) Mastitis (C, H).

10) Otitis media (H).

11) Cervical lymphadenitis (H).

12) Toothache (H).

13) Edema (J).

14) Melena (J).

15) Oppilation (K).
16) Constipation (K).
17) Pneumonia (K).
Side Effects: Overdose results in urinary incontinence, dilated pupil, respiratory arrest, and
blindness.

Flower
Local Drug Name: Jin-zhen-cai (C), Gum-jum (H), Kin-shin-sai (J).
Processing: Dry under the sun or steam with heat (H).
Method of Administration: Oral (decoction: J).
Folk Medicinal Uses:
                    1) Insomnia (H).

Scientific Research:
 Chemistry
   1) Amino acids: oxypinnatanine [1].
   2) Anthraquinones: chrysophanol [2], methyl rhein, 1,8-dihydroxy-3-methoxy-
      anthraquinone, rhein [3].
   3) Amines: choline [3].
 Pharmacology
   1) Antimicrobial effect [3].

Literature:
[1] Kruger, G. J. et al.: J. S. Afr. Chem. Inst. **1976**, 29, 24.
[2] Wang, Q. et al.: Zhongcaoyao **1990**, 21, 12.
[3] Sarg, T. M. et al.: Int. J. Crude Drug Res. **1990**, 28, 153.

[C.K. Sung]

366.   *Hosta longipes* **Matsumura**   (Liliaceae)

Iwa-giboshi (J), Bi-bi-chu (K)

Flower
Local Drug Name: Ja-ok-jam (K).
Processing: Dry under the sun (K).
Method of Administration: oral (K).
Folk Medicinal Uses:
                        1) Ulcer (K).
                        2) Uterus hemorrhage (K).
                        3) Antitussive (K).

Scientific Research:
 Chemistry
   1) Vitamin C [1].
   2) Fatty acids: linoleic acid [2].
   3) Saponin [3].

Pharmacology
 1) Anti-tumor effect [3].
Literature:
[1] Park, K. W. *et al.*: *Han'guk Wonye Hakhoechi* **1993**, 34(3), 191.
[2] Kato, M. *et al.*: *J. Am. Oil Chem. Soc.* **1981**, 58(9), 866.
[3] Mimaki, Y. *et al.*: *Chem. Pharm. Bull.* **1995**, 43, 1190.

[C.K. Sung]

367.   *Hosta plantaginea* **Aschers**   (Liliaceae)

Yu-zan (C), Maruba-tama-kanzashi (J), Ok-jam-hwa (K)

Flower
 Local Drug Name: Yu-zan (C), Gyoku-san-ka (J), Ok-jam-hwa (K).
 Processing: Dry in the shade (C, K).
 Method of Administration: Oral (decoction: J, K); Topical (decoction: C).
 Folk Medicinal Uses:
                1) Burns (C, K).
                2) Swelling and pain in throat (C, J).
                3) Difficult urination (C).
                4) Dysmenorrhea (C).
                5) Lymphadenitis (K).

Scientific Research:
 Chemistry
    1) Triterpenoid, polysaccharide, amino acid [1].
 Pharmacology
    1) Antineoplastic effect [2].
Literature:
[1] Anonymous: *Zhongcaoyao Youxiao Chengfande Yanjiu* **1972**, p.442.
[2] Ding, Z.Z. *et al.*: In: Wu, Z. Y. (Eds.) *Xinhua Bencao Gangyao,* Shanghai Science and
    Technology Press, Shanghai, **1991**, 2, 533.

[C.K. Sung]

368.   *Lilium lancifolium* **Thunb.**   (Liliaceae)
                   (L. tigrinum Ker-Gawl.)

Juan-dan (C), Cham-na-ri (K)

Related Plant: *Lilium brownii* F. E. Brown var.*veridulum* Baker: Bai-he (C), *L. pumilum* DC.:
       Xi-ye-bai-he (C).

Bulb (CP)
Local Drug Name: Bai-he (C), Bark-hup (H), Baek-hap (K).
Processing: Briefly dip in boiling water, dry under the sun (C, K).
Method of Administration: Oral (decoction: C, H, K).
Folk Medicinal Uses:

         1) Furuncle (K).
         2) Mastitis (K).
         3) Suppuration (C, K).
         4) Boil (K).
         5) Dislocation of the leg (K).
         6) Trauma (K).
         7) Insomnia (C, H).
         8) Restlessness (C, H).

Scientific Research:
Chemistry
  1) Carotenoids: sporopollenins [1–2], capsanthin, darpoxanthin, 6-epidarpoxanthin,
      lilixanthin [3].
  2) Carbohydrates [4, 9].
  3) Lignin [7].
  4) Pigment: β-carotene [8].
  5) Alkaloid [10].
  6) Flavonoid [10]

Literature:
[1] Heslop-Harrison, J.: *Symp. Soc. Exp. Biol.* **1971**, 25, 277.
[2] Manskaya, S. M. *et al.*: *Geokhimiya* **1976**, (1), 3.
[3] Maerki, F. E. *et al.*: *Helv. Chim. Acta* **1985**, 68, 1708.
[4] Fuwa, H. *et al.*: *Carbohydr. Res.* **1979**, 70, 233.
[5] Sugimoto, Y. *et al.*: *Denpun Kagaku* **1979**, 26, 182.
[6] Sugimoto, Y.: *Denpun Kagaku* **1980**, 27, 28.
[7] Manskaya, S. M. *et al.*: *Adv. Org. Geochem., Proc. Int. Conf., 6th*, **1973** (pub. 1974), 97.
[8] Togasawa, Y. *et al.*: *Nippon Nogei Kagaku Kaishi* **1967**, 41, 184.
[9] Motomura, Y. *et al.*: *Tohoku J. Agr. Res.* **1962**, 13, 237.
[10] Wu, H.B. *et al.*: *Xiandai Yingyong Kexue* **1962**, 13, 237.

                                               [C.K. Sung]

369.   *Scilla scilloides* **(Lindl.) Druce**   (Liliaceae)

Mian-zao-er (C), Min-jo-yee (H), Tsurubo (J), Mu-reut (K)

Related plant: *Scilla sinensis* (Lour.) Merr.

Bulb
Local Drug Name: Mian-zao-er (C), Min-jo-yee (H), Myeon-jo-a (K).
Processing: Dry under the sun (C, K) or use in fresh (C).

Method of Administration: Oral (decoction: C, K), topical (paste: C).
Folk Medicinal Uses:
>1) Traumatic injury (C, H).
>2) Toothache (C, H)
>3) Cardiac edema (C, H).
>4) Soreness and pain in waist and lower extremities (C).
>5) Mastitis (C, H, topical).
>6) Lumbago (H).
>7) Arthralgia (H).
>8) Carbunculosis (H, topical).
>9) Snake bites (H, topical).
>10) Antitussive (K).
>11) Chronic gastritis (K).
>12) Neuralgia (K).

Contraindications: pregnancy.

Scientific Research:
Chemistry
>1) Homoisoflavanones [1].
>2) Spirocyclic nortriterpenoids [2–3].

Literature:
[1] Kouno, I. *et al.*: *Tetrahedron Lett.* **1973**, (46), 4569.
[2] Sholichin, M. *et al.*: *Chem. Pharm. Bull.* **1985**, 33, 12756.
[3] Sholichin M.: *Heterocycles*, **1982**, 17(Spec. Issue), 251.

[C.K. Sung]

370. *Veratrum maackii* Regel var. *japonicum* T. Shimizu (Liliaceae)

Shuroso (J), Yeo-ro (K)

Rhizome
Local Drug Name: Ri-ro (J), Yeo-ro (K).
Processing: Dry under the sun (J, K).
Method of Administration: Oral (decoction: H, K); Topical (decoction: J).
Folk Medicinal Uses:
>1) Insect bite (J, K).
>2) Louse (J).
>3) Jaundice (H).
>4) Sputum (H).
>5) Skin disease (H).
>6) Pleurisy (K).
>7) Weakness after child-birth (K).

Side Effects: poisonous

Scientific Research:
Chemistry
>1) Steroids: (20R, 20S)-verazine [1].

2) Alkaloids: maackinine, germanitrine, angeloylzygadenine, verazinin, zygadenine, verazine [2–4].

Literature:

[1] Han, X. *et al.*: *Planta Med.* **1992**, 58, 449.
[2] Zhao, W. *et al.*: *Chem. Pharm. Bull.* **1989**, 37, 2920.
[3] To, I.K. *et al.*: *Wakan Iyaku Gakkaishi* **1988**, 5, 382.
[4] Zhao, W.J. *et al.*: *Zhongyao Tongbao* **1986**, 11, 294.

[C.K. Sung]

371.   *Lycoris radiata* **Herb.**   (Amaryllidaceae)

Shi-suan (C), Higanbana (J), Ga-eul-ga-jae-mu-reut (K)

Bulb
Local Drug Name: Shi-suan (C), Seki-san (J), Seok-san (K).
Processing: Fresh. Dry under the sun, or usedin fresh (C, J).
Method of Administration: Topical (paste: C; fomentation: J).
Folk Medicinal Uses:
          1) Edema (C, J, K).
          2) Mastitis (J).
          3) Suppuration (J, K).
          4) Food intoxication (oral, small piece, as emetics) (J, K).
          5) Furuncle (C).
          6) Rheumatic arthritis (C).
          7) Snake bite (C).
          8) Tuberculos lymphadenitis (C).
Side effects: Toxic, causing serious vomiting.

Scientific Research:
Chemistry
    1) Alkaloids: lycorine [1], lycoramine, galanthamine [2], tazettine [3], lycorenine, homolycorine, pluviine, caranine [4], pseudolycorine, demethylhomolycorine, norpluviine [5], 2-epigalanthamine, vittatine, haemanthamine, hippeastrine [6], haemanthidine, lycoricidinol, lycoricidine[7].
    2) Polysaccharide: lycorisin, higanbana-mannan [8].

Literature:

[1] Kotera, K. *et al.*: *Tetrahedron* **1968**, 24, 2463.
[2] Takagi, S. *et al.*: *Chem. Pharm. Bull.*, **1968**, 16, 1121.
[3] Irie, H. *et al.*: *J. Chem. Soc.* **1959**, 1446; Takagi, S. *et al.*: *Yakugaku Zasshi* **1968**, 88, 941.
[4] Kitagawa, T. *et al.*: *J. Chem. Soc.* **1959**, 3741; Nakagawa, Y. *et al.*: *J. Chem. Soc.* **1959**, 3736; Mizukami, S.: *Tetrahedron* **1960**, 11, 89; Hung, S. H. *et al.*: *Yueh Hsueh Hsueh Pao* **1964**, 11, 1.
[5] Uyeo, S. *et al.*: *J. Chem. Soc.* **1959**, 172.

[6] Boit, H. G. *et al.*: Chem. Ber., **1956**, 89, 1129; **1957**, 90, 369; Wildmann, W. C.: *J. Am. Chem. Soc.* **1958**, 80, 2567; Fals, H. M. *et al.*: *J. Am. Chem. Soc.* **1960**, 82, 197; Uyeo, S. *et al.*: *Chem. Pharm. Bull.* **1966**, 14, 793.
[7] Okamoto, T. et al: *Chem. Pharm. Bull.*, **1968**, 16, 1860.
[8] Mizuno, T.: *Nogei shi*, **1957**, 31, 29; **1957**, 31, 31; **1957**, 31, 138.

[T. Kimura]

372. *Narsissus tazetta* **L. var. *chinensis* Roem.** (Amaryllidaceae)

Shui-xian (C), Shui-sin (H), Suisen (J), Su-seon-hwa (K)

Flower
Local Drug Name: Sui-sen-ka (J), Su-seon-hwa (K).
Processing: Dry under the sun (K).
Method of Administration: Oral (decoction: K).
Folk Medicinal Uses:
>1) Female disease (J, K).
>2) Mastitis (K).
>3) Boil (K).
>4) Appendicitis (K).
>5) Diarrhea (K).

Bulb
Local Drug Name: Shui-xian (C), Shui-sin (H), Sui-sen-ken (J).
Processing: Dry under the sun (C, H), fresh (H, J: ground and mixed with wheat flour).
Method of Administration: Topical (paste: C, poultice: H, fomentation: J).
Folk Medicinal Uses:
>1) Mastitis (H, J).
>2) Parotitis (C, H).
>3) Boils (C, H).
>4) Abscesses (H).
>5) Suppuration (J).
>6) Swelling (J).

Scientific Research:
Chemistry
>1) Alkaloids: narcissus alkaloid [1], pretazettine, tazettine [5, 10], lycorine [6, 9–10, 14], pseudolycorine [9, 12, 14], choline [6], *O*-methylmaritidine [11].
>2) Polysaccharides: glucomannan [3, 7–8].
>3) Flavonoids: narcissin [4], rutin [5].
>4) Triterpenes: α-amyrin [5].
>5) Sterols: β-sitosterol [5].
>6) Fatty acids: stearic acid, linolenic acid [6].

Pharmacology
>1) Antiviral acitivity (alkaloid fraction) [2].
>2) Antileukemic acition (narcissus alkaloid) [1].

Literature:

[1] Furusawa, E. *et al.*: *Proc. Soc. Exp. Biol. Med.* **1972**, 140, 1034.

[2] Papas, T. S. *et al.*: *Biochem. Biophys. Res. Commun.* **1973**, 52, 88.

[3] Kato, K. *et al.*: *Carbohyd. Res.* **1973**, 29, 469.

[4] Nasudari, A. A. *et al.*: *Farm. Zh.(Keiv)* **1972**, 27, 86.

[5] Furusawa, E. *et al.*: *Chem. Pharm. Bull.* **1976**, 24, 336.

[6] El-Moghazy, A. M. *et al.*: *Egypt. J. Pharm. Sci.* **1976**, 17, 273.

[7] Tomoda, M. *et al.*: *Chem. Pharm. Bull.* **1980**, 28, 3251.

[8] Khamidkhodzhaev, S. A. *et al.*: *Uzb. Biol. Zh.* **1979**, (5), 42.

[9] Cao, R.-Q. *et al.*: *Chung Ts'ao Yao* **1981**, 12, 39.

[10] Bruno, S. *et al.*: *Plant. Med. Phytother.* **1985**, 19, 211.

[11] Tani, S. *et al.*: *Chem. Pharm. Bull.* **1981**, 29, 3381.

[12] Li, Q. *et al.*: *Zhongcaoyao* **1981**, 12, 502.

[13] Ohyama, T. *et al.*: *Nippon Dojo Hiryogaku Zasshi* **1986**, 57, 119.

[14] Cao, R. *et al.*: *Nanjing Daxue Xuebao, Ziran Kexue* **1984**, (2), 321.

[C.K. Sung]

373. *Commelina communis* **L.** (Commelinaceae)

Ya-zhi-cao (C), Ngap-jak-cho (H), Tsuyukusa (J), Dal-geui-jang-pul (K)

Whole plant (CP)

Local Drug Name: Ya-zhi-cao (C), Ngap-jak-cho (H), O-seki-so (J), Ap-Cheok-Cho (K).

Processing: Eliminate foreign matter, dry under the sun (C).

Method of Administration: Oral (decoction: C, H, J, K); Topical (decoction: C).

Folk Medicinal Uses:

1) Edema (C, H, J, K).

2) Influenza (C, H).

3) Acute tonsillitis, pharyngitis (C, H).

4) Genito-urinary infection (C, H).

5) Dysentery, enteritis (C, H, J).

6) Mumps (C).

7) Beriberi (C, J).

8) Oliguria (C, H).

9) Jaundice (C).

10) Epistaxis (C, J, K).

11) Hematuria (C, K).

12) Leukorrhea (C, K).

13) Traumatic injury (C, K).

14) Diabetes (K).

Contraindications: Spleen-stomach-deficiency.

Scientific Research

Chemistry

1) Alkaloids: 1-carbomethoxy-carboline, harman, norharman [1].

2) Anthocyanin: commelinin [2–5], flavocommelin [6].

3) (−)-loliolide, friedelin, β-sitosterol [7].

Pharmacology
1) Antibacterial effect [1].
2) Weak diuretic effect.
3) Antipyretic effect.

Literature

[1] Bae, K. W. *et al.*: *Arch. Pharmacal Res.* **1992**, 15(3), 220.
[2] Kondo, T. *et al.*: *Tennen Yuki Kagobutsu Toronkai Koen Yoshishu* **1991**, 33rd, 385.
[3] Kondo, T. *et al.*: *Bio. Ind.* **1992**, 9, 444.
[4] Mitsui, S. *et al.*: *Botan. Mag.* (Tokyo) **1959**, 72, 325.
[5] Mitsui, S. *et al.*: *Proc. Japan Acad.* (Tokyo) **1959**, 35, 169.
[6] Takeda, K. *et al.*: *Botan. Mag.* (Tokyo) **1966**, 79, 578.
[7] Baek, S. H. *et al.*: *Yakhak Hoechi* **1990**, 34(1), 64.

[P.P.H. But]

374. *Eriocaulon buergerianum* Koern. (Eriocaulaceae)

Gu-jing-cao (C), Guk-jing-cho (H), O-hosikusa (J)

Related plant: *Eriocaulon siebodianum* Sieb. et Zucc.: Gok-jeong-cho (K).

Flower (CP)
Local Drug Name: Gu-jing-cao (C), Guk-jing-cho (H), Koku-sei-so (J), Gok-jeong-cho (K).
Processing: Eliminate foreign matter, cut into sections (C, K).
Method of Administration: Oral (decoction: C, H, J, K).
Folk Medicinal Uses:
    1) Eye inflammation with photophobia and headache caused by wind-heat (C, H, J, K).
    2) Nebula (C, H, K).
Scientific Research:
 Chemistry
    1) Flavonoids [1].
 Pharmacology
    1) Antifungal effect [2–3].
    2) Antibacterial effect [4].
    3) Inhibitory effect on aldose reductase [5].
Literature:

[1] Bate-Smith, E. C. *et al.*: *Phytochemistry* **1969**, 8, 1035.
[2] Zhen, W. F. *et al.*: *Zhonghua Yixue Zazhii* **1952**, 38, 315.
[3] Cao, R. L. *et al.*: *Zhonghua Pifuke Zazhi* **1957**, (4), 286.
[4] Departments of Internal Medicine and Laboratory: *Weishengwu Xuebao* **1960**, 8(1), 52.
[5] Matsuda, H. *et al.*: *Biol. Pharm. Bull.* **1995**, 18, 463.

[J.X. Guo]

375. *Eriocaulon sieboldianum* Sieb. et Zucc. ex Steud. (Eriocaulaceae)

Sai-gu-jing-cao (C), Guk-jing-cho (H), Gok-jeong-cho (K)

Related plant: *Eriocaulon buergerianum* Koern.: Gu-jing-cao (J), O-hoshikusa (J)

Herb
Local Drug Name: Gu-jing-cao (C), Guk-jing-cho (H), Koku-sei-so (J), Gok-jeong-cho (K).
Processing: Dry under the sun (C, K).
Method of Administration: oral (decoction: C, H, J, K).
Folk Medicinal Uses:
> 1) Inflammation of the eye with photophobia (C, K).
> 2) Headache caused by wind-heat (C).
> 3) Nebula (C).
> 4) Conjunctivitis (H).
> 5) Corneal opacities (H).
> 6) Nyctalopia (H).
> 7) Central retinitis (H).
> 8) Eye diseases (J).
> 9) Headache (J).
> 10) Toothache (J).
> 11) Sore throat (J).

Scientific Research:
  Pharmacology
   1) Antibacterial effect [1].
   2) Antifungal effect [1].

Literature:

[1] Anonymous: *Zhongyao Dacidian*, Shanghai People Press, Shanghai, **1977**, 1, 1150.
[2] Matsui, A. *et al.*: *Med. Pharmacol. Exp.* **1967**, 16, 414.

[C.K. Sung]

376. *Coix lachryma-jobi* L. var. *ma-yuen* Stapf (Gramineae)

Yi-yi (C), Yi-might (H), Hatomugi (J), Yul-mu (K)

Caryopsis (CP, JP)
Local Drug Name: Yi-yi-ren (C), Yi-might (H), Yoku-i-nin (J), Eui-i-in (K).
Processing: 1) Dry under the sun (C, J).
           2) Stir-fry with bran until turnong pale yellow (C).
Method of Administration: Oral (decoction: C, H, J, K).
Folk Medicinal Uses:
> 1) Wart (H, J, K). Verruca plana (C).
> 2) Edema (C, H, J, K).
> 3) Beriberi (H, J, K).
> 4) Arthralgia (J, K). Arthritis with contracture of joints (C).

5) Pulmonary abscess (C, H, J).
6) Pneumonia (K).
7) Oliguria (C).
8) Diarrhea (C, H).
9) Appendicitis (H).
10) Chronic enteritis (H).
11) Leukorrhea (H).
12) Gastric cancer (H).
13) Cervical cancer (H).
14) Eczema (H).
15) Freckle (K).
16) Neurasthenia (K).

Root

Local Drug Name: Ng-gook-gee-gun (H).
Method of Administration: Oral (decoction: H).
Folk Medicinal Uses:
1) Urinary tract infection (H).
2) Urinary tract stones (H).
3) Jaundice (H).
4) Leukorrhea (H).
5) Ascariasis (H).

Scientific Research:

Chemistry
1) Steroids: *trans*-feruloyl stigmastanol, *trans*-feruloyl campestanol [1].
2) Glycans: coixan A, B, C [2].
3) Benzoxazinones [3].
4) Phthalides: coixinden A, B [4].
5) Coixenolide

Pharmacology
1) Depressing contraction of flog skeletal muscles (ether extract) [5].
2) Depressing blood sugar and blood calcium (ether extract) [5].
3) Antimicrobial effect (coixinden A, B) [4].
4) Increasing antibodies *in vitro* (acetone extract) [6].
5) Antitumor (methanol extract) [7].
6) Toxicity on Raji cell [8].
7) Inducing ovulation (feruloyl stigmastanol: feruloyl campestanol (9:1)) [9].
8) Depressing blood sugar (coixan A, B, C) [10].

Literature:

[1] Kondo, Y. *et al.*: *Chem. Pharm. Bull.* **1988**, 36, 3147.
[2] Takahashi, M. *et al.*: *Planta Med.* **1986**, 52, 64.
[3] Nagao, T. *et al.*: *Phytochemistry* **1985**, 24, 2959.
[4] Ishiguro, Y. *et al.*: *Nippon Nogei Kagaku Kaishi* **1993**, 67, 1405.
[5] Hano, K. *et al.*: *Yakugaku Zasshi* **1959**, 24, 2959.
[6] Kiyoguchi, Y. *et al.*: *Wakan Iyakugaku Zasshi* **1986**, 3, 170.
[7] Kosuge, *et al.*: *Yakugaku Zashi* **1985**, 105, 791.
[8] Konoshima, T. *et al.*: *Shoyakugaku Zasshi* **1987**, 41, 344.
[9] Kondo, Y. *et al.*: *Chem. Pharm. Bull.* **1988**, 36, 31.

[10] Takahashi. M., *et al.*: *Planta Med.* **1986**, 52, 64.
[11] Yamada, H. *et al.*: *Phytochemistry* **1986**, 25, 129.

[T. Kimura]

377.   *Imperata cylindrica* **(L.) Beauv.**   (Gramineae)
          I. cylindrica **Beauv. var. *major* (Nees) C. E. Hubb.**

Bai-mao (C), Bark-mow (H), Chigaya (J), Baek-mo (K)

Rhizome (CP, JP)
  Local Drug Name: Bai-mao-gen (C), Bark-mow-gun (H), Bo-kon (J), Baek-mo-geun (K).
  Processing: 1) Dry under the sun or stir-fry the sections until turning brown (C).
  Method of Administration: Oral (decoction: C, H, J, K).
  Folk Medicinal Uses:

                1) Anasarca (J, K).
                2) Nephritic edema (C, H, J).
                3) Urinary tract infection (C, H, J).
                4) Epistaxis (H).
                5) Hematemesis (C, H).
                6) Hematuria (C, H).
                7) Fever and febrile disease with thirst (C, H).
                8) Cough (H).
                9) Hypertension (H).
                10) Hemorrhage (K).
                11) Jaundice (C).

Scientific Research:
  Chemistry
    1) Triterpenoids: cylindrin [1–2, 6], arundoin[2–3, 6], fernenol, simiarenol, isoarborinol
         [4–6], arborinol, arborinone, friedelin, arborinol 3-methylether [6].
    2) Sesquiterpenoids: cylindrene [7].
    3) Phenolic compounds: cylindol A, cylindol B [8].
    4) Sugars: sucrose, glucose, fructose [5, 10].
    5) Dimethyl 4,4-dimethoxy-5,6,5,6-dimethylenedioxybiphenyl-2,2-dicarboxylate [10].
  Pharmacology
    1) Diuretic effect [9].
    2) Inhibition of vascular smooth muscle contraction (cylindrene) [7].
    3) Antiinflammatory effect, 5-lipoxygenase inhibitory (cylindol A, B) [8].

Literature:
  [1] Ohno, S. *et al.*: *Yakugaku Kenkyu* **1961**, 33, 238.
  [2] Ohmoto, T. *et al.*: *Chem. Pharm. Bull.*, **1965**, 13, 22.
  [3] Nishimoto, K. *et al.*: *Tetrahedron Lett.* **1965**, 2245.
  [4] Nishimoto, K. *et al.*: *Tetrahedron* **1968**, 24, 735.
  [5] Haginiwa, T. *et al.*: *Yakugaku Zasshi* **1956**, 76, 863.

[6] Ohmoto, T. *et al.*: *J. Chem. Soc. (D)* **1969**, 601; *Yakugaku Zasshi* **1969**, 89, 1682.

[7] Matsunaga, K. *et al.*: *J. Nat. Prod.* **1994**, 57, 1183.

[8] Matsunaga, K. *et al.*: *J. Nat. Prod.* **1994**, 57, 1290.

[9] Yamaguchi, I. *et al. Chosen Igaku Kaishi* **1928**, 86, 173; Haginiwa, T. *et al.*: *Shoyaku-gaku Zasshi* **1963**, 17, 6; Kanchanapee, P. *et al.*: *Shoyakugaku Zasshi* **1967**, 21, 65.

[10] Wang, M.L. *et al.*: *Shenyang Yaoke Daxue Xuebao* **1996**, 13, 153.

[T. Kimura]

378.   *Phyllostachys bambusoides* Sieb. et Zucc. (Gramineae)

Gang-zhu (C), Madake (J), Wang-dae (K)

Root
  Local Drug Name: Ban-zhu-gen (C), Ban-juk-geun (K).
  Method of Administration: Oral (decoction: C, K).
  Folk Medicinal Uses:
                1) Rheumatalgia (C).
                2) Sputum (C, K).
                3) Coughing (C, K).

Culm sheath
  Local Drug Name: Ben-zhu-ke (C), Ban-juk-gak (K).
  Method of Administration: Oral (decoction or ash: C).
  Folk Medicinal Uses:
                1) Feverish disease (C).
                2) Measles (C).

Flower
  Local Drug Name: Ban-zhu-hua (C), Ban-juk-hwa (K).
  Method of Administration: Oral (decoction: C, K).
  Folk Medicinal Uses:
                1) Scarlet fever (C, K).

Leaf
  Local Drug Name: Ban-zhu-ye (C), Wa-tan-chiku-yo (J).
  Method of Administration: Oral (decoction: C, J).
  Folk Medicinal Uses:
                1) Febrile diseases (C, J).

Scientific Research
  Chemistry
    1) Elements: Ag, Al, Ba, Ca, Cu, Fe, Ga, Mg, Mn, Ni, Pb, Si, Sn, Sr, Ti, Zn, Zr [1], Ca, K, N, P [2], Cd, Co [4].
    2) Abscisic acid [5].

Literature

[1] Zhou, Z. X.: *Tianran Chanwu Yanjiu Yu Kaifa* **1992**, 4(1), 44.

[2] Nishida, T.: *Bamboo J.* **1989**, 7, 1.

[3] Chen, Y. D. *et al.*: *Linchan Huaxue Yu Gongye* **1985**, 5(4), 32.

[4] Mori, M. *et al.*: *Sagami Joshi Daigaku Kiyo* **1978**, 42, 19.

[5] Oritani, T. *et al.*: *Nippon Sakumotsu Gakkai Kiji* **1971**, 40(1), 34.

[P.P.H. But]

379.　　　　　　　*Zea mays* **L.**　(Gramineae)

Yu-mi (C), Yuk-suk-shue (H), To-morokoshi (J), Ok-su-su (K)

Style

Local Drug Name: Yu-mi-xu (C), Suk-might-so (H), Nanba-mo (J), Ok-mi-su (K).

Processing: Eliminate foreign matter and dry.

Method of Administration: Oral (decoction: C, H, J, K).

Folk Medicinal Uses:

　　　　　　1) Nephritic edema (C, H, J, K).

　　　　　　2) Beriberi (C, H, J, K).

　　　　　　3) Urinary tract infection and stone (C, H, J, K).

　　　　　　4) Cirrhosis (C, H).

　　　　　　5) Ascites (C, H).

　　　　　　6) Cholecystitis (C, H).

　　　　　　7) Gall stone (C, H).

　　　　　　8) Hepatitis (C, H, J).

　　　　　　9) Hypertension (C, H, K).

　　　　　　10) Diabetes (C, H, J).

　　　　　　11) Mastitis (C).

　　　　　　12) Hematemesis (C).

　　　　　　13) Uterus cancer (K).

Cob core

Local Drug Name: Yu-mi-zhou (C), Suk-might-sum (H), Ok-chok-seo (K)

Processing: Eliminate remnanats of caryopses, dry under the sun.

Method of Administration: Oral (decoction, C, H, K)

Folk Medicinal Uses:

　　　　　　1) Edema (C, H, K).

　　　　　　2) Beriberi (C, K).

　　　　　　3) Dysentery (C, K).

　　　　　　4) Indigestion (C, H, K).

Scientific Research

Chemistry

1) Sitosterol: di-0-(indole-3-acetyl)-myo-inositol, tri-0-(indole-3-acetyl)-myo-inositol, 2-0-*trans*-*p*-couma-royl-(2S,3S)-hydroxycitric acid, 2-0-*trans*-feruloyl-(2S,3S)-hydroxy-citric acid, 2-0-*trans*-caffeoyl-(2S,3S)-hydroxycitric acid [1–3].

2) Xylans: arabinoglucuronoxylans [4].

3) Indole-3-acetic acid, 2-0-myoinositol ester [5].

4) Fatty acid methyl esters [6].

5) Carotenoids: β-carotene, ζ-carotene, β-zeacarotene, phytofluene, luteol, zeaxanthol, cryptoxanthol [7].

Pharmacology

1) Hypoglycemic effect [8].

Literature

[1] *Carbohydr. Res.* **1974**, 36, 1.

[2] *Agric. Biol. Chem.* **1977**, 41, 359.

[3] Nicholls, P.B. *et al.*: *Phytochemistry* **1971**, 10, 2207.

[4] Dutton, G.G.S. *et al.*: *Phytochemistry* **1972**, 11, 779.

[5] Nicholls, P.B.: *Planta* **1967**, 72, 258.

[6] Fathipour, A. *et al.*: *Biochim. Biophys. Acta* **1967**, 144, 476.

[7] Genevois, L. *et al.*: *Qual. Plant. Mater. Veg.* **1966**, 13, 78.

[8] Miura, T. *et al.*: *Natural Medicines* **1996**, 50, 363.

[P.P.H. But]

380.   *Areca catechu* L.   (Palmae)

Bing-lang (C), Bun-long (H), Binro (J), Bin-rang (K)

Seed   (CP, JP)

Local Drug Name: Bing-lang (C), Bun-long (H), Bin-ro-ji (J), Bin-rang-ja (K).

Processing: 1) Cut into slices, and dry in the shade (C, J, K).

2) Stir-fry the slices until turning yellow (C).

Method of Administration: Oral (decoction: C, H, J, K).

Folk Medicinal Uses:

1) Parasites (H, J, K).

2) Taeniasis (H, C, J, K).

3) Ascariasis (C).

4) Fasciolopsiasis (C).

5) Abdominal pain due to intestinal parasitosis (C, K).

6) Diarrhea and tenesmus due to accumulation of undigested food (C).

7) Edema (C, H).

8) Malaria (C).

9) Beriberi (H).

Pericarp (CP)

Local Drug Name: Da-fu-pi (C), Die-fuk-pay (H), Daifukuhi (J).

Method of Administration: Oral (decoction: C, H, J).

Folk Medicinal Uses:

1) Edema (C, H, J).

2) Beriberi (H).

3) Epigastric and abdominal distention (C).

Scientific Research:
Chemistry
  1) Alkaloids: arecoline, arecaidine, guvacine, guvacoline, isoguvacine [1]; arecolidine [2].
  2) Tannins [3]: proanthocyanidin A-1, A-4, A-5[10].
Pharmacology
  1) Parasympathomimetic activities. Sedative, drooling, epiphora, convulsion, tremor, atony, diarrhea (arecoline) [4].
  2) Central nervous system activities (arecoline) [5].
  3) Inhibition of angiotensin transferase prevention against hypertension (tannin) [6].
  4) Anthelmintic effect (tannins with fatty acids) [7].
  5) Inhibition of glucan production frrom sucrose (tannin) [8].
  6) Antitumor (tannin) [9].
  7) Antibacterial (fatty acids) [8].
  8) Inhibition of endogenous nitrosationin humans [11].
  9) Inhibition of cyclic AMP Phosphodiesterase [12].

Literature:
[1] Jahns: *Ber.* **1888**, 21, 3404; **1891**, 24, 2615; Hess: *Ber.* **1918**, 51, 1004.
[2] Dehmlow, E.V.: *Heterocycles* **1994**, 37, 355.
[3] Nishioka, I. *et al.*: *Chem. Comm.* **1981**, 781.
[4] Mon, Y.: *Nippon Yakubutsugaku Zasshi* **1938**, 29, 73; Snyder, S. H. *et al.*: *Fed. Proc.* **1975**, 34, 1915.
[5] Nieschulz, O.: *Arzneim.-Fotsch.* **1967**, 17, 1292; Sitaram, N. *et al.*: *Science* **1978**, 201, 274; Molinengo, L. *et al.*: *J. Pharm. Pharmacol.* **1988**, 40, 821.
[6] Inokuchi, J. *et al.*: *Life Sci.* **1986**, 38, 1375.
[7] Kiuchi, F. *et al.*: *Chem. Pharm. Bull.*, **1987**, 35, 2880.
[8] Hada, S. *et al.*: *Phytother. Res.* **1989**, 3, 140.
[9] Uchino, K. *et al.*: *Planta Med.* **1988**, 54, 419, 422.
[10] Nonaka, G. *et al.*: *Chem. Pharm. Bull.*, **1987**, 35, 149.
[11] Stich, H. F. *et al.*: *JNCI. J. Natl. Cancer Inst.* **1983**, 70, 1047.
[12] Nikaido, T. *et al.*: *Planta Med.* **1982**, 43, 18.

[T. Kimura]

381.   *Arisaema erubescens* **(Wall.) Schott.** (Araceae)

Tian-nan-xing (C), Tin-narm-sing (H), Du-ru-mi-cheon-nam-seong (K)

Related plants: *A. heterophyllum* Bl.: Yi-ye-tian-nan-xing (C); *A. amurense* Maxim.: Dong-bei-tian-nan-xing (C); *A. serratum* (Thunb.) Schott: Mamushi-gusa (J); *A. amurense* Maxim. var. *serratum* Nakai: Cheon-nam-seong (K).

Rhizome (CP)
Local Drug Name: Tian-nan-xing (C), Tin-narm-sing (H), Ten-nan-sho (J), Cheon-nam-seong (K).
Processing: 1) Eliminate foreign matter, wash clean, and dry (C, K).

2) Soak in water, and change water 2-3 times a day and add alum if necessary, until it only causes a numbing sensation to the tongue. Boil in water with ginger and alum, dry in air briefly, cut into thin slices, and dry thoroughly (C, K).

Method of Administration: Oral (decoction: C, H, K); Topical (powder mixed with vinegar or liqour: C, J, K).

Folk Medicinal Uses:

> 1) Intractable sputum with cough (C, H, J, K).
> 2) Vertigo (C, H, K).
> 3) Stroke with sputum in the throat, deviation of the eye and the mouth, and hemiplegia (C, H, K).
> 4) Epilepsy and convulsions (C, H, K).
> 5) Tetanus (C, H).
> 6) Boils, sores, snake and insect bite (C, H).
> 7) Shoulder discomfort (topical) (J).

Contraindications: Use with caution in pregnancy (C).

Scientific Research:

Chemistry

> 1) Cyanogenic glycoside: triglochinin [1].

Pharmacology

> 1) Expectorant effect [2].
> 2) Anticonvulsive effect [3].
> 3) Improving the recovery from anemia [4].

Literature:

[1] Nahrstedt, A.: *Phytochemistry* **1975**, 14, 2627.
[2] Gao, Y. D. *et al.*: *Zhonghua Yixue Zazhi* **1956**, 10, 959.
[3] Xue, G. H. *et al.*: *Xian Yixueyuan Xuebao* **1958**, 5, 22.
[4] Shin, C. S. *et al.*: *Koryo Taehakkyo Vikwa Taehak* **1980**, 17(1), 183.

[J.X. Guo]

382. *Homalomena occulta* **(Lour.) Schott** (Araceae)

Qian-nian-jian (C), Chin-gun-but (H)

Rhizome (CP)

Local Drug Name: Qian-nian-jian (C), Chin-gun-but (H).

Processing: Eliminate foreign matter, wash clean, soften thoroughly, cut into slices, and dry in the sun (C).

Method of Administration: Oral (decoction: C, H).

Folk Medicinal Uses:

> 1) Rheumatoid arthritis with pain and sensation in the loins and knees (C, H).
> 2) Muscular contracture and numbness of the lower extremities (C).
> 3) Traumatic injury (H).

Scientific Research:

Chemistry

1) Volatile oils: α-pinene, β-pinene, limonene, linalool, α-terpineol, nerol, geraniol, lugenol [1], myrcenal, β-terpineol, β-terpineol, terpinene-4-ol, pogostol, isoborneol [2].

Pharmacology

1) Toxic reaction [3].

Literature:

[1] Rui, H. K. *et al.*: *Zhongcaoyao* **1982**, 13(7), 43.
[2] Liu, G. S. *et al.*: *Yaoxue Tongbao* **1984**, 19(12), 22.
[3] Liao, Y. L. *et al.*: *Fujian Zhongyiyao* **1963**, 8(5), 28.

[J.X. Guo]

383.　　　　*Spirodela polyrhiza* **Schleider**　(Lemnaceae)

Zi-ping (C), Ukikusa (J), Gae-gu-ri-bap (K)

Herb (CP)

Local Drug Name: Fu-ping (C), Fu-hyo (J), Bu-pyung (K).
Processing: Dry under the sun (C, J, K).
Method of Administration: Oral (decoction: C, J, K); Topical (decoction: C).
Folk Medicinal Uses:

1) Urticaria with itching (C, K).
2) Measles without adequate eruption (C).
3) Edema with oliguria (C).
4) Rheumatism (J).
5) Anasarca (J).
6) Diuretic (K).
7) Dermatopathy (K).
8) Alcohol poisoning (K).

Scientific Research:

Chemistry

1) Flavonoids: flavone C- and O-glycoside [1].
2) Fatty acids: linolenic acid [12–13], linoleic acid [13].
3) Amino acids: L-valine, L-isoleucine, L-leucine [7–8], alanine, threonine, proline, serine, γ-aminobutyric acid, glutamine, aspartic acid, asparagine, glutamic acid [8].
4) Plant hormones: abscisic acid [2, 9, 16].
5) Anthocyans: malonyl cyanidin 3-monoglucoside [14].
6) Pigments: carotenoids and chlorophylls [3].
7) Phenols: hydroxycinnamic acid, quinic acid [11].
8) Proteins [4].
9) Carbohydrates [5].

Pharmacology

1) Radioprotective effect (abscisic acid) [2, 15].

Literature:

[1] Wallace, J. W.: *Phytochemistry* **1975**, 14, 1765.
[2] Magone, I. *et al.*: *Fiziol. Biokhim. Kul't. Rast.* **1973**, 5, 427.
[3] Adabra-Michanol, Y. *et al.*: *Physiol. Veg.* **1975**, 13, 619.
[4] Matasumoto, S.: *Kagaku to Seibutsu,* **1981**, 19, 594.
[5] Bytniewska, K. *et al.*: *Biochem. Physiol. Pflanz.* **1980**, 175, 172.
[6] Chang, S.-M. *et al.*: *Bull. Inst. Chem. Acad. Sin.* **1978**, 25, 19.
[7] Borstlap, A. C.: *Acta Bot. Neerl.* **1975**, 24, 203.
[8] Borstlap, A. C.: *Acta Bot. Neerl.* **1972**, 21, 404.
[9] Saks, Y. *et al.*: *Aust. J. Plant Physiol.* **1980**, 7, 73.
[10] Strack, D. *et al.*: *J. Chromatogr.* **1978**, 156, 359.
[11] Kraus, J.: *Z. Pflanzenphysiol.* **1978**, 88, 465.
[12] Lechevallier, D.: *Physiol. Veg.* **1977**, 15, 95.
[13] Le Pabic, C.: *Plant Sci. Lett.* **1980**, 17, 303.
[14] Krause, J. *et al.*: *Z. Pflanzenphysiol.* **1979**, 95, 183.
[15] Lysenko, N. I. *et al.*: *Deposited Doc.* **1974**, VINITI 3032-3074, 16 pp
[16] Smart, C. C. *et al.*: *Plant Cell Environ.* **1983**, 6, 507.

[C.K. Sung]

384. *Cyperus rotundus* L. (Cyperaceae)

Sha-cao (C), Heung-foo (H), Hama-suge (J), Hyang-bu-ja (K)

Rhizome (CP, JP)
Local Drug Name: Xiang-fu (C), Heung-foo-gee (H), Ko-bu-shi (J), Hyang-bu-ja (K).
Processing: 1) Remove fibrous matter and foreign matter, pound to pieces or cut into thin
 slices (C, K).
 2) Stir-fry with vinegar to dryness (C).
Method of Administration: Oral (decoction: C, H, J, K).
Folk Medicinal Uses:
 1) Stagnation of the liver qi characterized by distending pain in the chest,
 hypochondria and epigastrium (C, H, J).
 2) Indigestion (C, J, K).
 3) Feeling of stuffiness in the chest and epigastrium (C, H, J).
 4) Abdominal colic (C, H).
 5) Distending pain in the breast (C).
 6) Menstrual disorders (C, H, J, K).
 7) Amenorrhea or dysmenorrhea (C, H, J, K).
 8) Traumatic injury (H).
 9) Leukorrhea (K).
 10) Gastrointestinal disorder, gastric neurosis (J, K).
 11) Headache (J, K).
 12) Morning sickness (J)
 13) Miscarriage (J).

Scientific Research:

Chemistry

    1) Volatile oils: cyperene, β-seliene, α-cyperone, β-cyperone, patchoulenone, limonene, 1,8-cineol, β-pinene, camphene, *p*-cymene [1], cyperotundone [2], cyperolone [3], cyperol, isocyperol [4], sugenolacetate, sugenol [5], α-rotunol, β-rotunol [6], copadiene, epoxyguaiene, rotundone [7], sugetriol [8], 4α,5α-oxidoeudesm-11-en-3α-ol [9], caryophyllene [10], kobusone, isokobusone, patchoulenyl acetate, sugeonyl acetate [18].

    2) Tannins: leucocyanidin, leucocyanidin glucoside [11].

    3) Phenolic acids: *p*-cownaric acid, ferulic acid, vanillic acid, *p*-hydroxybenzoic acid, protocatechuic acid [11].

    4) Flavonol glycoside: rhamnetin 3-*O*-rhamosyl-(1→4)-rhamopyranoside [12].

Pharmacology

    1) Inhibition of the contraction of womb [13].

    2) Analgesic effect [14].

    3) Antifungal effect [15].

    4) Inhibitory effect on prostaglandin biosynthesis (cyperone) [16].

    5) Antihistaminic effect (ethanol extract) [17].

Literature:

[1] Motal, O. *et al.*: *Chem. Ind.* **1963**, 1284; *Tetrahedron Letters* **1964**, 1197; *Collection Czec. Chem. Communs.* **1964**, 29, 1675.

[2] Hikino, H. *et al.*: *Chem. Pharm. Bull.* **1965**, 13, 628; **1966**, 14, 890.

[3] Hikino, H. *et al.*: *Chem. Pharm. Bull.* **1966**, 14, 1439; **1967**, 15, 1349.

[4] Hikino, H. *et al.*: *Chem. Pharm. Bull.* **1967**, 15, 1929.

[5] Hikino, H. *et al.*: *Chem. Pharm. Bull.* **1968**, 16, 52.

[6] Hikino, H. *et al.*: *Tetrahedron Letters* **1969**, 2741.

[7] Kapadia, V. H. *et al.*: *Tetrahedron Letters* **1967**, 4661.

[8] Hikino, H. *et al.*: *Chem. Pharm. Bull.* **1968**, 16, 1900.

[9] Hikino, H. *et al.*: *Phytochemistry* **1976**, 15, 1265.

[10] Dhillon, R. S. *et al.*: *Plant Growth Regul.* **1993**, 13(1), 89.

[11] Komai, K. *et al.*: *Zasso Kenkyu* **1975**, 20(2), 66.

[12] Singh, N. B. *et al.*: *J. Indian Chem. Soc.* **1986**, 63, 450.

[13] Zhang, F. C. *et al.*: *Yaoli Yanjiu Baogao* **1935**, 1(2), 148.

[14] Deng, S. Z. *et al.*: *Guiyaang Yixueyuan Xuebao* **1959**, 113.

[15] Meguro, M. *et al.*: *Univ. Sao Poulo, Fac. Fil., Cienc, Letras, Bol. Bot.* **1969**, 24, 173.

[16] Kiuchi, F. *et al.*: *Chem. Pharm. Bull.* **1983**, 31, 3391.

[17] Itokawa, S. *et al.*: *Shoyakugaku Zasshi* **1983**, 37, 223.

[18] Komai, K. *et al.*: *Phytochemistry* **1989**, 28, 1883.

[J.X. Guo & T. Kimura]

385.   *Scirpus fluviatilis* **A. Gray**   (Cyperaceae)

Jing-san-len (C), Ukiyagara (J), Mae-ja-gi (K)

Rhizome

Local Drug Name: Jing-san-len (C), Koku-san-ryo (J), Hyeong-sam-reung (K).

Processing: Dry under the sun (C, J, K); process with vinegar (C).
Method of Administration: Oral (decoction: C, J, K).
Folk Medicinal Uses:

1) Amenorrhea (C).
2) Pain caused by blood stasis (C).
3) Abdominal distension or mass formation in the abdomen (C).
4) Menstrual disorder (J).
5) Blood stasis (J).
6) Chronic gastritis (K).
7) Hemorrhage (K).

Scientific Research:
Chemistry
1) Stilbene derivatives.: hydroxystilbene compounds I, II [1–2], stilbene trimer compound
I [3], scirpusin A, B [4].
Pharmacology
1) 5-Lipoxygenase inhibition effect (hydroxystilbene derivatives) [1–2].
2) Acetylcholine esterase inhibition effect [3].

Literature:

[1] Nakajima, K. *et al.*: *Jpn. Kokai Tokkyo Koho*, JP 04159279 A2 920602 Heisei, 8 pp.
[2] Nakajima, K. et al: *Jpn. Kokai Tokkyo Koho*, JP 04159280 A2 920602 Heisei, 6 pp.
[3] Akiyama, T. *et al.*: *Jpn. Kokai Tokkyo Koho*, JP 03294273 A2 911225 Heisei, 4 pp
[4] Nakajima, K. *et al.*: *Chem. Pharm. Bull.* **1978**, 26, 3050.

[C.K. Sung]

386.　　　*Alpinia chinensis* **Rosc.**　(Zingiberaceae)

Hua-shan-jiang (C), Wah-sarn-geung (H)

Rhizome
Local Drug Name: Hua-shan-jiang (C), Wah-sarn-geung (H).
Method of Administration: Oral (decoction: C, H); Topical (C, H).
Folk Medicinal Uses:

1) Gastralgia (C, H).
2) Rheumatalgia, arthralgia (C, H).
3) Cough and wheezing (C, H).
4) Irregular menses (C, H).
5) Traumatic injury (C, H).
6) Pyodermas (C, H).

Seed
Local Drug Name: Hua-shan-jiang (C), Wah-san-geung (H).
Method of Administration: Oral (decoction: C, H).
Folk Medicinal Uses:

1) Gastralgia (C, H).
2) Cough and wheezing (H).

Scientific Research
Chemistry
1) Volatile oil: (E,E)-α-farnesene, α-humulene, β-bisabolene, β-caryophyllene, γ-selinene, valencene, caryophyllene oxide, cineole, β-pinene [1-4].
2) Fatty acid: palmitic acid [4].
3) Flavonoid: alpinetin, izalpinin [5].

Literature
[1] Dung, N.X. *et al.*: *J. Essen. Oil Res.* **1994**, 6, 91.
[2] Dung, N.X. *et al.*: *J. Essen. Oil Res.* **1994**, 6, 637.
[3] Leclercq., P. A. *et al.*:. *J. Essen. Oil Res.* **1994**, 6, 401.
[4] Kimura, Y.: *J. Pharm. Soc. Japan* **1940**, 60, 145.
[5] Kimura, Y.: *J. Pharm. Soc. Japan* **1940**, 60, 151.

[P.P.H. But]

387.　　　　　*Alpinia galanga* **Willd.**　(Zingiberaceae)

Da-gao-liang-jiang (C), Hung-dou-kou (H), Nankyo-so (J), Hong-du-gu (K)

Fruit (CP)
Local Drug Name: Hong-dou-kou (C), Hung-dou-kou (H), Ko-zu-ku (J), Go-ryang-gang (K).
Processing: Collect when mature and dry in shade.
Method of Administration: Oral (decoction: C, H, J, K).
Folk Medicinal Uses:
　　　　　　1) Stomachache (C, H, J, K).
　　　　　　2) Nausea (C, H, J, K).
　　　　　　3) Stomach distention and pain (C, H, K).
　　　　　　4) Vomiting and diarrhea (C, H, K).
　　　　　　5) Indigestion (H, J, K).
　　　　　　6) Drunkenness (C).

Rhizome
Local Drug Name: Da-gao-liang-jiang (C), Die-go-leung-geung (H), Dai-ko-ryo-kyo (J)
Processing: Eliminate foreign matter and dry.
Method of Administration: Oral (decoction, C, H).
Folk Medicinal Uses:
　　　　　　1) Epigastic pain (C, H).
　　　　　　2) Nausea (C, H, J).

Scientific Research
Chemistry
1) Fruit contains cedrol, 1,8-cineole, eugenol, linalool, α-pinene, β-pinene [1], caryophyllene oxide, caryophyllenol-I, caryophyllenol-II, 1'-acetoxychavicol acetate, 1'-acetoxyeugenol acetate, fatty acid methyl esters, *trans*-4-methoxycinnamyl alcohol, *n*-7-heptadecene, *n*-pentadecane, *trans*-3,4-dimethoxycinnamyl alcohol, *trans*-4-hydroxycinnamaldehyde [2–3].

197

2) Rhizome contains borneol, isoborneol, bornyl acetate, camphene, Δ^3-carene, 1,8-cineol, *trans*-β-cymene, citronellol, *p*-cymene, α-fenchene, α-fenchol, geranial, geraniol, geranyl acetate, limonene, linalool, *trans*-2-*p*-menthen-1-ol, *cis*-2-*p*-menthen-1-ol, *cis*-β-ocimene, α-phellandrene, α-pinene, β-pinene, β- phellandrene, sabinene, *trans*-sabinene hydrate, α-terpinene, γ-terpinene, terpinen-4-ol, α-terpineol, myrcene, neral, terpinolene, α-thujene, β-thujone, tricyclene [4], α-bergamotent, β-bisabolene, butyl acetate, carveol I, carveol II, β-caryophyllene, caryophyllene oxide, chavicol, neryl acetate, chavicol acetate, citronellyl acetate, α-copaene, *p*-cymenol, *ar*-curcumene, eugenyl acetate, *trans*-β-farnesene, α-humulene, methyleugenol, 2-methypropyl acetate, pentadecane, santalene, β-sesquiphellandrene, tridecane [5], eugenol, [6], 1'-acetoxychavicol acetate, 1'-acetoxyeugenol acetate, 1'-hydroxychavicol acetate [7], *p*-hydroxy-cinnamaldehyde, [di-(*p*-hydroxy-*cis*-styryl)]methane [20].

3) Seed contains (E)-8(17),12-labddiene-15,16-dial, (E)-8β(17)-epoxylabd-12-ene-15,16-dial, galanals A-B, galanolactone [14].

Pharmacology

1) Antibacterial effect [8–11].
2) Antiprotozoal effect [8–9].
3) Antifungal effect [11, 14, 24].
4) Antiulcer effect [12–13, 26].
5) Hypotensive effect [8, 14–15].
6) CNS-depressant effect [8, 14–15].
7) Respiratory-depressant effect [8].
8) Expectorant effect [16].
9) Diuretic effect [15].
10) Spasmolytic effect [8].
11) Antineoplastic effect [3].
12) LD50 of rhizome oil 0.68 ml/kg IP in guinea pigs [9].
13) Protective effect against cytological and biochemical changes induced by cyclophosphamide [18].
14) Cytotoxic effect [19].
15) Nematocidal effect [25].

Literature

[1] Rui, H.K. *et al.*: *Zhongcaoyao* **1982**, 13, 331.
[2] Mitsui, S. *et al.*: *Chem. Pharm. Bull.* **1976**, 24, 2377.
[3] Itokawa, H. *et al.*: *Planta Med.* **1987**, 32.
[4] Scheffer, J.J.C. *et al.*: *Science and Pharmacy* **1981**, 49, 337.
[5] De Pooter, H.L. *et al.*: *Phytochemistry* **1985**, 24, 93.
[6] Trabaud, L.: *France Parfums* **1964**, 7, 141.
[7] Janssen, A.M. *et al.*: *Planta Med.* **1985**, 507.
[8] Chopra, I.C. *et al.*: *Indian J. Med. Res.* **1954**, 42, 385.
[9] Chopra, I.C. *et al.*: *Antibiotics and Chemotherapy* **1957**, 7, 378.
[10] Bhargava, A.K. *et al.*: *Indian J Pharm* **1968**, 30, 150.
[11] Scheffer, J.J.C. *et al.*: *Planta Med.* **1981**, 42, 140.
[12] Mitsui, S. *et al.*: *Chem. Pharm. Bull.* **1976**, 24, 2377.
[13] Ogiso, A. *et al.*: *Japan Kokai* 74 36,817, 05 Apr **1974**, Appl. 72 81,562, 15 Aug **1972**; 3pp.
[14] Bhakuni, D.S. *et al.*: *Indian J. Exp. Biol.* **1969**, 7, 250.
[15] Dhawan, B.N. *et al.*: *Indian J. Exp. Biol.* **1977**, 15, 208.
[16] Inamdar, M.C. *et al.*: *Indian J. Physiol. Pharm.* **1962**, 6, 150.

[17] But, P.P.H. *et al.*: *Abstr Chin Med (ACME)* **1987**, 1, 449.

[18] Qureshi, S. *et al.*: *Int. J. Pharmacog.* **1994**, 32(2), 171.

[19] Morita, H. *et al.*: *Planta Med.* **1988**, 54, 117.

[20] Barik, B.R. *et al.*: *Phytochemistry* **1987**, 26, 2126.

[24] Mishra, A.K. *et al.*: *Econ. Bot.* **1990**, 44, 530.

[25] Kiuchi, F. *et al.*: *Shoyakugaku Zasshi* **1989**, 43, 294.

[26] Al-Yahya, M.A. *et al.*: *Phytothery Res.* **1990**, 4, 112.

[27] Jitoe, A. *et al.*: *J. Agric. Food Chem.* **1992**, 40, 1337.

[P.P.H. But]

388. *Alpinia japonica* Miq.   (Zingiberaceae)

Shan-jiang (C), Sarn-geung (H), Hana-myoga (J), Ggot-yang-ha (K)

Seed
Local Drug Name: Tu-sha-ren (C), I-zu-shuku-sha (J), I-du-chuk-sa (K).
Processing: Dry under the sun (J, K).
Method of Administration: Oral (decoction: J, K).
Folk Medicinal Uses:
        1) Gastrointestinal disorder (J, K).

Rhizome
Local Drug Name: Shan-jiang (C), Sarn-geung (H).
Processing: Dry under the sun (C).
Method of Administration: Oral (decoction: C, H).
Folk Medicinal Uses:
        1) Rheumatic arthritis (C, H).
        2) Traumatic injury (C).
        3) Toothache (C).
        4) Stomachache (C).
        5) Abdominal distention (H).

Flower
Local Drug Name: Shan-jiang-hua (C), San-kyo-ka (J).
Processing: Dry under the sun.
Method of Administration: Oral.
Folk Medicinal Uses:
        1) Dyspepsia (J).
        2) Hang over (J).

Whole herb
Local Drug Name: Shan-jiang (C). Wa-san-kyo (J).
Processing: Dry under the sun (J).
Method of Administration: Oral (decoction: J).
Folk Medicinal Uses:
        1) Articular rheumatism (J).
        2) Food intoxcation (J).

Scientific Research:
Chemistry
  1) Flavonoids: alpinone, izalpinin [1], rhamnocitrin, kumatakenin [2].
  2) Monoterpenes: 1,8-cineole, camphor[3].
  3) Sesquiterpenes: halpinone, 10-epi-5-β-hydroperoxy-β-eudesmol, 10-epi-5α-
      hydroperoxy-β-eudesmol, 4,10-epi-5β-hydroxy-dihydroeudesmol, isohanalpinone,
      alpinenone, alpinolide peroxide, 6-hydroxy alpinolide, nerolidol, humulene epoxide
      II, 4α-hydroxydihydroagarofuran [4–5].
Pharmacology
  1) Spasmolytic effect [5].

Literature:

[1] Kimura, Y. *et al.*: *Yakugaku Zasshi* **1934**, 54, 47; 1935, 55, 229.
[2] Kimura, Y. *et al.*: *Yakugaku Zasshi* **1967**, 87, 1132.
[3] Kimura, Y. *et al.*: *Yakugaku Zasshi* **1933**, 53, 794; Fukui, K. *et al.*: *Kashi* **1965**, 86, 1079.
[4] Itokawa, H. *et al.*: *Chem. Pharm. Bull.* **1987**, 35, 1460, 2849.
[5] Morita, M. *et al.*: *Chem. Pharm. Bull,* **1996**, 44, 1603.

[T. Kimura]

389.   *Alpinia katsumadai* **Hayata**   (Zingiberaceae)

Cao-dou-kou (C), Cho-dou-kou (H), So-zu-ku (J), Cho-du-gu (K)

Seed (CP)
  Local Drug Name: Cao-dou-kou (C), Cho-dou-kou (H), So-zu-ku (J), Cho-du-gu (K)
  Processing: Eliminate foreign matter, break into pieces before use (C)
  Method of Administration: Oral (decoction: C, H, J, K).
  Folk Medicinal Uses:
              1) Epigastric pain (C, H, J, K).
              2) Eructation (C, H).
              3) Dysentery (C, H).
              4) Drunkenness (C, H, J).
              5) Nausea, dyspepsia (C, H, J, K).
              6) Vomiting and anorexia (C).

Scientific Research
Chemistry
  1) Seed oil contains alpinetin, cardamonin [1], bornyl acetate, camphor, carvotanacetone,
      1,8-cineol, *trans,trans*-farnesol, geranyl acetate, α-humulene, linalool, methyl
      cinnamate, terpinen-4-ol [2], *trans*-cinnamaldehyde, *trans,trans*-1,7-diphenyl-4,6-
      heptadien-3-one, (3S,5R)-3,5-dihydroxy-1,7-diphenylheptane, *trans*-1,7-diphenyl-5-
      hydroxy-1-heptene, *trans,trans*-1,7-diphenyl-5-hydroxy-4,6-heptadien-3-one,
      (3S,5S)-*trans*-1,7-diphenyl-3,5-dihydroxy-1-heptene, (5R)-*trans*-1,7-diphenyl-5-
      hydroxy-6-hepten-3-one, pinocembrin [3], aromadendrene, benzyl acetone, borneol,
      γ-cadinene, *d*-cadinene, calamenene, Δ³-carene, caryophyllene, α-copaene, limonene,
      p-cymene, methyl cinnamate, α-muurolene, α-pinene, β-pinene, sabinol, α-terpineol,
      γ-patchoulene, α-phellandrene, sabinyl acetate, thymol, 4-phenyl-butan-2-one [4, 9].

2) Stem and leaf oil contain α-pinene, β-pinene, myrcene, α-phellandrene,1,8-cineol, fenchone, geraniol [8].

3) Cd, Cu, Fe, Mn Ni, Zn [5].

Pharmacology

1) Pepsin-stimulant effect [6].

Literature

[1] Kimura, Y. *et al.*: *Yakugaku Zasshi* **1968**, 88, 239.

[2] Saiki, Y. *et al.*: *Phytochemistry* **1978**, 17, 808.

[3] Kuroyanagi, M. *et al.*: *Chem. Pharm. Bull.* **1983**, 31, 1544.

[4] Okugawa, K. *et al.*: *Shoyakugaku Zasshi* **1987**, 41, 108.

[5] Itokawa, H. *et al.*: *Shoyakugaku Zasshi* **1980**, 34, 155.

[6] Li, Z.L. *et al.*: *J. Trad. Chin. Med.* **1980**, 21, 148.

[7] But, P.P.H. *et al.*: *Abstr. Chin. Med. (ACME)* **1988**, 2, 135.

[8] Dung, N.X. *et al.*: *J. Essen. Oil Res.* **1990**, 2, 259.

[9] He, R.Y. *et al.*: *Yaimu Fenxi Zazhi.* **1995**, 15(Suppl.) 469.

[P.P.H. But]

390.   *Alpinia officinarum* **Hance**   (Zingiberaceae)

Gao-liang-jiang (C), Go-leung-geung (H), Ko-ryo-kyo(J), Go-ryang-gang (K)

Rhizome (CP)

Local Drug Name: Gao-liang-jiang (C), Go-leung-geung (H), Ko-rhy-kyo (J), Go-ryang-gang (K).

Processing: Eliminate foreign matter, cut into slices, and dry (C).

Method of Administration: Oral (decoction: C, H, J, K); Topical (C, H).

Folk Medicinal Uses:

        1) Epigastric pain (C, H, J, K).

        2) Nausea (C, H, J, K).

        3) Indigestion (C, H, J, K).

        4) Gastritis, gastric and duodenal ulcer (C, H).

        5) Gastroenteritis (C, H, J).

        6) Tinea versicolor infection (C, H).

Contraindication: Yin-deficiency with heat.

Scientific Research

Chemistry

1) Rhizome contains 7-(4"-hydroxyphenyl)-1-phenyl-4-hepten-3-one, 5-methoxy-1,7-diphenyl-3-heptanone, 5-methoxy-7-(4"-hydroxyphenyl)-1-phenyl-3-heptenone [1], octahydrocurcumin, (3R,5R)-1-(4-hydroxyphenyl)-7-phenylheptane-3,5-diol [2], 7-(4"-hydroxy-3"-methoxyphenyl)-1-phenyl-3,5-heptadione, 5-hydroxy-7-(4"-hydroxyphenyl)-1-phenyl-3-heptenone, 5-methoxy-7-(4"-hydroxy-3"-methoxy-phenyl)-1-phenyl-3-heptenone [4], yakuchinone [6].

Pharmacology

1) Antibacterial effect.

2) Nematocidal effect [3].

3) Inhibitory effect on prostaglandin synthetase [4, 6].
4) Enhancing sulfaguanidine absorption [5].

Literature

[1] Itokawa, H. *et al.*: *Chem. Pharm. Bull.* **1985**, 33, 4889.
[2] Uehara, S. *et al.*: *Chem. Pharm. Bull.* **1987**, 3298.
[3] Kiuchi, F. *et al.*: *Shoyakugaku Zasshi* **1989**, 43, 353.
[4] Kiuchi, F. *et al.*: *Chem. Pharm. Bull.* **1982**, 30, 2279.
[5] Sakai, K. *et al.*: *Yakugaku Zasshi* **1986**, 106, 947.
[6] Sankawa, U. *et al.*: *Igaku no Ayumi* **1983**, 126, 867.

[P.P.H. But]

391. *Alpinia oxyphylla* **Miq.** (Zingiberaceae)

Yi-zhi (C), Yik-gee (H), Yaku-chi (J), Ik-ji (K)

Fruit (CP)
Local Drug Name: Yi-zhi (C), Yik-gee (H), Yaku-chi (J), Ik-ji (K)
Processing: Eliminate foreign matter, and dry in shade (C).
Method of Administration: Oral (decoction: C, H, J, K)
Folk Medicinal Uses:

  1) Dyspepsia (C, H, J, K).
  2) Diarrhea (C, H, K).
  3) Abdominal pain (C, H, K).
  4) Spermatorrhea (C, H).
  5) 'Kidney' asthenia (C, H).
  6) Poor memory (C, H).
Contraindication: Yin-deficiency with heat, leukorrhea.

Scientific Research
Chemistry
  1) Fruit oil contains camphor, 1,8-cineol, pinene, zingiberene, zingiberol [1–3].
  2) Diarylheptanoids: yakuchinones A-B [4–5].
  3) Sesquiterpene: nootkatol [6].
  4) Ca, Cu, Fe, K, Mg, Mn, Na, Ni, P, Pb, Zn [7, 18].
Pharmacology
  1) Pungency [4–5].
  2) Antineoplastic effects [8].
  3) Calcium-antagonistic effect [6, 9–10].
  4) Vasodilating effect [11].
  5) Inhibitory effects on prostaglandin synthetase [12–13, 16].
  6) Antiulcer effect [15].
  7) Tyrosinase-inhibitory effect [17].

Literature

[1] Kariyone, T. *et al.*: *Yakugaku Zasshi* **1927**, 47, 674.

[2] Kimura, Y. *et al.*: *J. Jap. Bot.* **1966**, 41, 49.

[3] Akabori, Y. *et al.*: *21st Annual Meeting of the Pharmaceutical Society of Japan* **1965**, 382.

[4] Itokawa, H. *et al.*: *Phytochemistry* **1981**, 20, 769.

[5] Itokawa, H. *et al.*: *Phytochemistry* **1982**, 21, 241.

[6] Shoji, N. *et al.*: *J. Pharm. Sc.* **1984**, 73, 843.

[7] Itokawa, H. *et al.*: *Shoyakugaku Zasshi* **1980**, 34, 155.

[8] Itokawa, H. *et al.*: *Shoyakugaku Zasshi* **1979**, 33, 95.

[9] Wang, X. *et al.*: *J. Beijing Med. Univ.* **1986**, 18, 31.

[10] Shoji, N. *et al.*: *Planta Med.* **1984**, (2), 186.

[11] Mitsubishi Chemical Industries Co., Ltd.: *Chemical Abstract* **1984**, 100, 91345p.

[12] Kiuchi, F. *et al.*: *Chem. Pharm. Bull.* **1982**, 30, 754.

[13] Kiuchi, F. *et al.*: *Chem. Pharm. Bull.* **1982**, 30, 2279.

[14] But P. P. H. *et al.*: *Abstr Chin Med (ACME)* **1987**, 1, 601.

[15] Yamahara, J. *et al.*: *Chem. Pharm. Bull.* **1990**, 38, 3053.

[16] Sankawa, U. *et al.*: *Igaku no Ayumi* **1983**, 126, 867.

[17] Shirota, S. *et al.*: *Biol. Pharm. Bull.* **1994**, 17, 266.

[18] Wang, J. B. *et al.*: *Zhongguo Zhongyao Zazhi* **1990**, 15, 492.

[P.P.H. But]

392. *Amomum kravanh* Pierre ex Gagnep. (Zingiberaceae)

Bai-dou-kou (C), Bark-dou-kou (H)

Fruit (CP)
Local Drug Name: Dou-kou (C), Bark-dou-kou (H), Byaku-zu-ku (J)
Processing: Eliminate foreign matter, dry in shade, break into pieces before use (C).
Method of Administration: Oral (decoction: C, H, J)
Folk Medicinal Uses:
    1) Abdominal pain (J).
    2) Nausea (C, H, J).
    3) Dyspepsia (J).
    4) Indigestion, epigastric distention (C, H).

Scientific Research
Chemistry
  1) Cu, Fe, Mn, Ni, Pb [1].
  2) Volatile oil: 3,8,11-trioxa-tetracyclo[4,4,0^2,4,0^7,9]undecane(1α,2β,4β,6α,7β,9β), Δ^3-carene, α-terpineol, 4-terpinenol, thujone, and 47 other components [2].
Pharmacology
  1) Thiamin-inhibitory effect [3].

Literature
[1] Itokawa, H. *et al.*: *Shoyakugaku Zasshi* **1980**, 34, 155.
[2] Zhou, C. M. *et al.*: *Zhonguo Yaoxue Zazhi* **1991**, 26, 406.
[3] Rattanapanone, V. *et al.*: *Chiang Mai Med. Bull.* **1979**, 18(1), 9.

[P.P.H. But]

393.   *Amomum longiligulare* **T.L. Wu**   (Zingiberaceae)

Hai-nan-sha (C), Hae-nan-sa (K)

Fruit (CP)
Local Drug Name: Sha-ren (C), Shar-yun (H), Sa-in (K).
Processing: Eliminate foreign matter, break into pieces before use (C).
Method of Administration: Oral (fresh or decoction: C, H, K).
Folk Medicinal Uses:
  1) Epigastric distention (C, H).
  2) Nausea and vomiting (C, H, K).
  3) Diarrhea (C).
  4) Threatened abortion (C).
  5) Anorexia (K).
  6) Abdominal pain (K).

Scientific Research
Chemistry
  1) Volatile oil: β-farnesene, β-pinene, α-pinene, bornyl acetate, camphene, limonene, camphor, linalool, cineole, nerolidol, guaiol [1].

Literature
[1] Fang, H.J. *et al.*: *Zhongcaoyao* **1982**, 13, 197.

[P.P.H. But]

394.   *Amomum tsao-ko* **Crevost et Lemaire**   (Zingiberaceae)

Cao-guo (C), Cho-gwor (H), So-ka (J), Cho-gwa (K)

Fruit (CP)
Local Drug Name: Cao-guo (C), Cho-gwor (H), So-ka (J), Cho-gwa (K)
Processing: 1) Collect fruit when mature, dry; seed fried on low fire (C).
            2) Stir-fry the seeds with ginger juice to dryness (C).
Method of Administration: Oral (decoction: C, H, J, K)
Folk Medicinal Uses:
  1) Malarial diseases (C, H).
  2) Epigastric pain (C, H, J, K).
  3) Nausea (C, H, J, K).
  4) Vomiting (C, H, J, K).
  5) Dysentery (C, H, J, K).
  6) Maldigestion (C, H, K).
  7) Sputum (C, H).
  8) Acute gastritis (K).
Contraindications: Qi-deficiency or blood-asthenia with no cold-wet symptoms.

Scientific Research

Chemistry

1) Volatile oil: α-pinene, β-pinene, α-phellandrene, *p*-cymene, 1,8-cineole, limonene, 2-octen-1-al, citral, Δ³-carene, 1,4-cineole, nonan-2-one, fenchone, linalool, citronellol, myrcenol, thymol, α-terpineol, sabinol, terpinen-4-ol, 2-decen-1-al, geraniol, geranial, thymol, α-methyl cinnamaldehyde, geranyl acetate, 4-indanecarbaldehyde, 2-dodecen-1-al, γ-cadiene, elemol, nerolidol [1], *trans*-2-undecena [2].

Literature

[1] Okugawa, H. *et al*.: *Shoyakugaku Zasshi* **1987**, 41, 108.
[2] Li, S.C. *et al*.: *Zhongcaoyao Tongxun* **1977**, 8(2), 13.

[P.P.H. But]

395.   *Costus speciosus* **(Koen.) Smith**   (Zingiberaceae)

Bi-qiao-jiang (C), Bight-sour-geung (H), O-hozaki-ayame (J)

Rhizome

Local Drug Name: Zhang-liu-tou (C), Long-duk (H).
Processing: Dry under the sun and cut into slices.
Method of Administration: Oral (decoction, C, H).
Folk Medicinal Uses:

1) Edema (C, H).
2) Cirrhosis (C, H).
3) Urinary tract infection (C, H).
4) Pertussis (H).
5) Pliguria (C, H).
6) Dysuria (C, H).

Contraindications: Pregnancy.
Side effect: Poisonous if use when fresh.

Scientific Research

Chemistry

1) Alkaloid: [1]
2) Saponins: diosgenin [2], tigogenin [6], β-sitosterol glucoside [5], gracillin, dioscin [8], protodioscin, prosapogenins A-B of dioscin, furost-5-*n*-3β,26-diol, β-sitosterol-β-D-glucopyranoside, methyl protodioscin, 3-*O*-[α-L-rhamnopyranosyl (1→2)-β-D-glucopyranosyl]-26-*O*-[β-D-glucopyranosyl]-22α-methoxy-(25*R*) [10].
3) Methyl triacontanoate [9], methyl-3-(4-hydroxyphenyl)-2*E*-propenoate [11].

Pharmacology

1) Smooth muscle relaxant effect [1].
2) Antispasmodic effect [1].
3) Cardiotonic effect [1].
4) Hydrocholeretic effect [1].
5) Diuretic effect [1].
6) CNS depressant effect [1].
7) Estrogenic effect [3–4].

8) Uterotonic effect [5].
9) Hypotensive effect [7].
10) Bradycardiac effect [7].
11) Antifungal effect [11].

Literature

[1] Bhattacharya, S. K. *et al.*: *J. Res. Indian Med.* **1973**, 8(1), 10.
[2] Sarin, Y. K. *et al.*: *Curr. Sci.* **1974**, 43, 569
[3] Tewari, P. V. *et al.*: *Indian J. Pharm.* **1973**, 35(1), 35.
[4] Singh, S. *et al.*: *Indian J. Med. Res.* **1972**, 60(2), 287.
[5] Pandey, V.B. *et al.*: *Indian J. Pharm.* **1972**, 34(5), 116.
[6] Rathore, A.K. *et al.*: *Lloydia* **1978**, 41, 640.
[7] Banerji, R. *et al.*: *Indian Drugs* **1981**, 18(4), 121.
[8] Tschesche, R. *et al.*: *Phytochemistry* **1978**, 17, 1781.
[9] Gupta, M. M. *et al.*: *Phytochemistry* **1981**, 20, 2553.
[10] Singh, S. B. *et al.*: *J. Nat. Prod.* **1982**, 45, 667.
[11] Bandara, B. M. R. *et al.*: *Planta Med.* **1988**, 54, 477.
[12] Bandara, B. M. R. *et al.*: *J. Natl. Sci. Counc. Sri Lanka* **1989**, 17(1), 1.

[P.P.H. But]

396.   *Curcuma aromatica* **Salisb.**   (Zingiberaceae)

Yu-jin (C), Yuk-gum (H), Haru-u-kon (J), Ul-geum (K)

Root tuber
Local Drug Name: Yu-jin (C), Yuk-gum (H), Kyo-o (J), Ul-geum (K).
Processing: Eliminate foreign matter, clean, cut into sections, and dry (C).
Method of Administration: Oral (decoction or congee: C, H, J, K).
Folk Medicinal Uses:
> 1) Menstrual irregularities, amenorrhea, post-partum hematoma (C, H, J, K).
> 2) Oppresed feeling in chest and pain in hypochondrium (C).
> 3) Hematemesis (C).
> 4) Epigastric distention (C).
> 5) Urethremorrhage (C).
> 6) Jaundice, hepatitis (C, H, J, K).
> 7) Epilepsy (C).

Contraindications: Pregnancy.

Scientific Research
Chemistry
> 1) Volatile oil: α-pinene, β-pinene, camphene, 1,8-cineole, isofuranogermacrene, borneol, isoborneol, camphor, germacrone, tetramethylpyrazine [1].
> 2) Dipotassium magnesium dioxalate [2–3].

3) Sesquiterpene: isozedoarondiol, methylzedoarondiol, neocurdione, procurcumenol, zedoarondiol, germacrone, curdione, (4S,5S)-germacrone 4,5-epoxide, dehydro-curdione, curcumenone [4].

Pharmacology
   1) Antiarrhythmic effect [2–3].
   2) Antiinflammatory effect [5–7].

Literature

[1] Guo, Y. T. *et al.*: *Yao Hsueh Hsueh Pao* **1980**, 15, 251.
[2] Zeng, L. L. *et al.*: *Yaoxue Xuebao* **1982**, 17, 946.
[3] Chen, M. Z. *et al.*: *Zhongcaoyao* **1985**, 16, 312.
[4] Kuroyanagi, M. *et al.*: *Chem. Pharm. Bull.* **1987**, 35, 53.
[5] Chen, M. Z. *et al.*: *Yaoxue Tongbao* **1982**, 17, 396.
[6] Guo, X. Z. *et al.*: *Yaoxue Tongbao* **1982**, 17, 321.
[7] Dai, L. M. *et al.*: *Yaoxue Xuebao* **1982**, 17, 692.

[P.P.H. But]

397.   *Curcuma longa* **L.**   (Zingiberaceae)

Jiang-huang (C), Geung-wong (H), Ukon (J), Gang-hwang (K)

Related Plant: *Curcuma aromatica* Salisb.: Yu-jin (C), Haru-ukon (J), Ul-geum (K).

Rhizome (CP)
  Local Drug Name: Jiang-huang (C), Geung-wong (H), U-kon (J), Gang-hwang (K).
  Processing: After boil, dry under the sun (J, K). Cut into thick slices, and dry under the sun
        (C).
  Method of Administration: Oral (decoction: C, H, J, K); Topical (decoction: C).
  Folk Medicinal Uses:
         1) Gastrointestinal disorder (H, J, K).
         2) Cholecystitis (J, K).
         3) Choleithiasis (J, K).
         4) Hepatitis (J).
         5) Jaundice (J, K).
         6) Pricking pain in the chest and hypochndriac regions (C).
         7) Amenorrhea (C, H).
         8) Mass formation in the abdomen (C).
         9) Rheumatic pain of the shoulders and arms (C).
       10) Traumatic swelling and pain (C).
       11) Traumatic injury (H).

Root tuber (CP)
  Local Drug Name: Yu-jin (C), Yuk-gum (H).
  Processing: Dry under the sun after boiling in water. Soften throughly, cut into thin slices
        and dry, or break into pieces (C).
  Method of Administration: Oral (decoction: C, H).

Folk Medicinal Uses:
>1) Amenorrhea (C).
>2) Dysmenorrhea (C).
>3) Distending or pricking pain in the chest and abdomen (C).
>4) Impairment of consciousness in febrile diseases, epilepsy, mania (C).
>5) Jaundice with dark urine (C).

Scientific Research:
Chemistry
>1) Curcuminoids: curcumin-I, II, III [1], cyclocurcumin [2].
>2) Monoterpenes: d-camphene, d-camphor, 1,8-cineole, sabinene, borneol.
>3) Sesquiterpenes: l-α-curcumene, l-β-curcumene, turmerone, ar-turmerone.
Pharmacology
>1) Antiinflammatory effect.
>2) Cytotoxic effect [3].

Literature:
[1] Verghese, J.: *Flavour and Fragrance J.*, **1993**, 8, 315.
[2] Kiuchi, F. *et al.*: *Chem. Pharm. Bull.*, **1993**, 41, 1640.
[3] Takatsuki, S. *et al.*: *Natural Medicines*, **1996**, 50, 145.

[T. Kimura]

398.   *Hedychium coronarium* **Koen.**   (Zingiberaceae)

Jiang-hua (C), Geung-far (H)

Rhizome
Local Drug Name: Jiang-hua (C), Geung-far (H).
Processing: Dry under the sun (C).
Method of Administration: Oral (decoction or powder: C, H).
Folk Medicinal Uses:
>1) Traumatic injury (C, H).
>2) Common cold (C,H)
>3) Headache (C, H).
>4) Body ache (C, H).
>5) Rheumatism (C, H).

Fruit
Local Drug Name: Jiang-hua (C), Geung-far (H).
Processing: Dry under the sun (C).
Method of Administration: Oral (decoction or powder: C, H).
Folk Medicinal Uses:
>1) Gastric distention (C, H).
>2) Indigestion (C, H).
>3) Vomiting (C, H).
>4) Stomachache (C, H).

Scientific Research
Chemistry
1) Volatile oil: β-pinene, myrcene, limonene, cineole, *p*-cymene, camphor, borneol, methylsalicylate, eugenol, thylanthranilate [1], 2-methylbutanal oximes, 3-methylbutanal oximes, methyl epijasmonate, *trans*-ocimene, 2-*exo*-hydroxy-1,8-cineole, *cis*-jasmene lactone [6], linalool, methyl benzoate, *cis*-jasmone, eugenol, (E)-isoeugenol, methyl jasmonate [8].
2) Polysaccharide: starch [2].
3) Steroid: diosgenin [3].
4) Diterpenoid: coronarin A-F [4–5], coronarin-Dethylether, isocoronarin D [7].
Pharmacology
1) Cytotoxic effect [4].

Literature
[1] Haggag, M. Y. *et al.*: *Egypt. J. Pharm. Sci.* **1977**, 18, 465.
[2] Fujimoto, S. *et al.*:*Denpun Kagaku* **1984**, 31, 134.
[3] Carabot Cuervo, A. *et al.*: *Rev. Latinoam. Quim.* **1981**, 12(3-4), 132.
[4] Itokawa, H. *et al.*: *Planta Med.* **1988**, 54, 311.
[5] Itokawa, H. *et al.*: *Chem. Pharm. Bull.* **1988**, 36, 2682.
[6] Yamada, Y. *et al.*: *Koryo* **1991**, 171, 143.
[7] Singh, S. *et al.*: *Aust. J. Chem.* **1991**, 44, 1789.
[8] Matsumoto, F. *et al.*: *J. Essent. Oil Res.* **1993**, 5(2), 123.

[P.P.H. But]

399.   *Kaempferia galanga* L.   (Zingiberaceae)

Shan-nai (C), Sarn-noi (H), Ban-u-kon (J)

Rhizome (CP)
Local Drug Name: Shan-nai (C), Sha-geung (H), San-na (J).
Processing: Eliminate foreign matter, wash, cut into slices, dry under the sun (C).
Method of Administration: Oral (decoction: C, H, J); Topical (powder: C, H).
Folk Medicinal Uses:
1) Traumatic injury (C, H).
2) Dyspepsia (C, H, J).
3) Toothache (C, H, J).
4) Epigastric distention (C, H).

Scientific Research
Chemistry
1) Ethyl *p*-methoxy *trans*-cinnamate [1-2, 4-5], 3-caren-5-one [3], ethyl cinnamate, *p*-methoxycinnamic acid [4].
2) Cd, Cu, Fe, Mn, Ni, Pb, Zn [7].
Pharmacology
1) Monoamine oxidase inhibitory effect [2].
2) Insecticidal effect [4, 6].

Literature

[1] Chau, L. T. *et al.*: *Duoc Hoc* **1979**, (5), 9.
[2] Noro, T. *et al.*: *Chem. Pharm. Bull.* **1983**, 31, 2708.
[3] Kiuchi, F. *et al.*: *Phytochemistry* **1987**, 26, 3350.
[4] Kiuchi, F. *et al.*: *Chem. Pharm. Bull.* **1988**, 36, 412.
[5] Liu, B. M. *et al.*: *Fenxi Ceshi Xuebao* **1993**, 12(4), 45.
[6] Pandji, C. *et al.*: *Phytochemistry* **1993**, 34, 415.
[7] Itokawa, H. *et al.*: *Shoyakugaku Zasshi* **1980**, 34, 155.

[P.P.H. But]

400.　　　*Zingiber officinale* **(L.) Rosc.**　(Zingiberaceae)

Jiang (C), Geung (H), Shoga (J), Saeng-gang (K)

Rhizome (CP, JP)
Local Drug Name: Sheng-jiang (C), Sound-geung (H), Sho-kyo (J), Saeng-gang (K).
Processing:　Fresh
Method of Administration: Oral (decoction: C, H, J, K).
Folk Medicinal Uses:

　　　　1) Gastrointestinal disorder (H, J, K).
　　　　2) Dyspepsia (H, J, K).
　　　　3) Nausea, vomiting (C, H, J, K).
　　　　4) Pain (H, J, K).
　　　　5) Common cold (C, H, J, K).
　　　　6) Diarrhea (H, J, K).
　　　　7) Cough with expectoration of whitish thin sputum (C).

Rhizome (CP, JP)
Local Drug Name: Gan-jiang (C), Gon-geung (H), Kan-shokyo (J), Geon-saeng-gang (K).
Processing: Slice and dry under the sun.
Method of Administration: Oral (decoction: C, H, J).
Folk Medicinal Uses:

　　　　1) Epigastric pain with cold feeling (C, H).
　　　　2) Vomiting and diarrhea accompanied by cold exremities and faint
　　　　　　pulse (C, H).
　　　　3) Dyspnea and cough with copious expectoration (C, H).

Scientific Research:
Chemistry
　　1) Phenolic compounds: [6]-gingerol, [8]-gingerol, [10]-gingerol, dehydrogingerone,
　　　　(artefact; [6]-shogaol, zingerone) [1] .
　　2) Diarylhepatanoids: hexahydrocurcumin, desmethylhexahydrocurcumin [2–3].
　　3) Monoterpenes: α-pinene, *d*-camphene, myrcene, β-phellandrene, 1,8-cineole,
　　　　sabinene, borneol, neral, geranial, α-terpineol, borneol, neral, nerol, geranyl acetate,
　　　　sabinene [1].
　　4) Sesquiterpenes: α-curcumene, α-zingiberene, β-bisaborene, β-sesquiphellandrene [1].
　　5) Diterpenes: (E)-8β-17-epoxylabd-12-ene-15,16-dial, galanolactone [4].
　　6) Glycerols: gingerglycolipids A, B, and C [8].

7) 6-gingesulfonic acid, (+)-anaaagelicoidenol-2-*0*-β-D-glucopyranoside [8].
Pharmacology
    1) Pungency ([6]-, [8]-, [10]-gingerol, dehydrogingerone, shogaol, zingerone)
    2) Inhibition of vomiting (juice, pressed out) [5].
    3) Cholesterol biosynthesis inhibitory effect, blood circulation stimulant [6].
    4) Antirhinoviral effect (β-sesquiphellandrene) [7].
    5) Antiulcer effect (6-gingesulfonic acid) [8].

Literature:

[1] Nomura, H. *et al.*: *Sci. Rep. Tohoku Imp. Univ.* 1928, 17, 973; Xu, S. : *Chemistry* (The
    Chinese Chem. Taiwan) **1981**, 38, 63; Masada, Y. et al: *Yakugaku Zasshi* **1973**, 93,
    318; **1974**, 94, 735; Connel, D. W. *et al.*: *Aust. J. Chem.* **1969**, 22, 1033; Kiuchi, F. *et
    al.*: *Chem. Pharm. Bull.* **1982**, 30, 754; Kano, Y. *et al.*: *Shoyakugaku Zasshi* **1986**, 40,
    333; **1987**, 41, 277; **1989**, 43, 7.
[2] Connel, D. W. *et al.*: *Austr. J. Chem.* **1969**, 22, 1033; Murata, T., *et al.*: *Chem. Pharm.
    Bull.* **1972**, 20, 2291; Masada, Y. *et al.*: *Yakugaku Zasshi* **1973**, 93, 318; **1974**, 94, 735.
[3] Harvey, D. J.: *J. Chromatgr.* **1981**, 212, 75.
[4] Kano, Y. *et al.*: *Shoyakugaku Zasshi* **1990**, 44, 55; Tanabe, M. *et al.*: *Shoyakugaku
    Zasshi* **1991**, 45, 316.
[5] Yamada, Y.: *Gifu Ikadaigaku Kiyo* 1954, 1, 301.
[6] Tanabe, M. *et al.*: *Chem. Pharm. Bull.* **1993**, 41, 710.
[7] Denyer, C. V. *et al.*: *J. Nat. Prod.* **1994**, 57, 658.
[8] Yoshikawa, M. *et al.*: *Chem. Pharm. Bull.* **1994**, 42, 1226.

[T. Kimura]

INDEX TO SCIENTIFIC NAMES

中文索引　　（繁体字、簡体字、日字）(in Plant No.)

INDEX TO LOCAL HERB NAMES

222

INDEX TO DISEASES AND BIOACTIVITIES

Antiviral 252, 257, 259, 300, 311, 316, 328, 330, 340, 359, 362, 363, 372, 400
Apnea 335
Apoplexy 214, 267
Appendicitis 233, 270, 342, 376, 372, 344
Arachidonate lipoxygenase 251
Arteriosclerosis 219, 320, 351
Arthralgia 209, 216, 249, 232, 236, 240, 241, 244, 263, 318, 325, 327, 345, 347, 376, 369, 386
Arthritis 215, 221, 239, 241, 253, 270, 282, 271, 272, 273, 296, 313, 319, 332, 338, 342, 342, 343, 349, 352, 356, 376, 382, 371, 388
Ascariasis 201, 211, 221, 261, 348, 253, 350, 352, 376, 380, 360
Ascites 263, 275, 278, 304, 317, 325, 351, 358, 379
Ascorbic acid oxidase 250
Asthma 202, 202, 228, 269, 283, 285, 303, 326, 336
Ataxia 358
Atony 380
ATPase 247

Bad breath 329
Bed-wetting 364
Belching 285, 286, 303, 320
Beriberi 210, 248, 270, 312, 319, 376, 379, 380, 373
Bile duct disease 364
Bilirubin 340
Bleeding 204, 206, 207, 209, 212, 214, 215, 233, 233, 247, 258, 270, 285, 274, 277, 295, 298, 250, 314, 317, 320, 333, 338, 327, 343, 345, 347, 355, 385, 366
Blood stasis 385
Bloodshot eye 315
Blurred vision 266
Body ache 398
Boil 224, 226, 233, 235, 242, 245, 268, 270, 274,

280, 298, 300, 301, 250, 314, 315, 342, 307, 308, 351, 353, 358, 381, 363, 368, 372, 372
Bone lodged in throat 241, 267, 268
Bradycardia 335, 395
Bronchial dilatory 339
Bronchiectasic 202
Bronchitis 205, 208, 232, 252, 267, 268, 281, 282, 294, 295, 314, 333, 352, 363
Bruise 224, 237, 252, 262, 319, 339, 343, 343, 350
Burns 312, 214, 232, 295, 298, 300, 250, 328, 350, 362, 367

Calcification 269
Calcium antagonist 247, 318, 351, 391
Calcium channel bloker 263
Calculus 208, 222, 229, 279, 317, 376, 379
Calmative 202
Cancer 212, 217, 252, 285, 310, 376, 379, 362, 363
Carbuncle 201, 214, 228, 229, 232, 239, 256, 259, 268, 270, 274, 278, 280, 300, 301, 302, 314, 323, 337, 340, 342, 308, 353, 355, 356, 369
Carcinogenic 210, 212, 248, 273
Carcinostatic 228
Cardiac depressant 340, 346
Cardiac disorder 265, 364
Cardiotonic 251, 318, 331, 364, 395
Cardiovascular 202, 249, 241, 237, 257, 400
Caries 250
Cataleptogenic 227
Cataract 332
Catarrh 207
Catecholamine 242
Cathartic 221, 311, 362
Centipede bite 237, 358
Cervical erosion 342
Cholagogue 348, 354
Cholangitis 364

Cholecystitis 261, 379, 397
Cholecystokinin 263, 361
Choleithiasis 397
Choleretic 242, 340, 348, 349
Cholestasis 364
Cholesterol 232, 400
Chyluria 208
Cirrhosis 263, 317, 325, 358, 379, 395
Climacterium 351
CNS 321, 380
CNS depressant 249, 242, 346, 387, 395
CNS stimulant 237, 251
Coagulation 247, 255
Cold feeling 318, 351
Colic 216, 261, 273, 384
Colitis 274, 340
Common cold 208, 215, 229, 249, 237, 281, 282, 287, 290, 291, 298, 250, 251, 310, 314, 316, 329, 332, 333, 335, 338, 347, 353, 358, 360, 398, 400
Congelation 237, 328
Congestion 207, 245
Conjunctival congestion 207
Conjunctivitis 266, 321, 342, 353, 358, 374, 375
Constipation 201, 218, 224, 227, 228, 232, 254, 260, 265, 266, 268, 273, 275, 276, 278, 280, 299, 301, 304, 311, 341, 308, 362, 363, 365
Consumptive disease 261
Contraceptive 248, 296, 306, 328
Contracture 382
Contusion 213, 288, 250, 351, 360
Convulsion 259, 362, 380, 381
Corn 261, 292
Corneal opacity 332
Coronary disease 230
Corrosion 228
Corticosterone 293
Costalgia 245
Cough 202, 204, 214, 214, 218, 219, 220, 228, 249, 232, 243, 254, 257, 258, 261, 264, 265, 267, 268,

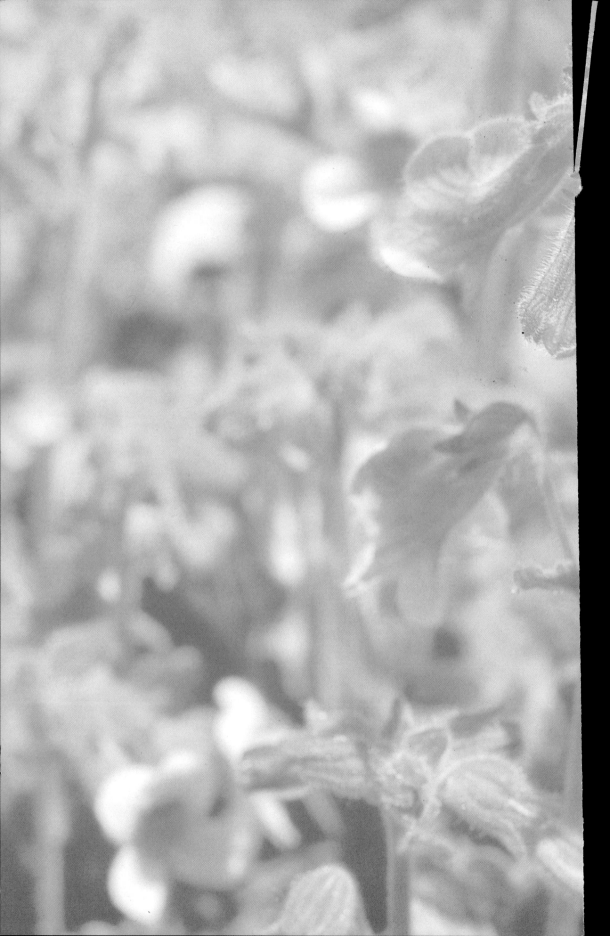